Vertebral Compression Fractures in Osteoporotic and Pathologic Bone

Afshin E. Razi • Stuart H. Hershman
Editors

Vertebral Compression Fractures in Osteoporotic and Pathologic Bone

A Clinical Guide to Diagnosis and Management

Springer

Editors
Afshin E. Razi
Vice Chair and Residency Program Director
Department of Orthopaedic Surgery
Maimonides Medical Center
Brooklyn, NY
USA

Stuart H. Hershman
Department of Orthopaedic Surgery
Massachusetts General Hospital
Harvard Medical School
Boston, MA
USA

ISBN 978-3-030-33860-2 ISBN 978-3-030-33861-9 (eBook)
https://doi.org/10.1007/978-3-030-33861-9

This Springer imprint is published by the registered company Springer Nature Switzerland AG
The registered company address is: Gewerbestrasse 11, 6330 Cham, Switzerland

Preface

Osteoporosis is a common condition experienced by an ever-growing segment of the population. While it is treated by many different medical disciplines, despite its prevalence, osteoporosis is frequently overlooked until it is a significant source of morbidity. Osteoporotic vertebral compression fractures serve as an example of one consequence that can occur as a result of untreated osteoporosis. All too often, vertebral compression fractures are the initial finding of osteoporosis, and while this situation occurs commonly, there is still much ambiguity regarding the subsequent management and treatment of these patients.

Due to a variety of reasons, there is a significant confusion among specialists as to the ideal management of osteoporotic compression fractures. While most conditions are treated by one group of specialists, osteoporotic compression fractures are treated by endocrinologists, rheumatologists, orthopedic surgeons, neurosurgeons, interventional radiologists, physiatrists, anesthesiologists, gynecologists, and primary care physicians. Physicians from these disciplines typically view the pathology through their own eyes, relying on their training and expertise to guide treatment. Unfortunately, it is virtually impossible to have all the knowledge and expertise of clinicians from other areas of medicine which could perhaps provide a more comprehensive treatment plan. One of our goals in writing this textbook was to help clarify the optimal management of these patients by presenting some of the latest literature published on the topic by experts in the various fields which treat these patients. By including authors from multiple disciplines, we hope to provide a more thorough treatment algorithm to help clinicians to better manage these patients, thereby minimizing clinical sequela from an otherwise preventable condition.

Brooklyn, NY, USA
Boston, MA, USA

Afshin E. Razi, MD
Stuart H. Hershman, MD

Contents

1 **Normal Bone Physiology** 1
Henock T. Wolde-Semait and Daniel Komlos

2 **Pathophysiology and Epidemiology of Osteoporosis** 9
Nicole M. Stevens and Sanjit R. Konda

3 **The Economic Burden of Osteoporosis** 21
Harold A. Fogel and Louis G. Jenis

4 **Evaluation and Medical Management of Vertebral Osteoporosis: Preventing the Next Fracture** 31
Faye N. Hant and Marcy B. Bolster

5 **Biomechanics of Vertebral Compression Fractures** 49
Peter J. Ostergaard and Thomas D. Cha

6 **Osteoporotic Vertebral Compression Fractures** 57
Ahmed Saleh and Michael Collins

7 **Pathologic Vertebral Compression Fractures: Diagnosis and Management** 63
Daniel G. Tobert and Joseph H. Schwab

8 **History, Physical Exam, and Differential Diagnosis of Vertebral Compression Fracture** 69
Michael Dinizo and Aaron Buckland

9 **Radiographic Diagnosis of Patients with Vertebral Compression Fractures** 75
R. Aaron Marshall and Mohammad Samim

10 **Natural History and Long-Term Sequelae of Vertebral Compression Fractures** 95
John A. Buza III and Emmanuel Menga

11 **Medical, Interventional, and Orthotic Management of Osteoporotic Vertebral Compression Fractures** 101
Kartik Shenoy and Yong H. Kim

12 **Outcomes of Non-operative Management and Vertebral Augmentation of Vertebral Compression Fractures** 109
Robert A. McGuire Jr and Joseph M. Zavatsky

13 Vertebroplasty Cement Augmentation Technique 115
A. Orlando Ortiz

14 Kyphoplasty Cement Augmentation Technique 137
Robert P. Norton

15 Management of Spinal Deformity in the Setting of Osteoporotic Vertebral Compression Fractures 145
Michael P. Kelly

16 Operative Treatment of Pathologic Compression Fractures of the Spine 153
Theodosios Stamatopoulos, Ganesh M. Shankar, and John H. Shin

17 Osteoporotic Vertebral Compression Fractures Adjacent to Previous Spinal Fusion 183
Peter G. Passias, Rivka C. Ihejirika-Lomedico, Hesham Saleh, Max Egers, Avery E. Brown, Haddy Alas, Katherine E. Pierce, Cole Bortz, and Yael Ihejirika

18 Surgical Strategies in Osteoporotic Bone 191
Joseph M. Zavatsky and Robert A. McGuire Jr

19 Sacral Insufficiency Fractures 205
Nicholas Shepard and Nirmal C. Tejwani

20 Future Treatment Strategies 221
Hai Le, Umesh Metkar, Afshin E. Razi, and Stuart H. Hershman

Index 229

Contributors

Haddy Alas, BS Department of Orthopedic Surgery, NYU Langone Orthopedic Hospital, NYU Langone Medical Center, New York, NY, USA

Marcy B. Bolster, MD Division of Rheumatology, Allergy, and Immunology, Massachusetts General Hospital, Harvard Medical School, Boston, MA, USA

Cole Bortz, BA Department of Orthopedic Surgery, NYU Langone Orthopedic Hospital, NYU Langone Medical Center, New York, NY, USA

Avery E. Brown, BS Department of Orthopedic Surgery, NYU Langone Orthopedic Hospital, NYU Langone Medical Center, New York, NY, USA

Aaron Buckland, MD Department of Orthopedic Surgery, NYU Langone Orthopedic Hospital, NYU Langone Medical Center, New York, NY, USA

John A. Buza III, MD, MS Department of Orthopedic Surgery, NYU Langone Orthopedic Hospital, NYU Langone Medical Center, New York, NY, USA

Thomas D. Cha, MD, MBA Department of Orthopaedic Surgery, Massachusetts General Hospital, Harvard Medical School, Boston, MA, USA

Michael Collins, MD Department of Orthopaedic Surgery, Maimonides Medical Center, Brooklyn, NY, USA

Michael Dinizo, MD Department of Orthopedic Surgery, NYU Langone Orthopedic Hospital, NYU Langone Medical Center, New York, NY, USA

Max Egers, BS Department of Orthopedic Surgery, NYU Langone Orthopedic Hospital, NYU Langone Medical Center, New York, NY, USA

Harold A. Fogel, MD Department of Orthopaedic Surgery, Massachusetts General Hospital, Harvard Medical School, Boston, MA, USA

Faye N. Hant, DO, MS CR Division of Rheumatology and Immunology, Medical University of South Carolina, Charleston, SC, USA

Stuart H. Hershman, MD Department of Orthopaedic Surgery, Massachusetts General Hospital, Harvard Medical School, Boston, MA, USA

Rivka C. Ihejirika-Lomedico, MD Department of Orthopedic Surgery, NYU Langone Orthopedic Hospital, NYU Langone Medical Center, New York, NY, USA

Yael Ihejirika, BA Department of Orthopedic Surgery, NYU Langone Orthopedic Hospital, NYU Langone Medical Center, New York, NY, USA

Louis G. Jenis, MD, MHCDS Department of Orthopaedic Surgery, Newton-Wellesley Hospital, Harvard Medical School, Newton, MA, USA

Michael P. Kelly, MD, MSc Department of Orthopedic Surgery, Washington University School of Medicine, Saint Louis, MO, USA

Yong H. Kim, MD Department of Orthopedic Surgery, NYU Langone Orthopedic Hospital, NYU Langone Medical Center, New York, NY, USA

Daniel Komlos, MD, PhD Department of Orthopaedic Surgery, Maimonides Medical Center, Brooklyn, NY, USA

Sanjit R. Konda, MD Department of Orthopedic Surgery, NYU Langone Orthopedic Hospital, NYU Langone Medical Center, New York, NY, USA

Hai Le, MD Department of Orthopaedic Surgery, University of California – Davis, Davis, CA, USA

R. Aaron Marshall, MD Department of Radiology, NYU Langone Orthopedic Hospital, NYU Langone Medical Center, New York, NY, USA

Robert A. McGuire Jr, MD Department of Orthopaedic Surgery, University of Mississippi Medical Center, Jackson, MS, USA

Emmanuel Menga, MD Department of Orthopaedic Surgery, University of Rochester Medical Center, Rochester, NY, USA

Umesh Metkar, MD Department of Orthopaedic Surgery, Beth Israel Deaconess Medical Center, Harvard Medical School, Boston, MA, USA

Robert P. Norton, MD Florida Spine Associates, Boca Raton, FL, USA

A. Orlando Ortiz, MD, MBA, FACR Department of Radiology, Jacobi Medical Center, Bronx, NY, USA

Peter J. Ostergaard, MD Department of Orthopaedic Surgery, Massachusetts General Hospital, Harvard Medical School, Boston, MA, USA

Peter G. Passias, MD Department of Orthopedic Surgery, NYU Langone Orthopedic Hospital, NYU Langone Medical Center, New York, NY, USA

Katherine E. Pierce, BS Department of Orthopedic Surgery, NYU Langone Orthopedic Hospital, NYU Langone Medical Center, New York, NY, USA

Afshin E. Razi, MD Department of Orthopaedic Surgery, Maimonides Medical Center, Brooklyn, NY, USA

Ahmed Saleh, MD Department of Orthopaedic Surgery, Maimonides Medical Center, Brooklyn, NY, USA

Hesham Saleh, MD Department of Orthopedic Surgery, NYU Langone Orthopedic Hospital, NYU Langone Medical Center, New York, NY, USA

Mohammad Samim, MD MRCS Department of Radiology, NYU Langone Orthopedic Hospital, NYU Langone Medical Center, New York, NY, USA

Joseph H. Schwab, MD Department of Orthopaedic Surgery, Massachusetts General Hospital, Harvard Medical School, Boston, MA, USA

Ganesh M. Shankar, MD PhD Department of Neurosurgery, Massachusetts General Hospital, Harvard Medical School, Boston, MA, USA

Kartik Shenoy, MD Department of Orthopaedic Surgery, Rothman Orthopaedic Institute, Philadelphia, PA, USA

Nicholas Shepard, MD Department of Orthopedic Surgery, NYU Langone Orthopedic Hospital, NYU Langone Medical Center, New York, NY, USA

John H. Shin, MD Department of Neurosurgery, Massachusetts General Hospital, Harvard Medical School, Boston, MA, USA

Theodosios Stamatopoulos, MD, MSc Department of Neurosurgery, Massachusetts General Hospital, Harvard Medical School, Boston, MA, USA

CORE-Center for Orthopedic Research at CIRI-AUTh, Aristotle University Medical School, Thessaloniki, Hellas, Greece

Nicole M. Stevens, MD Department of Orthopedic Surgery, NYU Langone Orthopedic Hospital, NYU Langone Medical Center, New York, NY, USA

Nirmal C. Tejwani, MD Department of Orthopedics, NYU Langone Orthopedic Hospital, NYU Langone Medical Center, New York, NY, USA

Daniel G. Tobert, M.D. Department of Orthopaedic Surgery, Massachusetts General Hospital, Harvard Medical School, Boston, MA, USA

Henock T. Wolde-Semait, MD Department of Orthopedic Surgery, NYU Long Island School of Medicine, NYU Langone Health, New York, NY, USA

Joseph M. Zavatsky, M.D. Spine and Scoliosis Specialists, Tampa, FL, USA

Normal Bone Physiology

1

Henock T. Wolde-Semait and Daniel Komlos

Throughout life, the bones of the human skeleton are perpetually remodeled. Changes in biomechanical forces and removal and replacement of old damaged bone with new bone all contribute to this process. There are four categories of bones – irregular, flat, long, and short. These categories are made up of the appendicular skeleton which has 126 bones, the axial skeleton which consists of 74 bones, 6 auditory ossicles, and a variable number of sesamoid bones. This number is not set at birth; typically newborns have about 270 bones; however, this gradually decreases to 206 [1] in the skeletally mature adult. While the primary function of the skeleton is structural support, it also functions critically in movement by providing levers for muscles, maintains hematopoiesis and acid-base balance, and serves as a reservoir for minerals, cytokines, and growth factors.

In general, bones are made up of two different regions, an outer dense, solid, cortical region and an inner loose honeycomb-like trabecular region. The ratio of each differs from bone to bone, with vertebrae being the most trabecular and the diaphysis of long bones containing the most cortical bone [2]. Periosteum covers the outside cortical bone, and an endosteum lines the inside – both layers nourish cortical bone through a dense network of blood vessels. Osteons contained within both cortical and trabecular bone each have a slightly different structure. Cortical osteons are also known as haversian systems and make up the functional unit of cortical bone. Each one is 4–10 mm long and about 0.2 mm in diameter and consists of 5–15 concentric layers or lamellae of compact bone that surrounds a central haversian canal [3]. Each canal in turn contains central blood vessels which nourish each system. Lamellae, whose circumferential layers look like rings of a tree and whose collagen fibrils are arranged in an orthogonal pattern contain within them, contain spaces or lacuna. Inside each lacuna is an osteocyte, a differentiated mature osteoblast. Osteocytes, while grossly may appear to be isolated within each lacuna, actually contact each other via long thin cytoplasmic processes which traverse within transverse tunnels known as canaliculi [4]. Osteocytes, along with osteoclasts and osteoblasts, play a significant role in bone growth and remodeling. Prior to examination of bone formation and remodeling, a basic overview of aforementioned cell types will be discussed.

Osteoclasts

The only cell known to be capable of resorbing bone, osteoclasts, is truly unique with respect to bone remodeling. They are derived from

H. T. Wolde-Semait (✉)
Department of Orthopedic Surgery, NYU Long Island School of Medicine, NYU Langone Health, New York, NY, USA

D. Komlos
Department of Orthopaedic Surgery, Maimonides Medical Center, Brooklyn, NY, USA
e-mail: dkomlos@maimonidesmed.org

A. E. Razi, S. H. Hershman (eds.), *Vertebral Compression Fractures in Osteoporotic and Pathologic Bone*, https://doi.org/10.1007/978-3-030-33861-9_1

mononuclear precursor cells that arise from a monocyte-macrophage lineage, and while found within many tissues, those which give rise to osteoclasts are thought to reside only in bone marrow [5]. Numerous transcription factors have been identified to play a role in osteoclast differentiation, many of which will be described below. PU.1 is an early transcription factor, which appears during myeloid differentiation and is essential for osteoclast development [5]. Likewise, c-Fos is essential for osteoclast development; mice lacking this transcription factor, like PU.1, develop osteopetrosis [6]. Interestingly, c-Fos-deficient mice still develop macrophages, while PU.1 knockout mice do not, implying c-Fos being secondary to PU.1 and PU.1 being necessary for early macrophage development [7]. Other transcription factors such as microphthalmia-associated transcription factor (MITF) and nuclear factor of activated T-cells cytoplasmic-1 (NFAT-1) are also required for osteoclast formation; however their roles are not as clearly defined [8]. RANKL and colony-stimulating factor-1 (CSF-1) are produced by osteoblasts and stromal cells of the bone marrow – these appear in both a cell surface and soluble form and play critical roles in mature osteoclast differentiation. Osteoprotegerin (OPG) functions to bind RANKL, thus leaving RANK receptors inactivated which decreases the maturation of osteoclasts. When mature, osteoclasts bind to bone matrix via integrin receptors to collagen, fibronectin, and laminin. This binding causes them to become polarized with their resorption surface developing the classic ruffled border, leading to the formation of vesicles containing cathepsin K and matrix metalloproteases. These vesicles are released into the extracellular space adjacent to the bone surface, and the acidic environment begins to digest organic matrix [9–11].

Osteoblasts

Osteoblasts develop from pluripotent mesenchymal stem cells and are controlled in part by the transcription factor RUNX2 – RUNX2 knockout mice have a complete lack of mineralized tissue [12]. The Wnt/Beta-catenin pathway has also been shown to be necessary for osteoblast formation with high expression being present within the embryonic skeleton. Osteoblasts form bone and play additional roles in the production of bone matrix proteins, bone mineralization, and the expression of osteoclastogenic factors [13]. They are a heterogeneous population – some respond one way to hormonal signals, while others have been shown to respond differently to similar signals within the axial and appendicular skeleton. When quiescent, osteoblasts exist in a flattened form which line both the endosteal surface as well as the undersurface of the periosteum. During bone remodeling they leave this state, become active and rounded, and move to areas of bone formation; they return to their flattened state once active bone growth is complete. Active forms secrete type I collagen and other matrix proteins and can be differentiated easily on microscopy due to their large single nucleus and prominent Golgi apparatus [14].

Osteocytes

Terminally differentiated osteoblasts are known as osteocytes and are found within lacunae inside bone matrix. Gap junctions allow for communication via filopodia and are required for osteocyte activity and survival. They function in mechanosensation and respond to various stresses placed on bone, a process which is thought to be mediated by cytoplasmic fluid flow [15]. Osteocytes live for decades, and the presence of empty lacunae in aging bone suggests apoptotic mechanisms, which has been shown to be regulated by estrogen deficiency. Estrogen treatment and bisphosphonates may function to prevent apoptosis and thus maintain bone health [16]. These three cell types are the most significant contributors to skeletal growth and remodeling – a brief overview will now be presented.

Bone Growth and Remodeling

Bone grows radially and longitudinally only during childhood and adolescence; however modeling occurs throughout life as bones make gradual adjustments based on changes in applied forces [17]. Bones normally widen with age, as new bone is deposited just deep to the periosteum and resorbed from the endosteum. It also thickens in certain regions based on the increased forces, a concept known as Wolff's law [18]. Bone remodeling allows bone to maintain its strength and mineral homeostasis capabilities. Unlike growth and modeling, which serve to increase the overall net amount of bone, remodeling can be thought of as keeping the overall amount of bone in a steady state [19]. It should be noted however that remodeling does increase slightly in aging men and women – this process occurs at a faster rate in postmenopausal women [20]. The remodeling cycle happens in four stages: activation, resorption, reversal, and formation. These stages occur sequentially. Fractures will initiate the remodeling cascade, otherwise the sites at which remodeling is initiated are seemingly random [20, 21].

Activation involves the production and detection of initiating signals. These signals can be direct mechanical strain placed on bone, hormones such as estrogen and PTH, or small molecules from underlying exposed matrix. Recruitment of osteoclast precursors occurs in response to detection of these signals, and once they arrive at the area of interest, they fuse to form multinucleated preosteoclasts [22]. Preosteoclasts then bind to the bone matrix via integrins and form annular "sealing zones" where bone resorption will occur [23, 24].

Resorption is the next phase of bone remodeling. It normally lasts about 2–4 weeks during each remodeling cycle and is a complex process regulated by numerous factors including RANKL, OPG, IL-1 and 6, CSF-1, PTH, calcitonin, and 1,25-dihydroxyvitamin-D [25, 27]. These factors are released by osteoblasts, and while each subtly functions to increase or decrease osteoclast activity, the collective net effect is an increase, and subsequent resorption, of bone [26]. IL-1 and 6 have been shown to induce osteoclast differentiation [27, 28] to their ready form, while CSF-1 promotes proliferation and survival of osteoclasts as well as increased osteoclast motility and cytoskeletal reorganization. RANKL promotes differentiation to mature cells and also increases resorption activity. Various hormones will then increase or decrease osteoclast activity based on what is required at the time. The actual mechanism of resorption involves the secretion of hydrogen ions via H+-ATPase proton pumps and Cl channels found within the osteoclast cell membranes. The enzymatic pH is generally around 4–5, a level at which bone matrix can easily be mobilized [29, 30]. Cathepsin K, matrix metalloproteinase 9, and tartrate-resistant acid phosphatase then become released from lysosomes and digest organic matrix. Once the inorganic and organic substances have been removed, a characteristic shallow bowl-shaped Howship's lacuna remains on the surface [31]. Once done, osteoclasts undergo apoptosis leading to the next phase of remodeling.

The reversal phase was so named because it is during this stage that bone resorption is reversed, leading to subsequent bone formation. Although osteoclasts have undergone apoptosis and are no longer present at lacuna, mononuclear precursor cells, preosteoblasts, and liberated osteocytes remain and begin the process of reversal and preparation [32]. While the exact signals that trigger the initiation of reversal are not yet known, TGF-Beta, IGF-1 and 2, and BMPs are thought to play significant roles [33, 34]. These factors promote the final removal of undigested matrix and prepare for the final phase, formation.

As the name suggests, formation involves all the steps needed to deposit and mineralize new bone and takes approximately 4–6 months to complete [34]. It is during this phase that osteoblasts synthesize new matrix composed of type I collagen and deposit it within the previously formed lacuna. Proteoglycans, alkaline phosphatase small integrin-binding ligand (SIBLING) proteins, and lipids make up the remaining minority of organic substance [35]. The remaining step is hydroxyapatite secretion and incorporation into collagen, and while that exact mechanism is unknown, nonspecific alkaline phosphatase and nucleotide pyrophosphatase phosphodiesterase are thought to create the optimal extracellular environment to allow for this mineralization process [35].

With the formation of new bone, the remodeling process concludes. Osteoclasts undergo apoptosis, while osteoblasts either follow a similar fate

Table 1.1 The microscopic physiology and anatomy of bone

Cell type	Compound	Function	Mutations
Osteoclasts	PU.1	Early transcription factor, responsible for hematopoiesis. Implicated in osteoclast development	Osteopetrosis
	C-Fos	Transcription factor, requires for macrophage-osteoclast lineage	Osteopetrosis
	MITF	Required for osteoclast-specific membrane channels	Waardenburg syndrome type 2
	NFAT-1	Required for osteoclast formation, exact function unknown	Breast cancer
	CSF-1	Osteoclast differentiation	Osteopetrosis
	Osteoprotegerin	Binds RANKL, decreases maturation of osteoclasts	Juvenile Paget disease
Osteoblasts	RUNX2	Transcription factor, required osteoblast differentiation, known as the "master regulator of bone"	Cleidocranial dysostosis, osteosarcoma
	Sp7	Transcription factor, thought to interact with RUNX2 to promote osteoblast differentiation, induces Col1a1, osteonectin, osteopontin	Osteogenesis imperfecta
	DLX5	Transcription factor, interacts with RUNX2 and DLX5	Hand and foot malformation syndrome
	FGF	Promotes osteoblast differentiation	Chondrodysplasias
	FosB	Released by mechanical stress, increases osteoblast formation	Short-rib thoracic dysplasia
Osteocytes	PHEX	Involved in bone mineralization, osteopontin is the substrate for PHEX	X-linked hypophosphatemic rickets
	MEPE	Involved in integrin recognition, highly expressed in osteocytes	Osteomalacia, osteoporosis
	DMP1	Highly expressed by osteocytes, required for bone mineralization	Autosomal recessive hypophosphatemia
	E11/gp38	Promotes cytoplastic process formation	Unknown
	Sclerostin	BMP antagonist, has anti-anabolic effect on bone	Van Buchem disease

(about 50–70% of the total pool) and revert to the bone-lining phenotype or become embedded within matrix and differentiate to osteocytes. Osteocytes live within their lacuna and maintain a healthy environment. The appearance of this bone is now the characteristic osteon, made up of both organic and inorganic matrix which is the final description of the microscopic physiology and anatomy of bone (Table 1.1).

Organic Bone Matrix

Type I collagen makes up 85–90% of collagenous protein, with types III, IV, and fibril-associated collagen with interrupted triple helices (FACIT) making up the remainder. The latter proteins are non-fibrillary collagens that are thought to serve as bridges and help stabilize and organize extracellular matrices; these members include collagens IX, XII, XIV, XIX, and XXI [36]. Non-collagenous proteins, such as proteoglycans, phosphatases, and growth factors, help regulate cellular activity and matrix mineralization. As mentioned above, osteoblasts are responsible for the synthesis and secretion of both collagenous and non-collagenous proteins. Alkaline phosphatase is the principle glycosylated protein present in the extracellular matrix and is also found bound to osteoblast surfaces. The most prevalent non-collagenous protein however is osteonectin, also known as secreted protein acid which is rich in cysteine (SPARC), and is a basement membrane protein that is thought to play a role in collagen fibril assembly, procollagen processing, osteoblast growth, and profileration [37].

Inorganic Bone Matrix

The overall composition of bone is about 50–70% mineral, 20–40% organic matrix, and 5–10% water, and the remainder is lipid. The overwhelming majority of mineral is hydroxyapatite

$[Ca_{10}(PO_4)_6(OH)_2]$, with the rest being carbonate, magnesium, and acid phosphates. Unlike their geological cousin, bone hydroxyapatite is smaller by weight, poorly crystallized, and more soluble. Alkaline phosphatase, osteocalcin, osteopontin, and bone sialoprotein all regulate bone mineralization via the amount of hydroxyapatite that is formed. Minerals are first deposited in zones between the ends of collagen fibrils and then subsequently filled [38]. As bone matures, hydroxyapatite crystals purify and enlarge through aggregation and individual crystal growth. While not mentioned earlier, vitamin D plays an important role in stimulating the mineralization of unmineralized bone. After GI absorption or skin production, vitamin D is converted to its active form via the liver and kidneys, to 1,25-dihydroxyvitamin-D. It is this compound that is responsible for maintaining serum calcium and phosphorus levels allowing for the passive mineralization of bone matrix. This is accomplished by promoting intestinal absorption of these ions, as well as differentiation of osteoblasts and osteoblast expression of osteocalcin, osteonectin, OPG, and numerous other cytokines. The description above provides a brief and classic overview of bone physiology; below will describe some advances in molecular biology that have helped further the understanding and function of bone.

Updates on Bone Physiology

Osteoclast function is complex – much of their regulation and function is still unknown. In recent years, attention has focused on preosteoclasts, the cells that will eventually form multinucleated osteoclasts. Recent evidence has shown that preosteoclasts are mobilized to blood by sphingosine-1 phosphate (S1P) and sphingolipid, which are secreted by erythrocytes and platelets. Preosteoclasts and osteoclasts express S1P receptors and are attracted by this chemokine, possibly helping to promote the fusion of the mononucleated precursors to their more mature multinucleated form. Additionally, S1P expression is negatively regulated by cathepsin K, which may posit a future role for its inhibitors as a bone stimulating agent [39, 40]. S1P levels are also increased in the synovial fluid of rheumatoid arthritis, which may attract preosteoclasts to affected joints [39], and calcitonin has been shown to inhibit osteoclast activity by way of S1P [41]. While still early, this may prove important with respect to potential future pharmacotherapeutic agents.

G-proteins and regulators of G-protein (RGS) act to enhance the action of G-protein signaling and represent another example of complex regulation which has been implicated in osteoblast physiology. RGS2 has been shown to play a role in osteoblast differentiation via upregulation of forskolin and PTH. RGS5 may play a role in the osteoblastic response to extracellular calcium and Axin, a member of the RGS family, which negatively regulates bone mass (Axin knockout mice have increased bone density as compared to their wild-type controls) [42].

Neurohormonal regulation is another emerging area in bone physiology with serotonin, leptin, and neuropeptide-Y all having effects on bone. Brain serotonin has been shown to stimulate proliferation of osteoblasts and inhibit bone resorption [43]. Interestingly, gut-derived serotonin has the opposite effect, with genetically modified mice with low levels of duodenal serotonin having increased bone density. This is supported by some clinical studies which have shown that patients treated with SSRIs have decreased bone mass and increased risk of osteoporotic hip fracture, while adolescents taking SSRIs have significantly decreased bone mineral density. This may be explained in part by the presence of serotonin transporters in bone, although the exact mechanism is yet to be fully elucidated [44].

Leptin has been shown to increase proliferation of osteoblasts, presumably through its action on the beta-1-adrenergic system and IGF-1 system [45, 46]. Conversely, it suppresses bone formation via its activity on beta-2-adrenergic receptors and inhibits brain serotonin release, implicating a complex role for this hormone.

Neuropeptide Y (NPY) has been shown to be produced by osteoblasts and osteocytes [47] in a negative regulatory fashion as NPY overexpression slows formation of endo- and periosteal bone, increases trabecular bone loss [48], and has been shown to be a modulator of leptin with respect to bone formation. Numerous other hormones, not typically associated with bone such as cannabinoids and norepinephrine, have also been shown to alter its physiology; however that is beyond the scope of this chapter and is merely mentioned to highlight the complexity of bone regulation.

Age-Related Changes in Bone

While peak bone age is achieved within relatively similar time frames, around 30 for both men and women, the point of maximal substantial bone loss differs significantly between the sexes. Cortical bone loss in women occurs in the years following menopause, while in men it occurs around 70–75 years of age. Trabecular bone loss by contrast occurs in both sexes at similar times with men experiencing 42% loss and women 37% loss by age 50 [64].

It was over 70 years ago that estrogen was first implicated in postmenopausal bone loss [49], and while initially unknown, it is now accepted that this mechanism acts through the RANKL/OPG system. Postmenopausal women have a threefold greater percentage of RANKL expressing cells as their premenopausal counterparts, and it seems that the reverse is true with the presence of estrogen suppressing bone resorption in both men and women [65]. Osteoporotic cortical and trabecular bone is thinner, although the mineral content per given area of tissue is actually increased, as is collagen linearity and carbonate content.

On a macroscopic scale, bone undergoes changes in shape throughout age in response to load, as described by Wolff's law. Additionally, it increases in cross-sectional area due to expansion of its outer diameter and thins at its cortical walls [50] – this pattern has been seen in both nonhuman and human models [51, 52]. With regard to trabecular bone, age-related loss is predominantly due to thinning of individual trabeculae in men, while in women, it is due to a loss of connectivity and a decreased complexity of networks [53]. Over time, resorption outweighs formation, and bone gradually thins – these macroscopic changes underlie the microscopic changes to individual populations of bone cells.

The major bone cell types have finite lifespans which are controlled by several external factors in addition to the replication cycles. It has been shown that osteoblast populations diminish due to decreases in their respective precursors [54]. A similar process happens in osteoclasts, with the number of hematopoietic precursor cells declining with age [55], while osteocytes are hypothesized to undergo apoptosis due to lack of mechanical stimulus or loss of canalicular networks [56]. At the next level of organization, proteins themselves undergo age-related changes.

There is evidence that bone's structural proteins undergo age-related changes as well, both in their modification and production, and perhaps the most important of these proteins is collagen. Appropriate function of collagen is essential for bone to maintain its strength, and if this is not maintained, bone can lose its integrity. A critical factor of collagen is its orientation and alignment with hydroxyapatite crystals. Collagen orientation becomes more linear with age (recall that it maintains its strength through its normally orthogonal orientation within lamellae), and this may have an effect on mineral crystallization as well as overall strength [56]. Enzymatic cross-linking of collagen is an important component of its posttranslational modification and adds to its strength; however nonenzymatic cross-linking has the opposite effect. There is evidence that nonenzymatic cross-linking of collagen increases with age and this leads to an overall decrease in bone's strength and toughness, which increases the risk of fracture [57, 58]. This type of cross-linking also affects the way collagen is mineralized which further alters its structural properties.

The mineral content of bone increases with age, and while this increases its breaking stress, it ultimately results in making it more brittle and decreasing toughness [59, 60]. Not only does the overall amount of inorganic substance change, but the composition changes as well. Hydroxyapatite crystals are their purest at around 25–30 years of age, over time, and they gain substitutions of carbonate for hydroxyl and phosphate within the apatite surface [61]. This, along with a concomitant decrease in acid phosphate content [62, 63], is thought to be a factor contributing to the decreased toughness of aging bone. A better understanding of these processes may help to give more insight into the factors that lead to age-related bone loss.

References

1. Musculoskeletal system. In: Standring S, editors. Gray's anatomy. 39th ed. New York: Elsevier; 2004. pp. 83–135.
2. Eriksen EF, Axelrod DW, Melsen F. Bone histomorphometry. New York: Raven Press; 1994. p. 1–12.
3. Kobayashi S, Takahashi HE, Ito A, Saito N, Nawata M, Horiuchi H, Ohta H, Ito A, Iorio R, Yamamoto N, Takaoka K. Trabecular minimodeling in human iliac bone. Bone. 2003;32:163–9.
4. Van Oers RFM, Wang H, Bacabac RG. Osteocyte shape and mechanical loading. Curr Osteoporos Rep. 2015;13(2):61–6.
5. Boyle WJ, Simonet WS, Lacey DL. Osteoclast differentiation and activation. Nature. 2003;423:337–42.
6. Tondravi MM, McKercher SR, Anderson K, Erdmann JM, Quiroz M, Maki R, Teitelbaum SL. Osteopetrosis in mice lacking haematopoietic transcription factor PU.1. Nature. 1997;386(6620):81–4.
7. Grigoriadis AE, Wang ZQ, Cecchini MG, Hofstetter W, Felix R, Fleisch HA, Wagner EF. c-Fos: a key regulator of osteoclast-macrophage lineage determination and bone remodeling. Science. 1994;266(5184):443–8.
8. Luchin A, Purdom G, Murphy K, Clark MY, Angel N, Cassady AI, Hume DA, Ostrowski MC. The microphthalmia transcription factor regulates expression of the tartrate-resistant acid phosphatase gene during terminal differentiation of osteoclasts. J Bone Miner Res. 2000;15(3):451–60.
9. Ross FP, Teitelbaum SL. V3 and macrophage colony-stimulating factor: Partners in osteoclast biology. Immunol Rev. 2005;208:88–105.
10. Teitelbaum SL, Abu-Amer Y, Ross FP. Molecular mechanisms of bone resorption. J Cell Biochem. 1995;59:1–10.
11. Vaananen HK, Zhao H, Mulari M, Halleen JM. The cell biology of osteoclast function. J Cell Sci. 2000;113:377–81.
12. Komori T, Yagi H, Nomura S, Yamaguchi A, Sasaki K, Deguchi K, Shimizu Y, Bronson RT, Gao YH, Inada M, Sato M, Okamoto R, Kitamura Y, Yoshiki S, Kishimoto T. Targeted disruption of Cbfa1 results in a complete lack of bone formation owing to maturational arrest of osteoblasts. Cell. 1997;89(5):755–64.
13. Karsenty G. Transcriptional control of skeletogenesis. Annu Rev Genomics Hum Genet. 2008;9:183–96.
14. Pittenger MF, Mackay AM, Beck SC, Jaiswal RK, Douglas R, Mosca JD, Moorman MA, Simonetti DW, Craig S, Marshak DR. Multilineage potential of adult human mesenchymal stem cells. Science. 1990;284:143–7.
15. Rubin CT, Lanyon LE. Osteoregulatory nature of mechanical stimuli: function as a determinant for adaptive bone remodeling. J Orthop Res. 1987;5:300–10.
16. Plotkin LI, Aguirre JI, Kousteni S, Manolagas SC, Bellido T. Bisphosphonates and estrogens inhibit osteocyte apoptosis via distinct molecular mechanisms downstream of extra- cellular signal-regulated kinase activation. J Biol Chem. 2005;280:7317–25.
17. Maggioli C, Stagi S. Bone modeling, remodeling, and skeletal health in children and adolescents: mineral accrual, assessment and treatment. Ann Pediatr Endocrinol Metab. 2017;22(1):1–5.
18. Bachrach LK. Acquisition of optimal bone mass in childhood and adolescence. Trends Endocrinol Metab. 2001;12:22–8.
19. Hemmatian H, Bakker AD, Klein-Nulend J, van Lenthe GH. Aging, osteocytes, and mechanotransduction. Curr Osteoporos Rep. 2017;15(5):401–11.
20. Klein-nulend J, Van Oers RFM, Bakker AD, Bacabac RG. Bone cell mechanosensitivity, estrogen deficiency, and osteoporosis. J Biomech. 2015;48(5):855–65.
21. Burr DB. Targeted and nontargeted remodeling. Bone. 2002;30:2–4.
22. Parfitt AM. Targeted and nontargeted bone remodeling: relationship to basic multicellular unit origination and progression. Bone. 2002;30:5–7.
23. Klein-Nulend J, Bakker AD, Bacabac RG, Vatsa A, Weinbaum S. Mechanosensation and transduction in osteocytes. Bone. 2013;54(2):182–90.
24. Babaji P, Devanna R, Jagtap K, et al. The cell biology and role of resorptive cells in diseases: a review. Ann Afr Med. 2017;16(2):39–45.
25. Raggatt LJ, Partridge NC. Cellular and molecular mechanisms of bone remodeling. J Biol Chem. 2010;285(33):25103–8.
26. Clarke B. Normal bone physiology. Clin J Am Soc Nephrol. 2008;3:S131–9.
27. Kim JH, Jin HM, Kim K, Song I, Youn BU, Matsuo K, Kim N. The mechanism of osteoclast differentiation induced by IL-1. J Immunol. 2009;183:1862–70.
28. Amarasekara DS, Yun H, Kim S, Lee N, Kim H, Rho J. Regulation of osteoclast differentiation by cytokine networks. Immune Netw. 2018;18:450–2.
29. Silver IA, Murrills RJ, Etherington DJ. Microelectrode studies on the acid microenvironment beneath adherent macrophages and osteoclasts. Exp Cell Res. 1988;175:266–76.
30. Reddy SV. Regulatory mechanisms operative in osteoclasts. Crit Rev Eukaryot Gene Expr. 2004;14:255–70.
31. Everts V, Delaissé JM, Korper W, Jansen DC, Tigchelaar-Gutter W, Saftig P, Beertsen W. The bone lining cell: its role in cleaning Howship's lacunae and initiating bone formation. J Bone Miner Res. 2002;17(1):77–90.

32. Hock JM, Centrella M, Canalis E. Insulin-like growth factor IGF-I has independent effects on bone matrix formation and cell replication. Endocrinology. 2004;122:254–60.
33. Locklin RM, Oreffo RO, Triffitt JT. Effects of TGFbeta and bFGF on the differentiation of human bone marrow stromal fibroblasts. Cell Biol Int. 1999;23:185–94.
34. Martin TJ, Sims NA. Osteoclast-derived activity in the coupling of bone formation to resorption. Trends Mol Med. 2005;11:76–81.
35. Robey P, Boskey A. In: Rosen C, editor. Primer on the metabolic bone diseases and disorders of mineral metabolism. 7th ed. 2008. pp. 32–8.
36. Chiquet M, Birk DE, Bönnemann CG, Koch M. Molecules in focus: Collagen XII: protecting bone and muscle integrity by organizing collagen fibrils. Int J Biochem Cell Biol. 2014;53:51–4.
37. Rosset EM, Bradshaw AD. SPARC/osteonectin in mineralized tissue. Matrix Biol. 2016;52:78–87.
38. Landis WJ. The strength of a calcified tissue depends in part on the molecular structure and organization of its constituent mineral crystals in their organic matrix. Bone. 1995;16:533–44.
39. Kikuta J, Iwai K, Saeki Y, Ishii M. S1P-targeted therapy for elderly rheumatoid arthritis patients with osteoporosis. Rheumatol Int. 2011;31:967–9.
40. Lotinun S, Kiviranta R, Matsubara T, Alzate JA, Neff L, Luth A, et al. Osteoclast-specific cathepsin K deletion stimulates S1P-dependent bone formation. J Clin Invest. 2013;123:666–81.
41. Keller J, Catala-Lehnen P, Huebner AK, et al. Calcitonin controls bone formation by inhibiting the release of sphingosine 1-phosphate from osteoclasts. Nat Commun. 2014;5:5215.
42. Jules J, Yang S, Chen W, Li Y-P. Role of regulators of G protein signaling proteins in bone physiology and pathophysiology. Prog Mol Biol Transl Sci. 2015;133:47–75.
43. Kode A, et al. FOXO1 orchestrates the bone-suppressing function of gut-derived serotonin. J Clin Invest. 2012;122:3490–503.
44. Zofkova I, Matucha P. New insights into the physiology of bone regulation: the role of neurohormones. Physiol Res. 2014;63:421–7.
45. Hamrick MW, Ferrari SL. Leptin and the sympathetic connection of fat to bone. Osteoporos Int. 2008;19:905–12.
46. Motyl KJ, Rosen CJ. Understanding leptin-dependent regulation of skeletal homeostasis. Biochemie. 2012;94:2089–96.
47. Matic I, et al. Bone-specific overexpression of NPY modulates osteogenesis. J Musculoskelet Neuronal Interact. 2012;12:209–18.
48. Franguinho F, Liz MA, Nunes AF, Neto E, Lamghari M, Sousa MM. Neuropeptide Y and osteoblast differentiation-the balance between the neuro-osteogenic network and local control. FEBS J. 2010;277:3664–7.
49. Albright F, Smith PH, Richardson AM. Postmenopausal osteoporosis. JAMA. 1941;116:2465–74.
50. Westerbeek ZW, Hepple RT, Zernicke RF. Effects of aging and caloric restriction on bone structure and mechanical properties. J Gerontol A Biol Sci Med Sci. 2008;63:1131–6.
51. Nagaraja S, Lin AS, Guldberg RE. Age-related changes in trabecular bone microdamage initiation. Bone. 2007;40:973–80.
52. Tommasini SM, Nasser P, Jepsen KJ. Sexual dimorphism affects tibia size and shape but not tissue-level mechanical properties. Bone. 2007;40:498–505.
53. Aaron JE, Makins NB, Sagreiya K. The microanatomy of trabecular bone loss in normal aging men and women. Clin Orthop Relat Res. 1987;(215): 260–71.
54. Lee CC, Fletcher MD, Tarantal AF. Effect of age on the frequency, cell cycle, and lineage maturation of rhesus monkey (*Macaca mulatta*) CD34+ and hematopoietic progenitor cells. Pediatr Res. 2005;8:315–22.
55. Szulc P, Seeman E. Thinking inside and outside the envelopes of bone: dedicated to PDD. Osteoporos Int. 2009;20:1281–8.
56. Rochefort GY, Pallu S, Benhamou CL. Osteocyte: the unrecognized side of bone tissue. Osteoporos Int. 2010;21(9):1457–69.
57. Banse X, Devogelaer JP, Lafosse A, Sims TJ, Grynpas M, Bailey AJ. Cross-link profile of bone collagen correlates with structural organization of trabeculae. Bone. 2002;31:70–6.
58. Viguet-Carrin S, Follet H, Gineyts E, Roux JP, Munoz F, Chapurlat R. Association between collagen cross-links and trabecular micro-architecture properties of human vertebral bone. Bone. 2010;46:342–7.
59. Currey JD. The relationship between the stiffness and the mineral content of bone. J Biomech. 1969;2:477–80.
60. Currey JD, Brear K, Zioupos P. The effects of ageing and changes in mineral content in degrading the toughness of human femora. J Biomech. 1996;29:257–62; *erratum* in J Biomech 30:1001, 1997.
61. LeGeros RZ. Properties of osteoconductive biomaterials: calcium phosphates. Clin Orthop Relat Res. 2002;395:81–98.
62. Loong CK, Rey C, Kuhn LT, Combes C, Wu Y, Chen S, et al. Evidence of hydroxyl-ion deficiency in bone apatites: an inelastic neutron-scattering study. Bone. 2000;26:599–602.
63. Rey C, Hina A, Tofighi A, Glimcher MJ. Maturational of poorly crystalline apatites – chemical and structural aspects *in vivo* and *in vitro*. Cells Mater. 1995;5:345–56.
64. Khosla S. Pathogeneiss of age-related bone loss. J Gerontol. 2013;68(10):1226–35.
65. Hannon R, Blumsohn A, Naylor K, Eastell R. Response of biochemical markers of bone turnover to hormone replacement therapy: impact of biological variability. J Bone Miner Res. 1998;13:1124–33.

Pathophysiology and Epidemiology of Osteoporosis

2

Nicole M. Stevens and Sanjit R. Konda

Key Points

1. Osteoporosis is an abnormality in the quantity, not the quality of bone.
2. The architecture of osteoporotic bone, including decreased trabecular number and caliber, and changes in cortical bone structure, predisposes elderly patients to fracture.
3. RANKL/RANK pathway, Wnt signaling pathway, and inflammatory cytokines all play a role in bone turnover and homeostasis.
4. Estrogen deficiency has multiple adverse effects on bone homeostasis, including increased osteoclastogenesis, increased rate of bone turnover, and decreased activation of osteoblasts.
5. There are multiple secondary causes of osteoporosis including systemic diseases and commonly prescribed medications.

Introduction

Osteoporosis is the most common disease of bone, and the surgeon general has defined it to be a major health problem affecting Americans [1]. As defined by the World Health Organization, osteoporosis is a bone mineral density (BMD) less than 2.5 standard deviations below the mean BMD in young healthy individuals measured in the vertebra or hip, or the occurrence of a documented fragility fracture.

The pathophysiology of osteoporosis is multifactorial, and not fully understood, but includes genetic predisposition, hormonal changes, abnormal inflammatory response, and variations in bony mechanics. This chapter will discuss the pathophysiology of osteoporosis as is known today and discuss the epidemiology and widespread implications of this common disease.

Definition of Osteoporosis

Osteoporosis is a complex disorder involving abnormalities in genetics, hormone regulation, inflammatory pathways, and mechanical loading of bone; ultimately this leads to a decrease in bone mineral density (BMD) and bone quantity [2]. BMD can be measured using a dual energy x-ray absorptiometry (DXA) scan. DXA scans take two dimensional images of bone in various parts of the body; the hip and vertebra are typically measured; however measurements of the

N. M. Stevens · S. R. Konda (✉)
Department of Orthopedic Surgery, NYU Langone Orthopedic Hospital, NYU Langone Medical Center, New York, NY, USA
e-mail: Nicole.stevens@nyulangone.org; sanjit.konda@nyulangone.org

A. E. Razi, S. H. Hershman (eds.), *Vertebral Compression Fractures in Osteoporotic and Pathologic Bone*, https://doi.org/10.1007/978-3-030-33861-9_2

distal radius and calcaneus have also been described. Normal is defined as the mean BMD in the vertebrae and hips of healthy young individuals at the time of peak bone mass. Osteopenia is defined as anything below 1 standard deviation of the mean, and osteoporosis is defined as anything below 2.5 standard deviations from the mean. DXA can also be used to compare an individual's bone mineral density against age-matched cohorts. While the DXA scan is a good marker for definition purposes, it is limited by its two dimensionality, and therefore does not fully describe the osteoporotic nature of the bone [3].

Bone Structure

The primary characteristic of osteoporotic bone is a decrease in bone *quantity*. This is distinctly different from osteomalacia, which is a decrease in bone *quality*. The actual mineralization of bone and its chemical composition is normal in osteoporosis. It is therefore important to describe normal bony architecture and to differentiate it from abnormal bony architecture. Normal bony architecture consists of two regions – cortical bone and cancellous bone. The two areas serve different functions. Cortical bone is a dense, highly organized, laminar network of osteons which provides structural integrity and strength. This structural bone is typically found on the outside, providing mechanical strength and leverage for many muscular attachments. The overlapping design of the osteons found in cortical bone, also helps to prevent fracture, since the "cement," or unmineralized cellular structure between each mineralized osteon, provides a cushion to absorb energy and prevent crack propogation [4]. Cortical bone is strong, but more brittle, given its highly organized nature, and has a bigger propensity to fail catastrophically – as seen in a typical long bone fracture.

Cancellous bone, in contrast, consists of a porous trabecular network of highly crosslinked bony bridges, which functions more as a sponge to provide flexibility. The cancellous portion acts more like a spring to absorb energy by deformation rather than breaking or cracking. Because each bridge of bone is a small structure, fracture of a single bridge typically does not require a huge amount of energy, nor does it result in catastrophic failure. Instead, when enough trabecular bridges are broken, fracture typically results in a collapse of the structure, as found in osteoporotic vertebral fractures. Cancellous bone is typically found within the medullary cavity of cortical bone. Its trabecular network also houses bone marrow, where mesenchymal stem cells are stored.

Each bone in the body has differing quantities of cortical versus cancellous bone to maximize the mechanical advantage. For example, long bones of the leg require thick cortices to act as levers and bear the weight of the body during ambulation. In contrast, vertebral bodies have a high quantity of cancellous bone, to account for the flexibility needed in the spine.

Bone is a dynamic structure and is constantly remodeling based on the forces it experiences. Remodeling occurs by a process of resorption and deposition. During skeletal growth, the rate of deposition surpasses that of resorption, resulting in net added bone mass. In early adulthood, typically between ages 18 and 25, homeostasis is achieved, such that resorption matches deposition. At this timepoint, the body has the greatest density of bone throughout its lifetime, which is defined as peak mineral density (PMD). Peak mineral density differs in individuals; genetics, diet, activity level, and various other factors have all been found to play a role. For example, Caucasians typically have lower peak mineral density than African Americans, and heavier individuals have higher PMD than lighter individuals. PMD is critically important because an individual's PMD is one of the factors defining an individual's risk for developing osteoporosis in the future. As much as 60–80% of PMD is defined by a person's genetics according to some studies [5].

As people age, and particularly after menopause in women, resorption starts to outpace deposition, and bone density declines. Rates are variable, but if resorption outpaces deposition enough, osteopenia and eventually osteoporosis results. This resorption is particularly troublesome if an individual starts with a lower PMD to begin with.

Biomechanics of Osteoporotic Bone

The changes in osteoporotic bony architecture are most profound in the cancellous region. As discussed earlier, the bony bridges are smaller to begin with – so lost mass is more profound. In addition, cancellous bony architecture and its fine network of trabeculae create a large surface area for bony turnover by osteoclasts and osteoblasts – the mechanism of which will be discussed later in the chapter. As resorption occurs, the dense trabecular network becomes more sparse, and the porosity of the bone increases. Normal cancellous bone has an interconnecting web of plate-like trabeculae, whereas osteoporotic bone has thinner, more rod-like trabeculae [6]. The trabecular network is critical to cancellous bone's strength. Studies have shown that the compressive strength of trabecular bone decreases by approximately 70% from age 25 to 75 [7]. This resorption and decreased surface area massively weakens the bone and increases the number of microfractures in the remaining trabeculae which are experiencing a greater proportion of force as the number of bridges declines. If enough microfractures occur, the bone will fracture on a macroscale, also known as a fragility or osteoporotic fracture.

Cortical bone is not immune to change either. Studies have shown that the elastic modulus of cortical bone, a measure of bone stiffness, decreases approximately 1–2% per decade beyond the age of 35 years [8, 9]. Strength was found to decrease 2–5% per decade; and toughness, which is a measure of energy required to fracture, decreases by 10% per decade [9]. There are a variety of factors playing into these changes in material properties. First, older cortical bone is more porous due to the mismatch in bone turnover and fewer collagen crosslinks [8]. Furthermore, as the porosity of cortical bone increases, the available surface area for bone turnover increases, thereby exacerbating the problem [3]. This increase in porosity also creates low energy pathways for fracture propagation. Finally, as the mismatch in resorption and deposition increases, the newly laid collagen does not have time to create structural crosslinks. These crosslinks are critical to bony strength as they connect the overlapping osteons. Long sheets of individual osteons do not have the strength or toughness of highly crosslinked osteon units, thereby increasing the risk of fracture.

The overall geometry of bone changes over time to compensate for changes in the microarchitecture. Numerous studies have shown that the cross-sectional area of vertebral bodies and long bones is positively correlated with age, particularly in men [10–12]. One study found a 15% increase in lumbar vertebra cross-sectional area in men from age 20 to 90 years [10]. This is likely a protective mechanism to increase bone strength and decrease risk of fracture. As the radius of the entire bone increases, the force applied to the skeleton is divided across a wider cross-sectional surface area, thereby distributing the stress. It is important to note that this phenomenon of increasing cross sectional area is found more consistently in males than in females, which correlates with females' increased risk of fracture [8].

In summary, bone's ability to resist fracture depends on both geometry and material properties. In this section, we discussed the geometric properties of osteoporotic bone; the next section will focus on its material properties and cellular makeup. By a combination of these factors, the compressive failure force of a vertebral body decreases by almost 80% from age 30 to 90 [13].

Pathogenesis

On a cellular level, there are several interconnecting pathways that lead to the increased absorption of bone in osteoporosis. Several pathways have been extensively studied and will be focused on here, but there are likely many pathways that are yet to be elucidated.

Bone resorption and deposition is primarily regulated by the receptor activator of nuclear factor kappa-B ligand (RANKL), a member of the tumor necrosis factor (TNF) receptor family. On a basic level, RANKL is produced by osteoblasts and their mature counterparts, osteocytes, in response to a number of signals and biologic states discussed later in this section. The RANKL binds to RANK on an osteoclast precursor cell – thereby activating it. Once activated, the osteoclast precursor forms a multinucleated cell which becomes an osteoclast. The osteoclast attaches to the surface of the bone, creating a tight seal, and secretes hydrochloric acid to dissolve the mineral bone and cathepsin K to dissolve the bony matrix. This creates a cavity in the bony surface. In normal bone turnover, this process is immediately followed by osteoblast activity, which lays down a new bone collagen matrix and is then mineralized, creating a new bone unit.

Another key receptor-ligand pair in osteoclast differentiation is macrophage – colony-stimulating factor (M-CSF) and CSF-1 receptor (c-Fms). C-Fms is expressed on osteoclast precursor cells. M-CSF is produced by pre-osteoblasts and stromal cells. When bound, they promote osteoclastogenesis. Of note, both the M-CSF/C-FMS and RANK/RANKL couplings are required for osteoclast differentiation, but RANK/RANKL is typically the rate-limiting step. There are still modulators that upregulate M-CSF production to create a pro-resorptive environment. These modulators include inflammatory cytokines like TNF-alpha and IL-1, produced by T cells [14].

The RANK/RANKL system is also policed by osteoprotegrin (OPG). OPG is a member of the TNF receptor superfamily but has unique characteristics, namely, that it is secreted as a soluble protein and lacks transmembrane and cytoplasmic domains. OPG blocks the RANK/RANKL coupling, thereby arresting osteoclast differentiation. It does this by acting as a decoy receptor, binding RANKL – to effectively sequester it from the system. OPG is produced by osteoblasts and stromal cells. It effectively shuts down osteoclast activity and is a strong protector of bone generation.

In abnormal, osteoporotic bone, as has been stated previously, the rate of resorption outpaces the rate of deposition. Therefore, the cavities in the bone created by the osteoclasts persist, creating increased porosity within the macro bone structure. It should also be noted that bone turnover can only occur in locations that already have bone, since the process works on the surface. So, in a fine trabecular network, where resorption is outpacing deposition, the trabeculae will become thinner and thinner, until they are completely resorbed. Ultimately, there is no surface for bony deposition to occur – leading to fewer and smaller trabeculae and increasing empty space.

Cellular signaling also changes based on mechanical load; the canonical Wnt signaling pathway is the most studied mechanical-cellular converter. The Wnt signal pathway is mediated primarily by osteocytes, which are the best suited cells to react to mechanical load, as they are encased within the bone. When Wnt is present, it prevents the breakdown of beta-catenin by binding to Frizzled and/or LRP5 or 6. Beta-catenin then translocates to the nucleus where it associates with transcription factors and regulates target genes like runx2 and WISP1. This ultimately leads to osteoblast differentiation and increased bone deposition. Wnt also inhibits osteoclastogenesis by inducing OPG, and likely other factors, to shut down osteoclast production. Therefore, upregulation of Wnt by increased mechanical loading leads to net positive bone formation. Wnt is antagonized by several proteins. Sclerostin is expressed by osteocytes and functions to limit Wnt signaling by binding to LRP5/6. It therefore inhibits bone formation and is primarily expressed when mechanical load is low or in hyperparathyroidism. Another inhibitor is Dickkopf-related protein 1 (DKK-1). DKK-1 binds with LRP-5/6 as well as a Kremen protein which inhibits the Wnt pathway [15]. In mice, neutralizing antibody blockade of either sclerostin or DKK-1 leads to increased BMD, trabecular volume, and osteoblast number [16–18] – therefore blocking these Wnt antagonists pharmacologically may prevent osteoporosis in humans.

Calcium and Vitamin D

Bone acts as a repository for calcium in the body and plays a critical role in calcium homeostasis. In low-calcium environments, such as inadequate dietary intake, impaired intestinal absorption, or vitamin D deficiency, bone is resorbed to release calcium from its stores and maintain appropriate serum levels. This process is primarily mediated by parathyroid hormone (PTH). When blood levels of calcium fall below a certain level, the parathyroid gland senses the drop and releases PTH. PTH then acts directly on bone units by activating stromal cells to produce RANKL and decrease OPG to ultimately increase osteoclastogenesis. This leads to bone resorption and serum calcium release. PTH also stimulates the kidneys to increase uptake of calcium and release activated vitamin D (1,25 dihydroxy vitamin D). The activated vitamin D travels to the intestines where it increases dietary absorption of calcium. The net result is increased serum calcium. Activated vitamin D also has an inhibitory effect on the parathyroid, decreasing parathyroid hormone production to prevent hypercalcemia [31].

When serum calcium levels are persistently low, hyperparathyroidism can result. At the bony level, this results in increased activation of the stromal cells and production of RANKL and inhibition of OPG, subsequently causing increased bone resorption. When there is decreased calcium intake, or impaired intestinal absorption, the bone is the only readily available source of calcium, and so pathologic resorption may take place, leading to osteoporosis.

Vitamin D3 is synthesized in the skin and converted to pre-vitamin D by UV light. Vitamin D3 can also be obtained from diet. Vitamin D is then oxidized first by the liver and transported to the kidney where it is oxidized once more thereby activating it. Activated vitamin D binds to vitamin D receptor (VDR) in several locations to affect calcium and phosphate homeostasis [32]. VDR is present in the intestine, as described above, and increases calcium absorption. It is also present in the bone, muscle, pancreas, and pituitary [31, 33–36]. Mutations in the VDR receptor can lead to severe osteomalacia and diseases like rickets, thereby highlighting its importance in bone homeostasis [32].

Low levels of vitamin D may also lead to a secondary hyperparathyroidism and eventually osteoporosis. Vitamin D deficiency impairs calcium absorption in the intestines. As above, if calcium is unable to be absorbed by the intestine, the body seeks out calcium in its only other repository, bone. Since vitamin D also plays an inhibitory role on PTH production, vitamin D deficiency leads to persistent activation of PTH. Persistent activation of PTH will result in upregulation of osteoclastogenesis and increased bony resorption [31, 33].

Estrogen Deficiency

Estrogen deficiency, the hallmark of menopause, increases the lifespan of osteoclasts and decreases the lifespan of osteoblasts [19]. This increases the rate of resorption, while decreasing the rate of formation. Not only is the net negative imbalance detrimental to bony architecture, but the rate of remodeling can increase the risk of fracture. Rapid remodeling removes bone before new bone can be laid down, leaving cavities that may be nidus points for fractures [20]. Furthermore, newly formed bone is less dense than the bone that was resorbed – this ultimately decreases the material stiffness, leading to greater flexibility and bending. Abnormal bending may lead to unusual load distribution, ultimately leading to fracture [21, 22]. Finally, new bone needs time to mature, primarily by creating crosslinks between collagen fibers. When the rate of remodeling is increased, the cross-linking process has less time to occur, weakening the overall structure [23]. Studies have shown that remodeling rates can as much as double 12 months after the last menstrual period and may remain persistently elevated over time, with rates being almost tripled 13 years after menopause has occurred [24].

The importance of the rate of remodeling can be shown by the effect of antiresorptive medications on reducing fracture risk in osteoporosis. Antiresorptive treatments, like bisphosphonates, have been shown to reduce fracture risk by almost 45%, but they only cause a bone mineral density (BMD) gain of approximately 20% [25]. Selective estrogen receptor modulators, like raloxifene, which have an estrogenic effect on bone and antiestrogenic effects on the uterus and breast, have also been shown to decrease fracture risk irrespective of changes in BMD.

The Multiple Outcomes of Raloxifene Evaluation (MORE) trial found that vertebral fracture risk was decreased by 40%, irrespective of change in bone mass, and also found that 96% of the fracture risk reduction was not related to a change in BMD [26].

Estrogen deficiency is also associated with decreased absorption of calcium in the intestine and increased excretion of calcium through the renal system. This may be due to increased serum calcium concentration from resorbed bone and a resulting decrease in parathyroid levels. The effects of calcium homeostasis are an important mediator of bone mineral density. As described above, decreased serum calcium, or the inability to absorb calcium, leads to an upregulation of osteoclasts and increased bone resorption.

Finally, estrogen has also been found to play a role in the inflammatory response modulating osteoporosis. Estrogen deficiency leads to T cell activation. These activated T cells produce cytokines, including TNFs and IL-1, which stimulate osteoclast activity, inhibiting apoptosis and osteoblasts [27–30]. This leads to an overall catabolic effect and increased bone resorption.

The rate of bone loss can be impressive – in the 5–7 years surrounding menopause, women can lose up to 12% of their bone mass [24, 27]. This is equivalent to one standard of deviation as measured by a DXA scan. This change begins even before menopause takes place, starting 1–2 years before menopause, when ovaries start producing less estrogen.

Epidemiology

According to the National Health and Nutrition Examination Survey III, conducted from 2005 to 2010, over 10.2 million adults had osteoporosis, and more than 43.4 million adults had low bone mass in the USA. As the baby boomer generation ages, this number will only become larger [37, 38]increasing both the rate of osteoporosis diagnoses and the risk of fracture . In the USA, the lifetime risk of fracture in Caucasian women over 50 years of age is 50%, while a Caucasian man has a 16–25% risk of low-energy fracture [27, 39, 40].

There are both heritable and nonheritable factors that play a role in the development of osteoporosis. Heritable factors primarily include genes, which may influence bone mass, size, macro- and micro-architecture, and intrinsic material properties, like the strength of the bone tissue. Many genes have been identified as possibly relating to the development of osteoporosis including transforming growth factor B1 (TGF-B1), bone morphogenetic proteins (BMPs), sclerostin (SOST), cathepsin K, type 1 collagen, chloride channel 7 (CLCN7), vitamin D receptor (VDR), estrogen receptors, and transcription factors including Runx2 [27].

Risk factors for primary osteoporosis and low bone mineral density include older age, female gender, smoking, prior wrist fracture, and spinal deformity [41]. The Women's Health Initiative found 11 clinical risk factors which were independent risk factors for 5-year hip fracture risk, having a hazards ratio greater than 1. These risks included age per year, self-reported health, height per inch, weight per pound, fracture after age 55, Caucasian vs African American race, low physical activity level, current smoking status, family history of osteoporotic fracture, steroid use, and diabetes [42]. It should be noted that these risk factors not only encompass the general health status and risk of osteoporosis but also reflect the likelihood of sustaining a low energy fall. There are several biochemical markers that also predict hip fracture independent of clinical risk factors, including low vitamin D, low bioavailable testosterone, and high pre-inflammatory cytokines [42].

There is also a plethora of secondary causes of osteoporosis – these include both medications and patient traits. These are important to screen for in at risk individuals, because their treatment may prevent or reverse osteoporosis.

Diseases Leading to Osteoporosis

Male Hypogonadism

Hypogonadism is a leading cause of osteoporosis in males, although the effects of testosterone on the bone mineral density have not been fully elucidated. Approximately 20% of men over the age of 60 have low testosterone levels, leading to an increased risk of osteoporosis and fragility fractures [43, 44]. There are a variety of causes of hypogonadism in men, including congenital defects, aging, pituitary disease, and medications leading to secondary hypogonadism [45]. Amory et al. demonstrated an increase in BMD in men treated with 36 months of testosterone – although this has not been shown to reduce fragility fractures [46].

Female Hypogonadism

As described above, estrogen plays a critical role in bone homeostasis, and the decreased levels of serum estrogen in menopause can have critical effects on bone turnover leading to osteoporosis. But even at a younger age, low estrogen states can significantly increase the risk of low bone mineral density. Amenorrheic women have been found to have BMD up to 8% less than control subjects regardless of their exercise state [47]. Furthermore, although the outcome is likely multifactorial, patients with anorexia nervosa associated with amenorrhea have a 90% chance of having low bone mineral density – in fact, 40% were osteoporotic [48].

Chronic Inflammatory Disease

There is a known correlation between many chronic inflammatory diseases such as rheumatoid arthritis (RA), inflammatory bowel disease, celiac disease, chronic obstructive pulmonary disease, and osteoporosis [49]. One study of patients which ulcerative colitis and Crohn's disease found that greater than 50% of patients had osteopenia orosteoporosis [50]. All of these diseases have an upregulation of inflammatory cytokines, many of which have been shown to have osteoclastogenic properties. In RA, infiltrating T cells and synovial cells have been shown to produce RANKL [51]. Chronic inflammatory diseases activate T cells, which produce pro-inflammatory cytokines such as IL-1, IL-6, and TNF-alpha, all of which act directly on stromal cells to increase RANKL and decrease OPG. They also affect the Wnt signaling pathway, by upregulating the Wnt inhibitors including sclerostin and DKK1 [49]. Nutritional status may also play a role in increased osteoporosis in this cohort, since many chronically ill patients are malnourished – which could negatively impact calcium homeostasis among other things.

Hematologic Disease

A variety of hematologic diseases, including multiple myeloma, leukemia, thalassemia, and lymphoma, have all been associated with low bone mineral density. The most studied of these disorders is multiple myeloma. The bone mineral density loss in multiple myeloma is primarily derived from pro-inflammatory cytokine secretion by the plasma cells characteristic of the disease [45]. Like many of the systemic diseases mentioned earlier, the pro-inflammatory cytokines upregulate RANK/RANKL signaling thereby increasing osteoclast activity.

Hyperthyroidism

Thyrotoxicosis is a known cause of osteoporosis and decreased bone mineral density. Interestingly, unlike many other causes of osteoporosis, it seems to primarily effect the cortices of bone rather than the trabecular bone. There are two mechanisms by which hyperthyroidism causes osteoporosis. First, T3, a thyroid hormone, interacts with bone nuclear receptor to accelerate bone remodeling. The rapid rate of remodeling, much like that caused in estrogen deficiency, leads to decreased bone mineral density, and weaker bone overall. The second mechanism is by decreasing levels of TSH. TSH reduces bony turnover; in hyperthyroidism TSH is low, leading to decreased inhibition, thereby exacerbating bone loss [52].

Diabetes Mellitus

Both type 1 and type 2 diabetes mellitus are associated with osteoporosis. Type 1 diabetes is associated with the typical pattern of osteoporosis, but like hyperthyroidism, type 2 diabetes is frequently associated with more cortical, rather than cancellous, porosity [53]. Unlike other secondary causes of osteoporosis, diabetes is associated with low bony turnover and decreased osteoblastic activity. Insulin may have an anabolic effect on bone, so type 1 diabetics may suffer from osteoporosis due to lack of insulin. Diabetic mice have also been shown to have upregulation in Wnt inhibitors including sclerostin and DKK1 [52].

Human Immunodeficiency Virus (HIV)

Up to 70% of patients with HIV have low bone mineral density, and the risk of osteoporosis seems to increase with anti-retroviral therapy [54]. The incidence of osteoporosis in HIV is likely multifactorial, and probably includes a systemic response to chronic disease, malnutrition, and the virus itself. HIV virus may upregulate the Wnt pathway, increasing bone turnover [52]. HAART has been shown to cause a 2–6% drop in BMD 2 years after its initiation, possibly due to upregulation of osteoclast activity [55]. Since people with HIV are living longer, recognizing and treating their osteoporosis is critical.

Glucocorticoid Excess

Exogenous or endogenous overproduction of steroids is one of the most common causes of secondary osteoporosis. Up to 50% of patients on chronic steroids will experience an osteoporotic fracture [56], and a similar risk is found in patients with Cushing's disease. Glucocorticoids affect several bone homeostasis pathways. First, glucocorticoids downregulate osteoblast differentiation by inhibiting the Wnt pathway through increasing the production of sclerostin and DKK1. Glucocorticoids also increase the rate of apoptosis of both osteoblasts and osteocytes. This weakens bone and decreases the rate of new bone production. While glucocorticoids decrease the lifespan of osteocytes and osteoblasts, they increase both the lifespan and the activity of osteoclasts. This is done by upregulating RANKL and suppressing OPG. Glucocorticoids quickly alter the homeostasis of bone metabolism. Within the first year of steroid use, bone mineral density can decrease by as much as 12% [52]. This is followed by a steady annual decline as steroid use continues.

Medications Causing Osteoporosis

Exogenous Steroids

One of the most commonly cited medications leading to osteoporosis is chronic exogenous steroid use. For a complete description of the effects of elevated glucocorticoids on bone mineral density and fracture risk, see the previous section.

Aromatase Inhibitors

Aromatase inhibitors are an effective means of decreasing the recurrence of breast cancer in women. Their mechanism of action is to reduce peripheral estrogen circulation by blocking the conversion of androgens to estrogens. This effectively lowers endogenous estrogen production by almost 90%. As described previously, decreased serum estrogen leads to adverse effects on bone mineral density. After 5 years of aromatase inhibitor therapy, studies have shown that bone mineral density in the spine and hip decrease by 6.05% and 7.25%, respectively [57]. Luckily, the decline in bone mineral density does seem to halt after stopping the medication [58].

Acid Suppressive Medications

Acid suppressive medications like proton pump inhibitors (PPIs) and H2 receptor antagonists are one of the most commonly prescribed medications worldwide. Several recent studies have shown an association between fracture risk and use of these medications, particularly in males with osteoporosis [59–62]. The data is more consistent that PPIs may lead to increased risk of fracture; H2 antagonist data is more inconsistent. The leading hypothesis for this correlation is that the acid suppressant impacts calcium homeostasis, although this has not yet born out in the literature.

Antiepileptic Drugs

Several cohort studies have shown a link between antiepileptic drugs and low bone mineral density and fracture risk [52, 63]. The pathophysiology is thought to be due to decreased circulation of pre-vitamin D caused by activation of the cytochrome P450 enzyme system in the liver and increased breakdown. Less pre-vitamin D leads to less activated vitamin D and ultimately, a secondary hyperparathyroidism leading to the activation of osteoclasts. In a randomized trial, Mikati et al. showed that high dose vitamin D supplementation in patients on antiepileptic drugs could help stabilize the bone mineral density as compared to a low-dose vitamin D regimen [64]. Newer antiepileptics, including gabapentin, topiramate, and levetiracetam, do not seem to decrease bone mineral density to the extent that older generation medications did [65].

Selective Serotonin Uptake Inhibitors (SSRIs)

SSRIs are widely prescribed for patients suffering from depression. While there has been a correlation found between patients with depression and low bone mineral density, several studies have found an increased risk of low bone mineral density and fracture in the subset of depressed patients taking SSRIs [52, 66]. There are other studies, however, which have not shown a correlation between low BMD and SSRI use. If SSRIs do have an impact on bone mineral density, the exact mechanism is unknown. One study proposed that serotonin has a direct effect on osteoblasts, reducing proliferation and thereby slowing bone deposition [67].

Lifestyle Factors

Smoking

Cigarette smoking is a well-known risk factor for low bone mass. Twin studies have suggested that smoking reduces peak bone mass, and in the perimenopausal period, smokers have a 5–10% decrease in their bone mineral density as compared to their nonsmoking twin counterparts [68]. The most likely cause of low bone mineral density in smokers is its effect on serum estrogen. Smoking increases hydroxylation of estradiol in the liver, leading to decreased active estrogen in the serum. Women who smoke typically have earlier menopause and lower serum estrogen concentrations than their peers [69].

There is likely also a direct effect on bone from smoking, but the mechanism has not yet been defined. The correlation between low bone mineral density in men and smoking has also been born out in the literature, although it has not yet been correlated with fracture risk.

Chronic Alcohol Abuse

Chronic alcohol abuse has been linked both to low bone mineral density and to osteopenia/osteoporosis. Ethanol has been found to have a direct effect on normal bone remodeling through the inhibition of osteoblast proliferation [70]. In chronic alcohol abuse, there is typically a decrease in the deposition of new bone, but resorption is typically normal or also decreased [71]. Unlike other secondary factors causing osteoporosis, chronic alcohol abuse has a decreased rate of bone turn over. Chronic alcohol consumption also has indirect effects on bone metabolism. Ethanol accelerates the clearance of testosterone leading to lower serum androgen levels which effects calcium homeostasis [72]. There is also likely a nutritional component as well, as chronic alcoholics typically have poor nutritional intake.

Recommended Screening for Osteoporosis

Given the number of secondary causes of osteoporosis, a workup of diagnosed osteoporosis should include a complete history, physical, and laboratory assessment of the patient to find modifiable causes. Typical blood tests include complete blood count (CBC), complete metabolic panel including liver tests (CMP), erythrocyte sedimentation rate (ESR), c-reactive protein (CRP), thyroid stimulating hormone (TSH) with reactive thyroid hormone tests if abnormal, and 24 hour urine calcium excretion. In men without an identifiable cause of osteoporosis, serum testosterone and 24 hours cortisol should be considered [69]. Any abnormality should be followed up, and if there is any concern for hematologic malignancy, a bone marrow biopsy should be considered.

Recognition of Patients at Risk

It should be noted that the orthopedic surgeon is often the first physician to encounter patients with osteoporosis when they present with an osteoporotic fracture. Studies have shown that less than 1/3 of patients presenting with osteoporotic fractures, which total over 1.5 million injuries a year, are effectively evaluated and treated for osteoporosis [41, 73, 74]. This lag represents an important area of recognition in the orthopedic and general medical community to better recognize and treat this widespread disease.

References

1. Cosman F, de Beur SJ, LeBoff MS, et al. Clinician's guide to prevention and treatment of osteoporosis. Osteoporos Int. 2014;25(10):2359–81.
2. Becker C. Pathophysiology and clinical manifestations of osteoporosis. Clin Cornerstone. 2008;9(2):42–50. http://dx.doi.org.ezproxy.med.nyu.edu/10.1016/S1098-3597(09)62038-X.
3. Osterhoff G, Morgan EF, Shefelbine SJ, Karim L, McNamara LM, Augat P. Bone mechanical properties and changes with osteoporosis. Injury. 2016;47:S11–20.. http://dx.doi.org.ezproxy.med.nyu.edu/10.1016/S0020-1383(16)47003-8
4. Seeman E, Delmas PD. Bone quality — the material and structural basis of bone strength and fragility. N Engl J Med. 2006;354(21):2250–61.
5. Pocock NA, Eisman JA, Hopper JL, Yeates MG, Sambrook PN, Eberl S. Genetic determinants of bone mass in adults. A twin study. J Clin Invest. 1987;80(3):706–10.
6. Akhter MP, Lappe JM, Davies KM, Recker RR. Transmenopausal changes in the trabecular bone structure. Bone. 2007;41(1):111–6. http://dx.doi.org.ezproxy.med.nyu.edu/10.1016/j.bone.2007.03.019.
7. Mosekilde L, Mosekilde L, Danielsen CC. Biomechanical competence of vertebral trabecular bone in relation to ash density and age in normal individuals. Bone. 1987;8(2):79–85. http://dx.doi.org.ezproxy.med.nyu.edu/10.1016/8756-3282(87)90074-3.
8. Silva MJ. Biomechanics of osteoporotic fractures. Injury. 2007;38(3):69–76. http://dx.doi.org.ezproxy.med.nyu.edu/10.1016/j.injury.2007.08.014.
9. Zioupos P, Currey JD. Changes in the stiffness, strength, and toughness of human cortical bone with age. Bone. 1998;22(1):57–66. http://dx.doi.org.ezproxy.med.nyu.edu/10.1016/S8756-3282(97)00228-7.
10. Riggs BL, Melton LJ, Robb RA, et al. Population-Based study of age and sex differences in bone volumetric density, size, geometry, and structure at different skeletal sites. J Bone Miner Res. 2004;19(12):1945–54.
11. Rühli FJ, Müntener M, Henneberg M. Age-dependent changes of the normal human spine during adulthood. Am J Hum Biol. 2005;17(4):460–9.
12. Duan Y, Seeman E, Turner CH. The biomechanical basis of vertebral body fragility in men and women. J Bone Miner Res. 2001;16(12):2276–83.
13. Ebbesen EN, Thomsen JS, Beck-Nielsen H, Nepper-Rasmussen HJ, Mosekilde L. Age- and gender-related differences in vertebral bone mass, density, and strength. J Bone Miner Res. 1999;14(8):1394–403.
14. Khosla S. Minireview: The OPG/RANKL/RANK system.
15. Rossini M, Gatti D, Adami S. Involvement of WNT/ß-catenin signaling in the treatment of osteoporosis. Calcif Tissue Int. 2013;93(2):121–32.
16. Li X, Ominsky MS, Warmington KS, et al. Sclerostin antibody treatment increases bone formation, bone mass, and bone strength in a rat model of postmenopausal osteoporosis. J Bone Miner Res. 2009;24(4):578–88.
17. Canalis E. Wnt signalling in osteoporosis: mechanisms and novel therapeutic approaches. Nat Rev Endocrinol. 2013;9:575–83.
18. Glantschnig H, Hampton RA, Lu P, et al. Generation and selection of novel fully human monoclonal antibodies that neutralize dickkopf-1 (DKK1) inhibitory function in vitro and increase bone mass in vivo. J Biol Chem. 2010;285(51):40135–47.
19. Raisz LG. Pathogenesis of osteoporosis: concepts, conflicts, and prospects. J Clin Invest. 2005;115(12):3318–25.
20. Lips P. Vitamin D physiology. Prog Biophys Mol Biol. 2006;92(1):4–8. https://doi.org/10.1016/j.pbiomolbio.2006.02.016.
21. Lips P. Vitamin D deficiency and secondary hyperparathyroidism in the elderly: Consequences for bone loss and fractures and therapeutic implications. Endocr Rev. 2001;22(4):477–501.
22. Norman AW, Roth J, Orci L. The vitamin D endocrine system: Steroid metabolism, hormone receptors,

and biological response (calcium binding proteins). Endocr Rev. 1982 Fall;3(4):331–66.
23. Reichel H, Koeffler HP, Norman AW. The role of the vitamin D endocrine system in health and disease. N Engl J Med. 1989;320(15):980–91.
24. Walters MR. Newly identified actions of the vitamin D endocrine system. Endocr Rev. 1992;13(4):719–64.
25. Manolagas SC. Birth and death of bone cells: Basic regulatory mechanisms and implications for the pathogenesis and treatment of osteoporosis. Endocr Rev. 2000;21(2):115–37.
26. Currey J, editor. Bones: structure and mechanics. Princeton: Princeton University; 2002.
27. Boivin G, Lips P, Ott SM, et al. Contribution of raloxifene and calcium and vitamin D3 supplementation to the increase of the degree of mineralization of bone in postmenopausal women. J Clin Endocrinol Metab. 2003;88(9):4199–205.
28. Boivin G, Meunier PJ. Changes in bone remodeling rate influence the degree of mineralization of bone. Connect Tissue Res. 2002;43(2–3):535–7.
29. Viguet-Carrin S, Garnero P, Delmas PD. The role of collagen in bone strength. Osteoporos Int. 2006;17(3):319–36.
30. Recker R, Lappe J, Davies K, Heaney R. Characterization of perimenopausal bone loss: a prospective study. J Bone Miner Res. 2000;15(10):1965–73.
31. Cummings SR, Karpf DB, Harris F, et al. Improvement in spine bone density and reduction in risk of vertebral fractures during treatment with antiresorptive drugs. Am J Med. 2002;112(4):281–9. http://dx.doi.org.ezproxy.med.nyu.edu/10.1016/S0002-9343(01)01124-X.
32. Sarkar S, Mitlak BH, Wong M, Stock JL, Black DM, Harper KD. Relationships between bone mineral density and incident vertebral fracture risk with raloxifene therapy. J Bone Miner Res. 2002;17(1):1–10.
33. Armas LAG, Recker RR. Pathophysiology of osteoporosis. Endocrinol Metab Clin N Am. 2012;41(3):475–86. http://dx.doi.org.ezproxy.med.nyu.edu/10.1016/j.ecl.2012.04.006.
34. Gilbert L, He X, Farmer P, et al. Inhibition of osteoblast differentiation by tumor necrosis factor-α. Endocrinology. 2000;141(11):3956–64.
35. Cenci S, Toraldo G, Weitzmann MN, et al. Estrogen deficiency induces bone loss by increasing T cell proliferation and lifespan through IFN-γ-induced class II transactivator. Proc Natl Acad Sci. 2003;100(18):10405–10.
36. Weitzmann MN, Roggia C, Toraldo G, Weitzmann L, Pacifici R. Increased production of IL-7 uncouples bone formation from bone resorption during estrogen deficiency. J Clin Invest. 2002;110(11):1643–50.
37. Wright NC, Looker AC, Saag KG, et al. The recent prevalence of osteoporosis and low bone mass in the United States based on bone mineral density at the femoral neck or lumbar spine. J Bone Miner Res. 2014;29(11):2520–6.
38. Carmona R. Bone health and osteoporosis, a report of the surgeon general. US department of health and human services: Rockville, MD; 2004.
39. Bilezikian JP. Osteoporosis in men. J Clin Endocrinol Metab. 1999;84(10):3431–34.
40. Cummings SR, Browner W, Cummings SR, et al. Bone density at various sites for prediction of hip fractures. Lancet. 1993;341(8837):72–5. http://dx.doi.org.ezproxy.med.nyu.edu/10.1016/0140-6736(93)92555-8.
41. Rozental TD, Shah J, Chacko AT, Zurakowski D. Prevalence and predictors of osteoporosis risk in orthopaedic patients. Clin Orthop. 2009;468(7):1765–72.
42. Jackson RD, Mysiw WJ. Insights into the epidemiology of postmenopausal osteoporosis: the women's health initiative. Semin Reprod Med. 2014;32(06):454–62.
43. Feldman HA, Longcope C, Derby CA, et al. Age trends in the level of serum testosterone and other hormones in middle-aged men: longitudinal results from the massachusetts male aging study. J Clin Endocrinol Metab. 2002;87(2):589–98.
44. Harman SM, Metter EJ, Tobin JD, Pearson J, Blackman MR. Longitudinal effects of aging on serum total and free testosterone levels in healthy men. J Clin Endocrinol Metab. 2001;86(2):724–31.
45. Hudec SMD, Camacho PM. Secondary causes of osteoporosis. Endocr Pract. 2013;19(1):120–8.
46. Amory JK, Watts NB, Easley KA, et al. Exogenous testosterone or testosterone with finasteride increases bone mineral density in older men with low serum testosterone. J Clin Endocrinol Metab. 2004;89(2):503-510.
47. Warren MP, Brooks-Gunn J, Fox RP, Holderness CC, Hyle EP, Hamilton WG. Osteopenia in exercise-associated amenorrhea using ballet dancers as a model: a longitudinal study. J Clin Endocrinol Metab. 2002;87(7):3162–8.
48. Grinspoon S, Thomas E, Pitts S, et al. Prevalence and predictive factors for regional osteopenia in women with anorexia nervosa. Ann Intern Med. 2000;133(10):790–4.
49. Montalcini T, Romeo S, Ferro Y, Migliaccio V, Gazzaruso C, Pujia A. Osteoporosis in chronic inflammatory disease: the role of malnutrition. Endocrine. 2013;43(1):59–64.
50. Ardizzone S, Bollani S, Bettica P, Bevilacqua M, Molteni P, Porro GB. Altered bone metabolism in inflammatory bowel disease: there is a difference between crohn's disease and ulcerative colitis. J Intern Med. 2000;247(1):63–70.
51. Ferrari-Lacraz S, Ferrari S. Do RANKL inhibitors (denosumab) affect inflammation and immunity? Osteoporos Int. 2011;22(2):435–46.
52. Emkey GR, Epstein S. Secondary osteoporosis: pathophysiology & diagnosis. Best Pract Res Clin Endocrinol Metab. 2014;28(6):911–35. https://doi-org.ezproxy.med.nyu.edu/10.1016/j.beem.2014.07.002.
53. Burghardt AJ, Issever AS, Schwartz AV, et al. High-resolution peripheral quantitative com-

puted tomographic imaging of cortical and trabecular bone microarchitecture in patients with type 2 diabetes mellitus. J Clin Endocrinol Metab. 2010;95(11):5045–55.
54. Brown TT, Qaqish RB. Antiretroviral therapy and the prevalence of osteopenia and osteoporosis: a meta-analytic review. AIDS. 2006;20(17):2165.
55. de Barbosa M, Marques EG, de FJA P, Machado AA, de Assis Pereira F, Barbosa F, Navarro AM. Impact of antiretroviral therapy on bone metabolism markers in HIV-seropositive patients. Bone. 2013;57(1):62–7. https://doi-org.ezproxy.med.nyu.edu/10.1016/j.bone.2013.07.019.
56. Steinbuch M, Youket TE, Cohen S. Oral glucocorticoid use is associated with an increased risk of fracture. Osteoporos Int. 2004;15(4):323–8.
57. Eastell R, Adams JE, Coleman RE, et al. Effect of anastrozole on bone mineral density: 5-year results from the anastrozole, tamoxifen, alone or in combination trial 18233230. JCO. 2008;26(7):1051–7.
58. Bouvard B, Soulié P, Hoppé E, et al. Fracture incidence after 3 years of aromatase inhibitor therapy. Ann Oncol. 2014;25(4):843–7.
59. Vestergaard P, Rejnmark L, Mosekilde L. Proton pump inhibitors, histamine H2 receptor antagonists, and other antacid medications and the risk of fracture. Calcif Tissue Int. 2006;79(2):76–83.
60. Gray SL, LaCroix AZ, Larson J, et al. Proton pump inhibitor use, hip fracture, and change in bone mineral density in postmenopausal women: results from the women's health initiative. Arch Intern Med. 2010;170(9):765–71.
61. Yu EW, Blackwell T, Ensrud KE, et al. Acid-suppressive medications and risk of bone loss and fracture in older adults. Calcif Tissue Int. 2008;83(4):251–9.
62. Yang Y, Lewis JD, Epstein S, Metz DC. Long-term proton pump inhibitor therapy and risk of hip fracture. JAMA. 2006;296(24):2947–53.
63. Lee RH, Lyles KW, Colón-Emeric C. A review of the effect of anticonvulsant medications on bone mineral density and fracture risk. Am J Geriatr Pharmacother. 2010;8(1):34–46.
64. Mikati M, Dib L, Yamouy B, Sawaya R, Rahi A, Fuleihan G. Two randomized vitamin D trials in ambulatory patients on anti-convulsants: impact on bone. Neurology. 2006;67(11):14.
65. Lee RH, Lyles KW, Sloane R, Colón-Emeric C. The association of newer anticonvulsant medications and bone mineral density. Endocr Pract. 2012. https://doi.org/10.4158/EP12119.OR.
66. Diem SJ, Blackwell TL, Stone KL, et al. Use of antidepressants and rates of hip bone loss in older women: the study of osteoporotic fractures. Arch Intern Med. 2007;167(12):1240–5.
67. Yadav VK, Ryu J, Suda N, et al. Lrp5 controls bone formation by inhibiting serotonin synthesis in the duodenum: An entero-bone endocrine axis. Cell. 2008;135(5):825–37.
68. Hopper JL, Seeman E. The bone density of female twins discordant for tobacco use. N Engl J Med. 1994;330(6):387–92.
69. Harper KD, Weber TJ. Secondary osteoporosis: diagnostic considerations. Endocrinol Metab Clin N Am. 1998;27(2):325–48. https://doi-org.ezproxy.med.nyu.edu/10.1016/S0889-8529(05)70008-6.
70. Klein RF. Alcohol-induced bone disease: impact of ethanol on osteoblast proliferation. Alcohol Clin Exp Res. 1997;21(3):392–9.
71. Díez A, Puig J, Serrano S, et al. Alcohol-induced bone disease in the absence of severe chronic liver damage. J Bone Miner Res. 1994;9(6):825–31.
72. Gordon GG, Altman K, Southren AL, Rubin E, Lieber CS. Effect of alcohol (ethanol) administration on sex-hormone metabolism in normal men. N Engl J Med. 1976;295(15):793–7.
73. Smith MD, Ross W, Ahern MJ. Missing a therapeutic window of opportunity: an audit of patients attending a tertiary teaching hospital with potentially osteoporotic hip and wrist fractures. J Rheumatol. 2001;28(11):2504.
74. Kamel HK, Hussain MS, Tariq S, Perry HM, Morley JE. Failure to diagnose and treat osteoporosis in elderly patients hospitalized with hip fracture. Am J Med. 2000;109(4):326–8.

The Economic Burden of Osteoporosis

3

Harold A. Fogel and Louis G. Jenis

Introduction

United States' healthcare is experiencing a paradigm shift in recent years. In response to national health expenditures rising at unsustainable rates, the reimbursement system is moving from a fee-for-service framework that incentivizes ordering more tests and performing more procedures to a value-based payment structure with goals of optimizing outcomes while controlling costs. In other words, US healthcare is evolving from volume-based to value-based medicine [1, 2].

From a healthcare perspective, value can generally be defined as a ratio of health outcomes achieved per dollars spent on care [1]. Based on this equation, the value of healthcare can be increased by either improving clinical outcomes at similar costs or reducing total costs while maintaining the quality of outcomes. Achieving high-value care at a population level is a monumental challenge. To do so, healthcare providers and policy experts must identify and critically evaluate the various medical needs of the modern patient.

One of the most widespread public health problems today is osteoporosis. Osteoporosis is the most common metabolic bone disorder and, through its prevalence as well as morbidity and mortality on those afflicted, places an enormous medical and economic burden on the healthcare system. The manifestation of osteoporosis on the skeletal system is well-known, and the spine is often one of the most affected areas. From physiological changes in posture to vertebral fragility fractures to weakened points of fixation, osteoporosis presents numerous challenges in the spine patient. Managing these patients, either operatively or nonoperatively, can result in high health expenditures over several months and years. It is crucial to understand the financial implications of osteoporotic spine disease in order to provide high-value spine care.

Epidemiology and Implications of Osteoporotic Spine Disease

The World Health Organization (WHO) defines osteoporosis as a bone mineral density (BMD) score of at least 2.5 standard deviations below the normal mean for a young adult (T-score < −2.5 SD) and osteopenia, or low bone mass, as a BMD score between 1 and 2.5 standard deviations below the young-adult normal mean (T-score −1.0 to −2.5 SD) [3, 4]. According to the National Osteoporosis Foundation (NOF), 12 million Americans in 2010 qualified for the diagnosis of

H. A. Fogel (✉)
Department of Orthopaedic Surgery, Massachusetts General Hospital, Harvard Medical School, Boston, MA, USA
e-mail: hfogel@mgh.harvard.edu

L. G. Jenis
Department of Orthopaedic Surgery, Newton-Wellesley Hospital, Harvard Medical School, Newton, MA, USA
e-mail: ljenis@partners.org; http://nwh.org/

A. E. Razi, S. H. Hershman (eds.), *Vertebral Compression Fractures in Osteoporotic and Pathologic Bone*, https://doi.org/10.1007/978-3-030-33861-9_3

osteoporosis, and another 43.4 million adults greater than the age of 50 had low bone mass [5, 6]. Since decreased bone mass is primarily an age-related consequence, the incidence and prevalence of osteoporosis and osteopenia is expected to rise dramatically with the aging US population. By 2025, the number of Americans 50 years or older is expected to increase by 60% compared to 2000, hitting a high of over 121 million [7]. Moreover, the disease becomes even more common as one gets older. Osteoporosis will affect approximately 10% of women aged 60, 20% of women aged 70, 40% of women aged 80, and 67% of women aged 90 [8, 9].

The obvious and direct consequence of an aging population, and thus larger pool of people with low bone mass, is the rising frequency of fragility fractures due to osteoporosis. Worldwide, an osteoporotic fracture occurs every 3 seconds; one in three women and one in five men over age 50 will sustain an osteoporotic fracture in their lifetime [10–13]. In the United States alone, more than two million new osteoporotic fractures occur annually, and the most common type is a vertebral compression fracture (VCF), with an estimated incidence between 700,000 and 750,000 annually. Once a person sustains their first VCF, they are at increased risk for more fragility fractures, commonly referred to as the *fracture cascade*. After a VCF, there is a fivefold increased risk of a second VCF occurring and a four- to fivefold increased risk of a hip fracture [14–16]. In fact, one in five women will sustain their second VCF within 1 year of the first [17].

Osteoporosis impacts the spine in ways other than fragility fractures; however this is much harder to quantify in terms of population numbers. The quality of the patient's bone, and thus the interface for spinal hardware, is a potential cause of complications. Pedicle screws obtain up to 40% of their stability in the cancellous bone of the vertebral body, the same bone that is disproportionately affected in osteoporosis [18, 19]. Not surprisingly then, pedicle screws have a high rate of loosening in osteoporotic patients, with some reports citing an incidence as high as 12.9% [20]. Weaker vertebral endplates can also be responsible for the loosening or subsidence of interbody or motion sparing devices [21–23]. Even if a successful surgery is performed, the osteoporotic bone adjacent to a prior fusion is at increased risk for a compression fracture, spondylolisthesis, or proximal junctional kyphosis (Fig. 3.1). Supplemental fixation in the form of laminar hooks, polymethyl methacrylate (PMMA), and both anterior and posterior instrumentation can be used to minimize the surgical complications from osteoporotic bone; however techniques simultaneously add to the complexity and overall cost of the surgery.

Direct and Indirect Medical Costs of Osteoporotic Spine Disease

The burden of osteoporotic spine disease can be broken down into direct costs and indirect costs. While the nomenclature is simple, often identifying and quantifying these direct and indirect costs are not. In the case of an osteoporotic vertebral compression fracture, the direct costs are a compilation of the patient's medical care, and this can be further broken down into in-hospital direct costs and post-hospitalization direct costs (this is also often categorized as acute and post-acute care). In-hospital costs will include the emergency room visit, diagnostic imaging, room charges if the patient is admitted, and then all intervention prior to the discharge, such as medication, therapy evaluation, and any related procedures or tests. Post-hospitalization costs can span several months or even greater than a year and include follow-up physician visits, home health providers or nursing home expenses, and outpatient medication. While the inpatient portion may be more labor intensive, previous research has shown there to be an almost even split in cost between acute and post-acute care [24]. Indirect costs, meanwhile, are more abstract than direct costs and are therefore much harder to quantify. These costs reflect lost time at work by the patient while they recover from their injury and also extend to family members and friends that may be assisting in their care. While health economists agree that productivity loss should be factored into the economic burden of

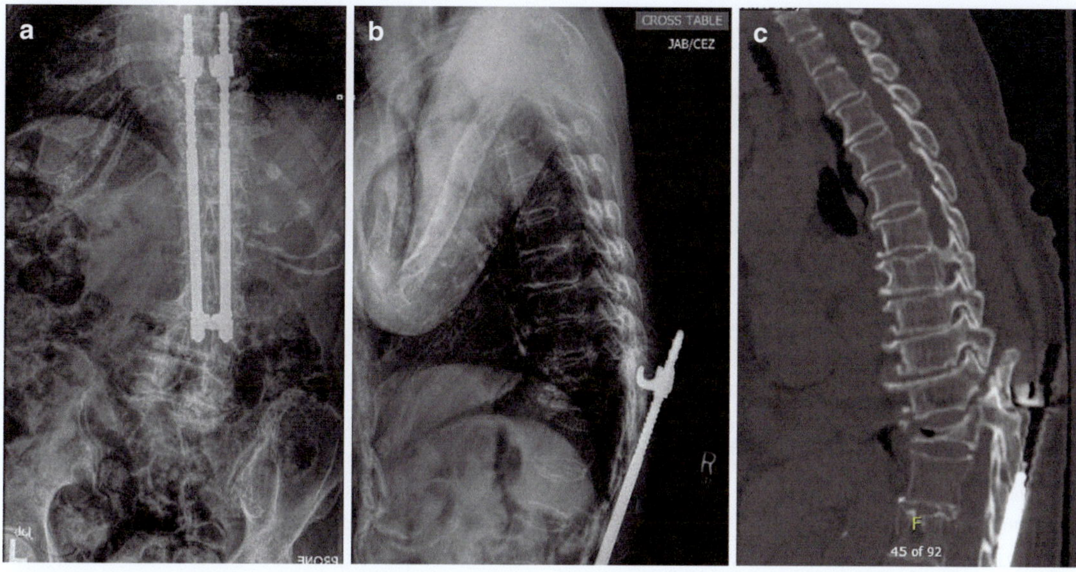

Fig. 3.1 AP (**a**) and lateral (**b**) radiographs of a 74-year-old female who sustained an osteoporotic compression fracture above previous hardware after a fall from standing height. While there were no prior radiographs for comparison, it was assumed that the Harrington rod fixation loosened and displaced as a result of the fracture. A CT scan (**c**) clearly identified a three-column fracture and the resultant kyphotic deformity. The patient subsequently underwent removal of hardware and T4 to ilium posterior spinal fusion with pedicle screw instrumentation and multilevel posterior column osteotomies

osteoporosis, there is disagreement as to how exactly it should be incorporated into a cost-effectiveness or cost-utility analysis. Sasser et al. calculated that women with osteoporosis have $4000 in loss productivity compared to $2300 for women without osteoporosis [25]. On a national scale, the total costs of osteoporosis, including direct and indirect costs, may be $34 billion or greater [26].

Numerous studies have attempted to calculate the direct costs of osteoporotic fractures. Most attempts thus far have utilized claims databases from commercial insurers, and as expected, there is great variability. Current estimates place the total direct cost of osteoporosis and related fractures between $17 billion and $20.3 billion dollars. For comparison, the total cost of breast cancer is $13 billion while heart disease is approximately $19 billion [27–32]. With the growing size and rising average age of the US population, this number is projected to exceed $25 billion per year by 2025. Women will account for 71% of all fragility fractures and 75% of associated costs, and while costs will go up for every demographic, the annual costs for people of Latin descent will increase the most – 175% from 2005 to 2025 based on population trends [7].

Studies that have estimated the direct cost of a single osteoporotic fracture accomplish this by comparing healthcare expenditures for affected individuals against matched controls, and then comparing costs for the year after a fracture to costs in the year prior to fracture. By this method, research from the Mayo Clinic identified a median incremental cost for any kind of osteoporotic fracture to be $2390. The highest incremental increase was for distal femur fractures (median $11,756) and hip fractures (median $11,241) while the lowest was for rib fractures (median $213). The median incremental cost for a vertebral fracture was $1955, or 17% of a hip fracture [33, 34]. A separate retrospective study of nearly 50,000 patients in a commercially insured US population between 2005 and 2008 reported a median post-fracture cost of $19,223 for hip fractures (mean incremental increase $16,663) and $10,605 for vertebral fractures (mean incremental increase $14,049) for the 6-month period post-fracture. Hospitalizations made up 64% and 72% of total direct costs for vertebral and hip fractures, respectively [35]. When compared to the Mayo Clinic study and adjusted for inflation, the hip fracture costs are comparable between the two studies; however a noticeable difference exists in vertebral fracture costs. Subgroup analysis in the latter study identified that the vertebral fracture patients were likely sicker than the hip fracture patients and thus accumulated higher medical costs. To illustrate this point, Orsini et al. performed a retrospective review of a commercial claims database which highlighted the significant role that comorbidities play in driving up healthcare costs in the setting of an osteoporotic fracture. Comorbid conditions in this patient population are frequently present and can be exacerbated by the traumatic incident (Fig. 3.2). In their study, Orsini et al. compared healthcare expenditures in osteoporotic patients with an osteoporotic fracture, osteoporotic patients without a fracture, and matched patients with neither a diagnosis of osteoporosis nor a fracture. Their findings showed that osteoporotic patients with a concurrent fracture incurred healthcare costs more than twice that of osteoporotic patients without fracture ($15,942 vs $6,476) and nearly three times the costs of the control group ($15,942 vs $4,658). The fracture group had significantly more comorbidities than the other two groups. In terms of overall healthcare costs, 75% of expenditures incurred because of the patient's comorbidities and not because of osteoporosis or the osteoporotic fracture itself. Even more, only 7% of total direct costs were attributable to osteoporosis in the osteoporosis, non-fracture cohort [36]. This clearly underscores the point that patients with osteoporosis and osteoporotic fractures are medically complex patients, and the fracture is simply a surrogate for their medical frailty.

When a VCF occurs, treatment options typically include medical management alone or medical management with cement augmentation, either in the form of vertebroplasty or kyphoplasty. Multiple studies have shown that the

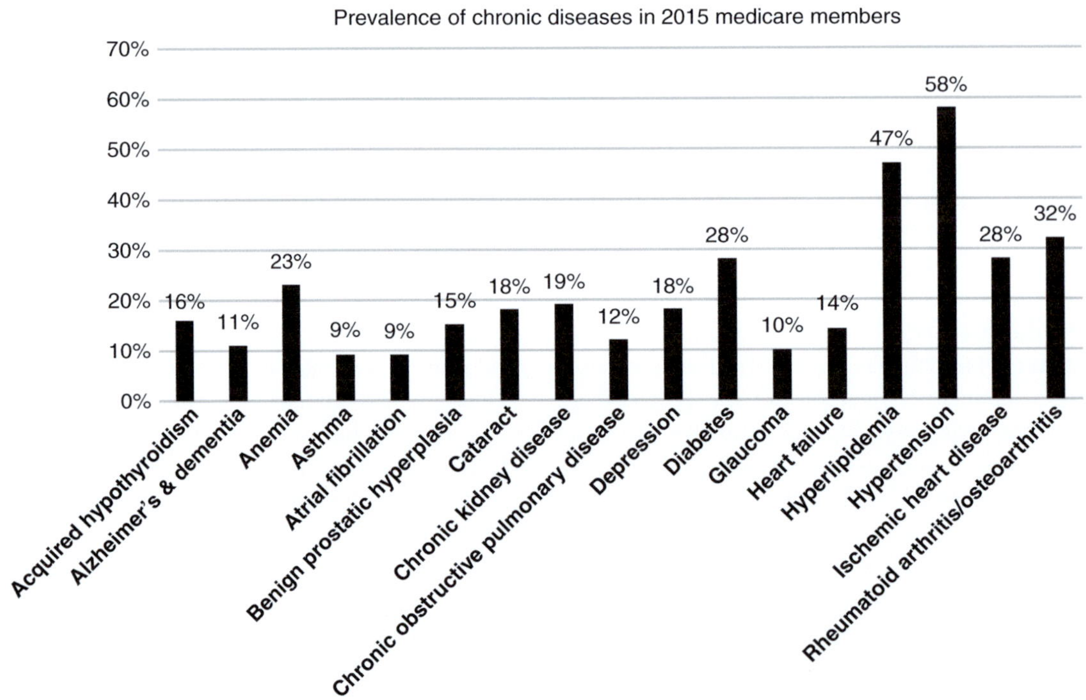

Fig. 3.2 Prevalence of chronic diseases in 2015 medicare members (citizens 65 years and older). (Source: Centers for Medicare and Medicaid Services. Chronic Conditions Data Warehouse. Medicare Chronic Condition Charts)

injection of PMMA into the fractured vertebral body reliably relieves fracture pain and improves the patient's mobility and functional outcomes both in the short-term and long-term post-injury. Cost-analysis of medical management versus cement augmentation demonstrates a significant difference in healthcare expenses. As expected, cement augmentation can be substantially higher than medical treatment alone. One study determined a vertebroplasty was more than 1.5 times greater cost than nonoperative medical care, while kyphoplasty was almost four times greater [37]. In a review of the Nationwide Inpatient Sample database, Zampini et al. found that total charges for a kyphoplasty was $37,231 compared to $20,112 for nonoperative care; the patients who underwent kyphoplasty also had a statistically significant 0.7 days longer hospital stay [38]. The limitation to such a cost-analysis, however, is that it does not encompass the entire episode of care. While the initial costs may be more expensive, if the kyphoplasty does indeed provide the intended clinical relief then it will likely lead to cost savings down the road and thus be an overall more cost-effective treatment choice. That same study found that 55% of kyphoplasty patients were discharged home with or without home care services, while only 33.3% of patients that received nonoperative care were discharged home. Long-term cost studies that follow the patient through the entire episode of care are needed to more accurately determine the full-term cost of each treatment option.

It is worth noting, though, that any present data on healthcare costs related to osteoporosis, including the aforementioned studies, has been met with skepticism and doubt. The defense for this criticism is multifactorial. Firstly, as previously described, most of the data used to calculate the direct costs for treatment of osteoporotic fractures is from commercial insurance claims databases. This therefore leaves out patients covered by Medicare and Medicaid, which by one estimate annually pays out close to 75% of all relevant medical expenditures for osteoporotic fractures [28]. This percentage is likely even larger now with the expansion of these programs under the Affordable Care Act. Moreover, the cost incurred in the commercially insured patient populations is not necessarily translatable to the Medicare and Medicaid populations. Medicare and Medicaid patients are on average more medically complex and have longer inpatient hospital stays, and thus their total in hospital direct costs tend to be higher [39]. A second critique of current cost estimates is exemplified by the wide range in numbers put forth by different studies. Very simply, yet for complex reasons, hospital charges and reimbursements for the same medical treatment vary greatly by the geographical location and practice setting in which patients are seen. Lastly, and perhaps most importantly, some believe that current cost estimates are inaccurate because the current costing methods are inherently inaccurate. As suggested by Professors Porter and Kaplan from the Harvard Business School, measuring what doctors' charge or how much insurance plans pay is extraordinarily misleading; in other words, charges and reimbursements do not equal costs. Until the system by which costs are measured is fundamentally changed, the true cost of caring for osteoporotic fractures will not be understood.

Determining Outcomes in the Treatment of Osteoporosis.

Determining the value of care for osteoporotic fractures requires a thorough evaluation of patients' outcomes, both in the short- and long-term. Focusing only on cost reduction while ignoring the utility of an intervention is a risk for *false savings* – short-term savings that is negated by long-term expenses because of inadequate care. While outcomes are the best tool to measure a provider's quality of care, there is no consensus on what outcomes we should be measuring and how we should measure them. In many cases, outcomes are chosen because they reflect the immediate results of a treatment intervention or simply because it's the easiest outcome for an institution to track. As proposed by Professor Porter, outcomes should incorporate three essential characteristics: the inclusion of health circumstances most relevant to the patient, addressing both near- and long-term health, and consideration of risk factors or initial conditions to allow for risk-adjustment [1].

The variety of outcome measurements reported for osteoporotic spine disease epitomizes the lack of consensus on how we should be evaluating the end result of care (either via treatment or natural history). Some studies focus on radiographic surrogates, such as if the fracture is healed or how well overall spinal alignment is maintained, to assess the utility of bracing. Others use guidelines from the Centers for Medicaid and Medicare Services (CMS), including survival, 30-day readmission, and complications. As discussed earlier, percutaneous cement augmentation is one of the most common interventions for VCFs, and multiple studies have attempted to determine its effectiveness. Two randomized controlled trials published in the New England Journal of Medicine in 2009 failed to show better clinical outcomes when comparing vertebroplasty to sham procedures in patients with painful osteoporotic VCFs [40, 41]. Primary outcomes in both studies were patient reported outcome measures, including the Roland-Morris Disability Questionnaire (a validated assessment of physical disability due to back pain) and a numerical scale for intensity of back pain. Following the results of these studies, the American Academy of Orthopedic Surgeons updated its clinical practice guidelines the following year to *strongly* recommend against vertebroplasty for such patients [42]. Kyphoplasty, meanwhile, has emerged as an alternative form of treatment with cement augmentation. Lee et al. performed a prospective study that compared conservative treatment to balloon kyphoplasty. While patients who underwent kyphoplasty showed better clinical outcomes at 1-month post-injury, there were no significant differences in Oswestry Disability Index and visual analog scale scores at 3, 6, or 12 months, and thus the utility of kyphoplasty may be minimal over the long-term. It's important to note, however, that certain patient subpopulations did not experience the same results. In fact, risk factors for failed conservative treatment were older age, severe osteoporosis, larger collapse rates, and being overweight. The authors therefore recommended kyphoplasty over conservative treatment in these particular patients, underscoring the importance of risk-adjustment when evaluating outcomes [43].

The Value of Preventative Care in Osteoporosis.

The enormous clinical and economic burden of osteoporosis places incredible importance on the prevention of this disease and its associated consequences. The critical question to answer in this scenario is whether preventive measures are more cost-effective in the long-term over doing nothing at all and subsequently treating the consequences of the disease. The first step in prevention is public awareness. Osteoporosis is a silent disease without symptoms, and thus many men and women do little to address it until after they reach a critically low bone mass and sustain their first fragility fracture. While osteoporosis is recognized as an age-related disease that affects the elderly, the decline in bone mass actually starts at a much younger age. Studies have shown peak bone mass to occur between the age of 25 and 30, and those with a higher peak bone mass are less likely to suffer from the natural biologic changes that can lead to osteoporosis later in life. Moreover, there are multiple risk factors for osteoporosis. Lifestyle choices such as smoking, drinking, unbalanced diets, and lack of exercise are all known risk factors for various medical problems, including low bone mass. Genetics, comorbidities, and various medications also represent a host of other risk factors. Despite knowing the wide range of risk factors, many of which are modifiable, detection and preventive treatment rates remain low. Almost 50% of women that meet guidelines for screening do not undergo testing, and this rate can be as low as 10% for high-risk populations [44, 45]. Detecting patients at an earlier time point can produce dramatic cost-savings and lower morbidity later in life, and thus it behooves the healthcare system to improve these efforts.

Once a diagnosis of osteoporosis is made, different medications can be prescribed in an effort to control the disease and ultimately, prevent an osteoporotic fracture from occurring. Calcium and vitamin D supplementation has historically been a first-line treatment option; however recent evidence has questioned its utility. In a 2017 meta-analysis of randomized clinical trials, Zhao et al. found that supplementation with calcium, vitamin D, or both did not reduce the risk of hip, non-vertebral, vertebral, or total fractures in community-dwelling adults over the age of 50 [46]. If the primary outcome of preventative treatment is to reduce the incidence of fractures, then, based on this study, vitamin D and calcium supplementation is a low-value treatment option. To the contrary, other medications have demonstrated effectiveness in preventing fragility fractures. Pharmacologic treatment with alendronate, risedronate, zoledronic acid, or denosumab have all shown some capacity to decrease the risk of fragility fractures, by as much as 50% [47, 48]. It is no surprise then that the 2017 American College of Physicians Clinical Practice Guidelines gave a *strong* recommendation to prescribing one of these medications in women with osteoporosis [49].

Another form of preventive treatment with potentially high value is patient enrollment in a fracture prevention program, often referred to as a fracture liaison service (FLS). As described earlier, after a patient sustains their first osteoporotic fracture, the subsequent risk of an additional fracture rises dramatically. A significant reason for this is that a majority of these patients, as much as 80%, are not properly identified and treated for osteoporosis [50]. In other words, the fragility fracture is managed acutely, but the underlying disease, osteoporosis, is never addressed. A FLS utilizes a team-based model dependent on care coordination and communication between multiple specialists, including orthopedic surgeons, endocrinologists, and the primary care physicians. Very simply, once a patient presents with a fragility fracture, they are automatically enrolled into this program, and osteoporotic treatment is initiated. Early results of such programs have been very promising, identifying a 30–40% reduction in refracture rates [51]. While there are obviously upfront costs in creating a FLS (e.g., healthcare providers, office space, care coordination), the potential for long-term savings and reduction in patient morbidity and mortality is what qualifies a FLS as a high-value care model. Moreover, as the healthcare system transitions into a value-based reimbursement structure with various quality-care incentives, hospitals and practices gain to benefit financially from a successful FLS.

The Future of Treating Osteoporosis.

The current medical and economic burden of osteoporosis is enormous and will only continue to grow. As the healthcare system evolves from a volume-based to a value-based system, it is imperative for providers and healthcare policy makers to develop cost-effective treatment strategies that rein in costs while optimizing outcomes. This will require in-depth analysis of current costing methods to more accurately identify where and how the money is being spent and also a new approach to medicine, where patients are identified at earlier time points and interventions are initiated proactively instead of reactively. Healthcare providers and the outcomes that we use to evaluate success will have to evolve and adapt around the patient's needs and concerns. Only then can we identify real areas for improvement and implement methods for providing the highest value of care possible. Reimbursements based on quality of care and patient outcomes will help drive this change in the future.

References

1. Porter ME. What is value in health care? N Engl J Med. 2010;363(26):2477–81.
2. Kaplan RS, Porter ME. How to solve the cost crisis in health care. Harv Bus Rev. 2011;89:46–52.
3. World Health Organization. Assessment of fracture risk and its application to screening for postmenopausal osteoporosis, WHO technical report series 843. Geneva: WHO; 1994.
4. Buist DS, LaCroix AZ, Manfredonia D, Abbott T. Identifying postmenopausal women at high risk of

fracture in populations: a comparison of three strategies. J Am Geriatr Soc. 2002;50:1031–8.
5. National Osteoporosis Foundation. Prevalence report [online]. Available from URL: http://www.nof.org/advocacy/resources/prevalencereport. Accessed 17 Sept 2017.
6. Wright NC, Looker AC, Saag KG, Curtis JR, Delzell ES, Randal S, et al. The recent prevalence of osteoporosis and low bone mass in the United States based on bone mineral density at the femoral neck or lumbar spine. J Bone Miner Res. 2014;29(11):2520–6.
7. Burge R, Dawson-Hughes B, Solomon DH, Wong JB, King A, Tosteson A. Incidence and economic burden of osteoporosis-related fractures in the United States, 2005–2025. J Bone Miner Res. 2006;4(22): 465–75.
8. Day JC. Population projections of the United States by age, sex, race, and hispanic origin: 1995 to 2050. Washington, D.C.: U.S. Government Printing Office; 1996.
9. World Health Organization Technical Report: Assessment of Osteoporosis at the Primary Health Care Level [online]. Available from URL: https://www.sheffield.ac.uk/FRAX/pdfs. Accessed 17 Sept 2017.
10. Johnell O, Kanis JA. An estimate of the worldwide prevalence and disability associated with osteoporotic fractures. Osteoporos Int. 2006;17(12):1726–33.
11. Melton LJ 3rd, Atkinson EJ, O'Connor MK, O'Fallon WM, Riggs BL. Bone density and fracture risk in men. J Bone Miner Res. 1998;13(12):1915–23.
12. Melton LJ 3rd, Chrischilles EA, Cooper C, Lane AW, Riggs BL. Perspective. How many women have osteoporosis? J Bone Miner Res. 1992;7(9):1005–10.
13. Kanis JA, Johnell O, Oden A, Sembo I, Redlund-Johnell I, Dawson A, et al. Long-term risk of osteoporotic fracture in Malmo. Osteoporos Int. 2000;11(8):669–74.
14. Kim DH, Vaccaro AR. Osteoporotic compression fractures of the spine: current options and considerations for treatment. Spine J. 2006;6(5):479–87.
15. Compston J. Osteoporosis: social and economic impact. Radiol Clin N Am. 2010;48(3):477–82.
16. Ismail AA, Cockerill W, Cooper C, Finn JD, Abendroth K, Parisi G, et al. Prevalent vertebral deformity predicts incident hip though not distal forearm fracture: results from the European Prospective Osteoporosis Study. Osteoporos Int. 2001;12(2):85–90.
17. Lindsay R, Silverman SL, Cooper C, Hanley DA, Barton I, Broy SB, et al. Risk of new vertebral fracture in the year following a fracture. JAMA. 2001;285:320–3.
18. Hirano T, Hasegawa K, Takahashi HE, Uchiyama S, Hara T, Washio T, et al. Structural characteristics of the pedicle and its role in screw stability. Spine. 1997;22(21):2504–9.
19. Richardson ML, Genant HK, Cann CE, Ettinger B, Gordan GS, Kolb FO, et al. Assessment of metabolic bone diseases by quantitative computed tomography. Clin Orthop Relat Res. 1985;(195):224–38.
20. Wu ZX, Gong FT, Liu L, Ma ZS, Zhang Y, Zhao X, et al. A comparative study on screw loosening in osteoporotic lumbar spine fusion between expandable and conventional pedicle screws. Arch Orthop Trauma Surg. 2012;132(4):471–6.
21. Truummees E, Demetropoulos CK, Yang KH, Herkowitz HN. Failure of human cervical endplates: a cadaveric experimental model. Spine. 2003;28(19):2204–8.
22. Hasegawa K, Abe M, Washio T, Hara T. An experimental study of the interface strength between titanium mesh cage and vertebra in reference to vertebral bone mineral density. Spine. 2001;26(8):957–63.
23. Jost B, Cripton PA, Lund T, Oxland TR, Lippuner K, Jaeger P, et al. Compressive strength of interbody cages in the lumbar spine: the effect of cage shape, posterior instrumentation, and bone density. Eur Spine J. 1998;7(2):132–41.
24. Levy P, Levy E, Audran M, Cohen-Solal M, Faredllone P, Le Parc JM. The cost of osteoporosis in men: the French situation. Bone. 2002;30(4):631–6.
25. Sasser AC, Rousculp MD, Birnbaum HG, Oster EF, Lufkin E, Mallet D. Economic burden of osteoporosis, breast cancer, and cardiovascular disease among postmenopausal women in an employed population. Womens Health Issues. 2005;15(3):97–108.
26. Vanness DJ, Tosteson AN. Estimating the opportunity costs of osteoporosis in the United States. Top Geriatr Rehabil. 2005;21:4–16.
27. Ray NF, Chan JK, Thamer M, Melton LJ 3rd. Medical expenditures for the treatment of osteoporotic fractures in the United States in 1995: report from the National Osteoporosis Foundation. J Bone Miner Res. 1997;12(1):24–35.
28. Hoerger TJ, Downs KE, Lakshmanan MC, Lindrooth RC, Plouffe L Jr, Wendling B, et al. Healthcare use among U.S. women aged 45 and older: Total costs and costs for selected postmenopausal health risks. J Womens Health Gend Based Med. 1999;8(8):1077–89.
29. Chrischilles E, Shireman T, Wallace R. Costs and health effects of osteoporotic fractures. Bone. 1994;15(4):377–86.
30. Phillips S, Fox N, Jacobs J, Wright WE. The direct medical costs of osteoporosis for American women aged 45 and older, 1986. Bone. 1988;9(5):271–9.
31. Holbrook TL, Grazier K, Kelsey JL, Stauffer RN. Frequency of occurrence, impact and cost of selected musculoskeletal conditions in the United States. Chicago: American Academy of Orthopedic Surgeons; 1998.
32. Truumees E. Osteoporosis. Spine. 2001;26:930–2.
33. Melton LJ 3rd, Gabriel SE, Crowson CS, Tosteson AN, Johnell O, Kanis JA. Cost-equivalence of different osteoporotic fractures. Osteoporos Int. 2003;14(5):383–8.
34. Gabriel SE, Tosteson ANA, Leibson CL, Crowson CS, Pond GR, Hammond CS, Melton LJ 3rd. Direct

medical costs attributable to osteoporotic fractures. Osteoporos Int. 2002;13(4):323–30.
35. Viswanathan HN, Curtis JR, Yu J, White J, Stolshek BS, Merinar C, et al. Direct healthcare costs of osteoporosis-related fractures in managed care patients receiving pharmacological osteoporosis therapy. Appl Health Econ Health Policy. 2012;10(3):163–73.
36. Orsini LS, Rousculp MD, Long SR, Wang S. Health care utilization and expenditures in the United States: a study of osteoporosis-related fractures. Osteoporos Int. 2005;16(4):359–71.
37. Licata AA. Cost analysis of medical and surgical treatment of vertebral fractures. In: Szpalski M, Gunzburg R, editors. Vertebral osteoporotic compression fractures. Philadelphia: Lippincott Williams & Wilkins; 2003. p. 257–60.
38. Zampini JM, White AP, McGuire KJ. Comparison of 5766 vertebral compression fractures treated with or without kyphoplasty. Clin Orthop Relat Res. 2010;468(7):1773–80.
39. Gehlbach SH, Burge RT, Puleo E, Klar J. Hospital care of osteoporosis-related vertebral fractures. Osteoporos Int. 2003;14:53–60.
40. Kallmes DF, Comstock BA, Heagerty PJ, Turner JA, Wilson DJ, Diamond TH, et al. A randomized trial of vertebroplasty for osteoporotic spinal fractures. N Engl J Med. 2009;361(6):569–79.
41. Buchbinder R, Osborne RH, Ebeling PR, Wark JD, Mitchell P, Wriedt C, et al. A randomized trial of vertebroplasty for painful osteoporotic vertebral fractures. N Engl J Med. 2009;361(6):557–68.
42. New guideline recommends against use of vertebroplasty [online]. Available from URL: https://www.aaos.org/AAOSNow/2010/Oct/cover/cover1/?ssopc=1. Accessed 17 Jan 2018.
43. Lee HM, Park SY, Lee SH, Suh SW, Hong JY. Comparative analysis of clinical outcomes in patients with osteoporotic vertebral compression fracture (OVCFs): conservative treatment versus balloon kyphoplasty. Spine J. 2012;12(11):998–1005.
44. Morris CA, Cabral D, Cheng H, Katz JN, Finkelstein JS, Avorn J, et al. Patterns of bone mineral density testing: current guidelines, testing rates, and interventions. J Gen Intern Med. 2004;19(7):783–90.
45. Amarnath AL, Franks P, Robbins JA, Xing G, Fenton JJ. Underuse and overuse of osteoporosis screening in a regional health system: a retrospective cohort study. J Gen Intern Med. 2015;30(12):1733–40.
46. Zhao JG, Zeng XT, Wang J, Liu L. Association between calcium or vitamin D supplementation and fracture incidence in community-dwelling older adults: a systematic review and meta-analysis. JAMA. 2017;318(24):2466–82.
47. Black DM, Thompson DE, Bauer DC, Ensrud K, Musliner T, Hochberg MC, et al. Fracture risk reduction with alendronate in women with osteoporosis: the Fracture Intervention Trial. J Clin Endocrinol Metab. 2000;85(11):4118–24.
48. Harris ST, Watts NB, Genant HK, McKeever CD, Hangartner T, Keller M, et al. Effects of risedronate treatment on vertebral and nonvertebral fractures in women with postmenopausal osteoporosis: a randomized controlled trial. Vertebral Efficacy with Risedronate Therapy (VERT) Study Group. JAMA. 1999;282(14):1344–52.
49. Qaseem A, Forciea MA, McLean RM, Denberg TD, Clinical Guidelines Committee of the American College of Physicians. Treatment of low bone density or osteoporosis to prevent fractures in men and women: a clinical practice guideline update from the American College of Physicians. Ann Intern Med. 2017;166(11):818–39.
50. Nguyen TV, Center JR, Eisman JA. Osteoporosis: underrated, underdiagnosed and undertreated. Med J Aust. 2004;180(5 Suppl):S18–22.
51. Nakayama A, Major G, Holliday E. Evidence of effectiveness of a fracture liaison service to reduce the re-fracture rate. Osteoporos Int. 2016;27(3):873–9.

Evaluation and Medical Management of Vertebral Osteoporosis: Preventing the Next Fracture

4

Faye N. Hant and Marcy B. Bolster

Introduction

Osteoporosis is a frequently silent, systemic disease defined by both low bone mineral density and changes in the microstructure of the skeleton, both of which lead to an increased risk for fragility fractures. A fragility fracture is defined by a fracture sustained from a fall from a standing height or less, or a fall out of bed. Additionally, a fragility fracture is one that occurs when a fracture otherwise would not have been expected, such as resulting from a slip on ice. Osteoporosis is the most common bone disease in humans and is a major public health concern. Vertebral compression fractures (VCFs) are the most common types of osteoporotic fractures. These fractures are often asymptomatic making them challenging to diagnose and are associated with increased risk of subsequent fracture as well as increased morbidity and mortality. This chapter both discusses the societal impact of and provides guidance for the evaluation and medical management of vertebral osteoporosis.

F. N. Hant (✉)
Division of Rheumatology and Immunology, Medical University of South Carolina, Charleston, SC, USA
e-mail: hant@musc.edu

M. B. Bolster
Division of Rheumatology, Allergy, and Immunology, Massachusetts General Hospital, Harvard Medical School, Boston, MA, USA
e-mail: mbolster@mgh.harvard.edu

Epidemiology

In the USA, ten million people over the age of 50 years carry a diagnosis of osteoporosis, and 34 million additional people have low bone mass [1, 2]. In those affected by osteoporosis, 1.5 million annual fragility fractures have been noted; half of these are VCFs – this is twice the rate of hip fractures [1, 2]. It is estimated that VCFs occur in up to 50% of people over the age of 50 years, and the incidence increases with age [3, 4]. It is difficult to estimate the true incidence of vertebral fractures, particularly as compared to other fragility fractures. Limitations in these estimates are affected by several factors including the fact that two-thirds to three-fourths of VCFs are asymptomatic, and <10% of patients are hospitalized related to the fracture [4–7]. Access to healthcare and the specific definition of a VCF also play a role in the reliability of this estimate. Vertebral fractures are diagnosed clinically, as when a patient presents with a painful spine fracture, or radiographically (the latter is termed a "morphometric" fracture), and this relationship is not well-defined, as few studies have prospectively compared the agreement between an incident radiographic VCF and an incident clinically recognized, radiographically confirmed VCF in the same person at the same vertebral level [6]. Spinal fractures may remain under-recognized as based on morphometric diagnosis: (1) they may be overlooked on imaging, (2) they may be recorded as "age indeterminate," or (3) they may

A. E. Razi, S. H. Hershman (eds.), *Vertebral Compression Fractures in Osteoporotic and Pathologic Bone*, https://doi.org/10.1007/978-3-030-33861-9_4

not be recorded in the patient's medical record – all three of scenarios likely result in treatment not being initiated at that time [4, 7].

A recent study provides a robust analysis of the worldwide prevalence and incidence of vertebral insufficiency fractures while acknowledging the paucity of quality data on this most common osteoporotic fracture, mostly due to its silent presentation in many [4]. Ballane and colleagues report that the assessment of vertebral fracture incidence and prevalence between distinct countries and areas is most reliable when vertebral fractures are defined morphometrically [4]. They found the prevalence of morphometric fractures in Europe to be lowest in Eastern Europe and highest in Scandinavia (18% vs. 26%, respectively), and in North America the prevalence rates are 20–24% in Caucasian women ≥50 years of age, with a Caucasian/African American ratio of 1.6 [4]. Prevalence rates in women ≥50 years old in Latin America are 11–19% and are lower than in North America and Europe. In Asia, rates in women ≥65 years old are lowest in Indonesia and highest in Japan (9% and 24%, respectively) [4]. Incidence data are scarce and heterogeneous, but these authors report that age-standardized incidence rates in studies that combine ambulatory and hospitalized VCFs are highest in Hong Kong, the USA, and South Korea and lowest in the UK [4]. In the USA, incidence rates in Caucasian patients are ~ fourfold higher than in African American patients [4].

The European Vertebral Osteoporosis Study (EVOS) is a multinational, multicenter population survey of vertebral osteoporosis, whose aim was to determine the prevalence of radiographically (morphometrically) defined "vertebral deformity" as a marker of vertebral osteoporosis by age and sex in different areas and populations of Europe [8]. EVOS revealed an overall increased prevalence of vertebral deformity in women compared with men, and this increased with age (from 5% at 50 years of age to 25% at 75 years of age in women compared with 10% at 50 years of age to 18% at 75 years of age in men) [8]. Notably the prevalence of vertebral deformity was higher in the younger age groups of men than women possibly due to a higher incidence of traumatic injury in men and is therefore less likely to be representative of a fragility fracture in men. It is also noted that men have higher bone density and after age 50 have a slower rate of bone loss compared with women, thereby corroborating the lower prevalence of vertebral deformity in men with increasing age [8].

Risk Factors for Vertebral Fracture

Bone remodeling is a continuous process whereby a healthy skeleton is preserved by removing older bone (resorption), and replacing it with new bone (formation). When this balance is altered, and more bone is removed than replaced, bone loss occurs. In older adults, bone mass equals the peak bone mass achieved by age 18–25 years minus the amount of bone subsequently lost [9]. The attainment of peak bone mass is determined by genetics as well as influences by multiple factors, including physical activity, nutrition, medication use, and endocrine status [9, 10]. With advancing age, and in women with menopause, the rate of bone remodeling increases, and an imbalance occurs leading to changes in skeletal architecture and an increased risk for fracture [9]. Cancellous bone, as is found in the vertebrae, undergoes changes with loss of individual plates of trabecular bone resulting in a weakened structure with diminished bone mass. There is an associated increased fracture risk related to the microarchitecture changes which is compounded by other age associated declines in function including but not limited to visual impairment, increased frailty, sarcopenia, and falls [9]. There are numerous risk factors and conditions (see Table 4.1) associated with an increased risk of osteoporotic fractures, and these can be categorized into areas such as endocrine, gastrointestinal, hematologic, neurologic and rheumatic diseases, as well as lifestyle factors, and medications [9, 11].

Table 4.1 Selected risk factors for osteoporosis and related fractures

Medications	Glucocorticoids Selective serotonin reuptake inhibitors Aromatase inhibitors Hypoglycemic agents: thiazolidinediones Proton pump inhibitors Antiepileptics Anticoagulants: heparin and oral agents Loop diuretics Antiretroviral agents Calcineurin inhibitors Androgen deprivation therapy Depot medroxyprogesterone acetate
Lifestyle	Tobacco use Excessive alcohol use Inadequate exercise Low calcium intake Immobilization Thin body habitus High salt intake
Gastrointestinal disease	Gastric bypass Malabsorption Inflammatory bowel disease Celiac disease
Endocrine disease	Thyrotoxicosis Diabetes mellitus (Type 1 and 2) Hyperparathyroidism Cushing's disease
Hematologic disease	Multiple myeloma Sickle cell disease Leukemia and lymphoma
Hypogonadal states	Anorexia nervosa Athletic amenorrhea Premature menopause (<40 years); Early menopause (<45 years) Panhypopituitarism
Rheumatologic disease	Rheumatoid arthritis Ankylosing spondylitis Systemic lupus erythematosus
Neurologic disease	Epilepsy Multiple sclerosis Parkinson's disease Muscular dystrophy
Genetic disease	Porphyria Hemochromatosis Parental history of hip fracture Osteogenesis imperfecta
Miscellaneous	Sarcoidosis Posttransplant bone disease Weight loss Amyloidosis Hypercalciuria AIDS/HIV

Adapted from Cosman et al. [9] and The Surgeon General's Report [11]

Societal Impact of Osteoporosis and Vertebral Fractures

As the most common bone disease in humans, osteoporosis and its fracture consequences carry a significant economic burden and profoundly affect individual morbidity and mortality. The Surgeon General Report reveals that in the USA, each year, two million fractures are related to osteoporosis leading to 2.5 million medical office outpatient visits, 432,000 hospital admissions, and ~ 180,000 nursing home admissions [11]. It is projected that between the years 2000 and 2025, the US population of 50 years of age and older will increase by 60% (to 121.3 million) [12].

A study designed to predict the US burden of osteoporosis-related fractures and costs yielded interesting results for clinicians, healthcare organizations, and policy makers and demonstrated the importance of interventions to reduce the burdens of this disease [13]. This study estimated, using a validated model, incident fractures and costs by age, race/ethnicity, sex, and skeletal site for the US population ≥50 years of age for 2005 through 2025. In 2005, there were more than two million incident fractures at an economic cost of $17 billion; this amount rose to more than $19 billion if costs of prevalent fractures were included [13]. The study predicted that by 2025, the healthcare burden of fragility fractures in the USA is anticipated to grow by approximately 50% to >three million fractures and equate to $25.3 billion annual in healthcare expenditures [13]. In addition, by race/ethnicity, the model estimated a 2.7-fold increase in fracture costs and incidence for Hispanic and other nonwhite populations [13]. The combined cumulative cost of both incident and prevalent fractures is projected to increase from $215 billion from 2006 to 2015 to $259 billion in the next decade, 2016–2025 [13]. Interestingly, men accounted for 25% of these costs and represented 29% of these fractures, recognizing that osteoporosis is not only a "woman's disease" [13]. The authors note that in 2005, the model predicts total incident fractures by skeletal site were vertebral (27%), wrist (19%), hip (14%), pelvis (7%), and other sites (33%), and that total costs by fracture type were vertebral (6%), wrist (3%), hip (72%), pelvis (5%), and other sites (14%) [13]. Thus, non-vertebral fractures accounted for 73% of the fractures and 94% of the costs [13]. Although there is a lower proportion of vertebral fractures estimated with lower cost burden, vertebral fractures remain the most common type of fracture, are under-detected, and are predictive of frailty, morbidity, and future fractures, thus vertebral fractures are an important fracture burden with high impact.

Diagnostic Approach

In 2015, the International Society for Clinical Densitometry (ISCD) released its official position for indications for BMD testing as a guide to clinicians, and these are summarized in Table 4.2 [14]. The dual-energy x-ray absorptiometry (DXA) scan provides the gold standard for assessment of bone mineral density (BMD). The DXA scan measures BMD at the lumbar spine, hip, and/or forearm. The World Health Organization (WHO) defines osteoporosis as a T-score at the lumbar spine, forearm, or hip which is less than or equal to −2.5, and this equates to at least 2.5 standard deviations below the mean BMD of a young-adult reference population. Severe osteoporosis is represented by a T-score less than or equal to −2.5 in the presence of an established fragility fracture. Osteopenia or low bone mass is defined by a T-score between −1.0 and −2.5, and normal BMD is a T-score of −1.0 or above (Table 4.3). Although the risk for osteoporosis is highest when there is a lower BMD, the majority of fragility fractures occur in patients with low bone mass/osteopenia rather than in those with T-scores in the osteoporosis range [9, 15].

In addition to the bone density definition of osteoporosis, the presence of a vertebral insufficiency fracture or a hip fragility fracture defines the presence of osteoporosis, and hence increased subsequent fracture risk. Asymptomatic VCFs require proactive imaging to diagnose, as their presence would change a patient's diagnostic bone health classification, affect treatment decisions,

Table 4.2 Indications for testing bone mineral density

1. Women age 65 years and older
2. Men age 70 years and older
3. Adults with a fragility fracture
4. Adults with a condition/disease known to be associated with bone loss or low bone mass
5. Adults taking a medication associated with bone loss or low bone mass
6. Postmenopausal women <65 years old with risk factors for low bone mass such as:
Prior fracture
High risk medication
Low body weight
Disease/condition associated with bone loss
7. Men <70 years old with risk factors for low bone mass such as:
Prior fracture
High risk medication
Low body weight
Disease/condition associated with bone loss
8. Perimenopausal women with clinical risk factors for fracture such as:
Prior fracture
High risk medication
Low body weight
9. Anyone being considered for pharmacologic therapy
10. Anyone being treated to monitor treatment effect
11. Anyone not receiving therapy in whom bone loss would lead to starting treatment
12. Women discontinuing estrogen

Adapted from The International Society for Clinical Densitometry (ISCD) [14]

Table 4.3 WHO definitions based on bone mineral density (BMD)

Classification	BMD	T-Score
Normal	Within 1 SD of the mean level for a young-adult reference population	T-score at −1.0 and above
Low bone mass (osteopenia)	Between 1.0 and 2.5 SD below that of the mean level for a young-adult reference population	T-score between −1.0 and −2.5
Osteoporosis	2.5 SD or more below that of the mean level for a young-adult reference population	T-score ≤ −2.5
Severe or established osteoporosis	2.5 SD or more below that of the mean level for a young-adult reference population with fractures	T-score ≤ −2.5 with one or more fractures

Adapted from Cosman et al. [9]

and impact future fracture risk [9, 16]. Independent of age, BMD, and other clinical risk factors, radiographically established vertebral fragility fractures define poor underlying bone strength and bone quality in addition to predicting increased risk for both subsequent vertebral and non-vertebral fractures [9].

Having a single VCF increases the risk of subsequent fractures fivefold and the risk for hip and other fractures two to threefold [9, 17]. After a vertebral fracture, the risk for subsequent vertebral fractures begins in the first year following the incident fracture. Vertebral imaging can be achieved using traditional diagnostic lateral (thoracic and lumbar) spine radiographs or, alternatively, the vertebral fracture assessment (VFA) software on the DXA scan. The VFA provides a lateral image of the thoracic and lumbar spine as a separate image on the DXA scan report. The ISCD, in its position paper, recommends use of VFA at the time of densitometric spine imaging to assist with the detection of vertebral fractures, acknowledging that VFA was designed to detect vertebral fractures and not other spinal abnormalities [14]. As VCFs are highly prevalent in the elderly and are most often asymptomatic (vide supra), there are recommendations for vertebral imaging (by standard radiography or VFA) listed in Table 4.4 that should be utilized in clinical practice [9, 14].

In an effort to determine the fracture probability in individuals with osteopenia (T-score between −1.0 and −2.4), the fracture risk assessment tool (FRAX®) was developed by the WHO Collaborating Centre for Metabolic Bone Disease at Sheffield, UK, and introduced in 2008 [15, 18]. The FRAX® tool estimates the 10-year probability of a hip fracture and of a major osteoporotic fracture (defined as a hip, forearm, proximal humerus, or vertebral fracture) and includes important clinical risk factors shown in Table 4.5, with or without the femoral neck BMD in the model [15]. The thresholds for treatment vary by country, and in the USA, treatment is recommended if the FRAX score for a 10-year probability of a hip fracture is ≥3% and/or a 10-year probability of a major osteoporosis-related fracture is ≥20% [15].

Table 4.4 Recommendations for vertebral imaging

[a]*Consider vertebral imaging tests for the following groups:*
1. All women 70 years and older and all men 80 years and older if BMD T-score is ≤ −1.0 at the spine, total hip, or femoral neck
2. Women 65–69 years old and men 70–79 years old, if BMD T-score is ≤ −1.5 at the spine, total hip or femoral neck
3. Postmenopausal women and men ≥50 years old with one of the following risk factors:
Historical height loss of 1.5 inches/4 cm or more[b]
Prospective height loss of 0.8 inches/2 cm or more[c]
Low-trauma fracture as an adult (age ≥ 50 years old)
Recent or ongoing long-term glucocorticoid treatment [equivalent to ≥5 mg of prednisone or equivalent per day for ≥3 months

Adapted from Cosman et al. [9] and The International Society for Clinical Densitometry (ISCD) [14]

[a]In the absence of BMD, vertebral imaging may be considered based solely on age

[b]Historical height is defined as current height compared to peak height during young adulthood

[c]Prospective height is defined as height loss measured during serial interval medical assessments

Table 4.5 Clinical risk factors utilized in the FRAX® calculation tool [18]

1. Current age
2. Gender
3. Prior osteoporotic fracture (includes asymptomatic VCFs and clinical fractures)
4. Weight
5. Height
6. Rheumatoid arthritis
7. Current smoking
8. Alcohol intake (3 or more units of alcohol daily)
9. Parental history of hip fracture
10. Use of oral glucocorticoids
Current exposure to oral glucocorticoids or ever exposure to oral glucocorticoids for more than 3 months at a dose of prednisone of 5 mg daily or more (or equivalent doses of other glucocorticoids)
11. Femoral neck BMD
12. Secondary causes of osteoporosis
Type I (insulin dependent) diabetes, chronic malnutrition, osteogenesis imperfecta in adults, hypogonadism or premature menopause (<45 years), untreated long-standing hyperthyroidism, malabsorption, and chronic liver disease)

The FRAX algorithm can be applied using different modalities including newer DXA machines, DXA software upgrades (provide the

FRAX® scores on the bone density report), or can be calculated by the clinician, with the FRAX calculator being found at the National Osteoporosis Foundation website (www.nof.org) or online at www.shef.ac.uk/FRAX. The FRAX tool is specific to a country and takes into account outcomes for fractures and associated morbidity and mortality [9]. This tool has been shown to improve fracture risk assessment compared to BMD alone [9, 19]. It is also important to note the application of FRAX® in the USA is intended for use in specific situations: in postmenopausal women and in men age ≥ 50; it is not meant to be used in patients currently or recently treated (within the last 2 years) with pharmacotherapy for osteoporosis [20]. Application of the BMD (femoral neck BMD) is preferred to use over the reported T-score in calculation [9, 18].

There are limitations to use of the FRAX® tool. Most importantly, the therapeutic thresholds are meant for clinical guidance and are not absolute "guidelines." This leaves treatment decisions to the provider emphasizing the importance of taking into consideration clinical judgment, individual patient factors, other risk factors not captured in FRAX® (such as falls, frailty, lumbar BMD), recent decline in BMD, and other factors that overestimate or underestimate fracture risk [9]. In addition, FRAX® underestimates fracture risk in patients with multiple osteoporotic fractures, those with recent fractures, and those at high risk for falls; it is most useful in those with low femoral neck BMD [9]. The use of FRAX® in patients with normal or low femoral neck BMD and lower lumbar spine BMD will underestimate the risk of fracture, as FRAX® is not validated for incorporation and does not utilize lumbar BMD in its calculation [9].

Risk Factor Modification

Risk factors that affect a person's underlying bone health should be assessed and modified as appropriate.

Regular weight-bearing and muscle strengthening exercise should be recommended to all patients to prevent falls as these can improve strength, posture, agility, and balance [9, 21–24]. Weight-bearing exercise refers to "exercise where the bones and muscles work against gravity as the lower extremities bear the body's weight," and the National Osteoporosis Foundation (NOF) strongly advocates for physical activity at all ages for overall health and osteoporosis prevention and recognizes that when exercise is stopped, its benefits are lost [9]. Examples of weight-bearing exercise recommendations include, but are not limited to, walking, hiking, dancing, stair climbing, tennis, and jogging. Examples of muscle strengthening exercises include, but are not limited to, weight training and resistive exercise such as pilates, use of resistive bands, yoga, and boot camp programs [9]. It is imperative to avoid a "one-size-fits-all" approach and to counsel patients individually about the most appropriate exercise programs to meet their needs based on their comorbidities and abilities.

Many patients with osteoporosis may benefit from physical and/or occupational therapy evaluations to assess balance and fall risk, to assist with walking aids and other assistive devices, and to provide balance and core strengthening programs. These modalities are discussed in more detail in other chapters.

Home environment assessment for fall prevention is an important intervention as more than 50% of falls in community-dwelling older adults occur in or around the home [25, 26]. A home health nursing visit can identify common environmental hazards whose modification may significantly reduce the risk for falling. These include, but are not limited to, improving dim lighting or glare with use of night lights and motion lighting, placement of handrails on the stairs and grab bars in the bathroom near toilets and showers, reviewing obstacles, removing clutter and tripping hazards, and improving slippery or uneven surfaces by placement of bathtub non-skid mats and removal of throw rugs and other non-stick floor coverings [27]. Additional research is needed in the areas of high-risk populations such as people who live in long-term care facilities, as these residents fall more frequently than community-dwelling individuals [28]. The astute clinician should also be aware of the many factors that put patients at risk for falls including but not limited to medications, poor vision, deconditioning, balance impairment, and environmental risk factors such as clutter and low level lighting and make appropriate modifications if possible [29].

Tobacco and alcohol represent other modifiable risk factors, and targeted counselling in patient encounters is important. The deleterious effects of tobacco on skeletal metabolism via hormonal changes and direct toxicity on bone are well-known, and BMD is lower in current and ever smokers than in never smokers, regardless of gender [30, 31]. The NOF strongly encourages an active smoking cessation program as part of a comprehensive osteoporosis management program [9]. Ethanol has both direct and indirect effects on bone cells. It decreases BMD and bone mass directly in both cortical and trabecular bone mainly via a decrease in bone formation as well as indirectly, through malnutrition leading to weight loss, decreased fat and lean mass, and hormonal alterations that may change bone cell activity [32]. Recommendations from work by Maurel and colleagues include counselling patients with excessive alcohol as defined by greater than two drinks a day for women and three drinks for men. The detrimental effects of alcohol on bone health include increased fall risk; for patients with recurrent falls, inquiry into the possibility of excessive alcohol use should be approached to improve safety [32].

In summary, the following recommendations should be made to the general public in an effort to preserve bone strength, and these include lifelong muscle-strengthening and weight-bearing exercise, tobacco cessation, treatment of excessive alcohol use, fall risk reduction, and sufficient intake of calcium and vitamin D.

Diet, Calcium and Vitamin D Intake

Adequate lifelong calcium intake is vital to attaining peak bone mass and maintaining bone health; a balanced diet rich in fruits, vegetables, and low-fat dairy products is fundamental [9].

Approximately 99% of the body's calcium stores are in the skeleton, and when the exogenous supply is limited, bone resorption occurs to maintain a steady level of serum calcium. Consumption of calcium and vitamin D is a safe and cost-effective way to reduce fracture risk in patients with osteoporosis with controlled trials demonstrating that this combination reduces the risk of fracture [9, 33]. Interestingly, while there are strong data to support the benefit of calcium and vitamin D supplementation in the management of osteoporosis, a meta-analysis performed by Zhao and colleagues revealed no fracture risk reduction with calcium and vitamin D supplementation in community-dwelling adults over the age of 50 years [34]. While of interest, these data should not be extrapolated to a population of patients with known osteoporosis requiring treatment or to a population of elderly subjects in an institution with increased fracture risk.

The NOF and the National Academy of Medicine recommend that men 50–70 years of age consume 1000 mg/day of calcium and that men ≥71 years old and women ≥51 years old consume 1200 mg/day of calcium [9, 35]. There is no evidence that higher doses are advantageous in regard to bone health, and doses above 1200–1500 mg/day may increase the risk for the development of cardiovascular disease, stroke, and renal stones, although this remains an area of debate [9, 36–39]. A study by Xiao et al. found that calcium supplementation of 1500 mg daily or higher was associated with increased cardiovascular risk in men; however this was not found in women, and additionally, lower supplementation doses were not associated with increased cardiovascular disease or strokes in men or women [40]. Sufficient dietary calcium intake is recommended first line, with judicious use of supplements added when adequate dietary consumption cannot be accomplished. Calcium supplementation can be provided with the use of calcium citrate or calcium carbonate and should be taken in divided doses throughout the day. Calcium citrate can be taken with or without food, not requiring an acidic environment, and is thus the supplement of choice in patients using proton pump inhibitors, while calcium carbonate requires food intake for adequate absorption.

Vitamin D also plays an essential role in bone health by enhancing calcium absorption, balance, and muscle performance and by reducing fall risk. The NOF recommendations are vitamin D 800–1000 IU daily in adults ≥50 years of age [9]. The National Academy of Medicine recommends vitamin D in a dose of 600 IU daily for adults to the age of 70 and 800 IU daily for adults ≥71 years of age [35]. The sun is a good source of vitamin D; dietary sources include salt water fish, liver, fortified milk (400 IU/quart), and some fortified cereals and juices (~40–50 IU/serving) [9]. Those at risk for vitamin D deficiency are patients with limited sun exposure, such as housebound and chronically ill patients, those with malabsorption or other gastrointestinal (GI) diseases (i.e., inflammatory bowel disease, celiac sprue, gastric bypass surgery), patients with renal insufficiency, dark skin pigmented individuals, and the obese [9]. Measurement of serum 25-OH-vitamin D should be undertaken in all patients at risk for deficiency and in those patients with osteopenia/osteoporosis, with supplementation recommended in amounts adequate to bring the serum 25-OH-vitamin D level to greater than 30 ng/ml (75 nmol/L) and a daily dose to maintain this level, especially in patients with osteoporosis [9].

It should be noted that many patients with osteoporosis will need more supplementation than the 800–1000 IU daily, and the National Academy of Medicine recommends the safe upper limit for vitamin D intake for the general adult population as 4000 IU daily [35]. If adults are noted to be vitamin D deficient, treatment with higher daily doses of Vitamin D3 supplementation are recommended, such as 4000–5000 IU daily, for 8–12 to achieve a 25-OH-vitamin D level of 30 ng/ml or higher, followed by a maintenance does of vitamin D3, 1500–2000 IU daily or a dose appropriate to maintain the target blood level [9, 41, 42].

Studies to date looking at high-dose vitamin D to reduce fall risk are inconclusive and warrant further study, with a recent study showing that a high-dose bolus vitamin D supplementation of 100,000 IU of vitamin D3/cholecalciferol monthly over 2.5–4.2 years did not prevent falls or fractures in a healthy, ambulatory, adult population [43]. Another study among older community-dwelling women, a single annual oral dose of 500,000 IU of vitamin D3/cholecalciferol resulted in an increased risk of falls and fractures [44].

Medical Management

When patients suffer from a VCF, treatment goals should be twofold: (1) to provide pain relief and (2) to assess and manage the underlying osteoporosis with appropriate pharmacologic therapies [2].

The acute pain arising from a new VCF usually improves over the course of 6–12 weeks, and throughout this interval, analgesics should be prescribed to decrease pain and to encourage movement [2, 45]. First-line analgesics should include acetaminophen or salicylates and nonsteroidal anti-inflammatory drugs (NSAIDs) [46]. Salicylates and NSAIDs should be used with caution in elderly patients with comorbidities due to the risk of gastric and/or renal adverse effects. Patients who fail initial management with these agents could be considered for opioid therapy; however these have considerable side effects especially in the elderly population, such as reduced GI motility and respiratory drive, urinary retention, and cognitive depressive effects. Opiate use in the elderly can lead to loss of balance and increased fall risk [47]. Short-term use of muscle relaxants for the first 1–2 weeks after vertebral fracture may be helpful to alleviate paravertebral muscle spasm associated with a VCF although side effects such as dizziness and drowsiness are potential concerns [2, 48]. In addition, the use of calcitonin agents for patients with acute pain from recent osteoporotic vertebral fractures is supported as an effective analgesic based on several randomized double-blind placebo-controlled trials, likely relating to an endorphin effect from this agent [2, 49].

Use of bracing remains largely opinion-based but can play a conservative role in many patients with VCFs. The main role of bracing in the management of osteoporosis-related VCFs is to prevent pain from movement by stabilizing the spine, and in addition, it leads to less back fatigue and allows for decreased bed rest with early mobilization following an acute fracture [2, 50, 51]. Ideally, if warranted based on the patient's clinical status, braces should be easy to put on, comfortable and lightweight, and prevent abdominal compression and respiratory effects [2]. Long-term use of back bracing may lead to core muscle weakness and further deconditioning [9]. Specific types of braces (corset, back brace, posture training support devices, etc.) used for VCFs will be covered in other chapters within this textbook.

After a short period of bed rest, patients should begin an early mobilization process with rehabilitation exercises with the goals of fall prevention, reduction of the development of kyphosis, corrective spinal alignment, and axial muscle strengthening [2]. It has been shown that spinal extensor strengthening and dynamic proprioceptive programs result in increased bone density and reduce the risk of VCFs [52–54]. Back extensor exercises improve spinal strength leading to reduction in kyphotic deformity and better dynamic-static posturing; the correction in kyphosis increases mobility, improves pain, and improves quality of life [55]. Physical therapy including core strengthening exercises as well as balance, gait analysis, fall risk evaluation, and spine protective practices (such as how to avoid leaning over to perform activities) have an important role in the medical management of these patients leading to pain relief and improvement in physical function [56].

Patients with painful, recent VCFs that fail the aforementioned conservative therapy may be candidates for intervention with kyphoplasty or vertebroplasty. Considerations for use of these procedures will be discussed in a different chapter in this textbook.

Pharmacologic Management

The following patients, postmenopausal women and men ≥50 years old, should be considered for pharmacologic treatment with a (1) history of hip or vertebral fracture (clinically or morphometric VCF); (2) T-score ≤ −2.5 at the total hip, femoral neck, or lumbar spine (or 1/3 radius if hip or spine BMD is unavailable or unreliable due to instrumentation or spinal deformity); and (3) low bone mass (T-score between −1.0 and −2.5 at the femoral neck or lumbar spine) and increased calculated FRAX® risk [9].

All patients who have had a vertebral insufficiency fracture should be counselled on risk factor reduction, the importance of calcium and vitamin D intake, fall prevention, and exercise as part of a comprehensive treatment strategy. Prior to starting pharmacologic treatment, an individual's risk factors and comorbidities should be addressed, and, as appropriate, patients should undergo a metabolic evaluation for secondary causes of bone loss. Although not requisite to determine the need for osteoporosis treatment, a patient with a VCF should undergo BMD measurement via DXA scanning to determine baseline BMD which can be used for assessing treatment response.

The available FDA-approved drugs for the prevention and treatment of postmenopausal osteoporosis include antiresorptive agents such as bisphosphonates (alendronate, risedronate, ibandronate, zoledronic acid), estrogens (estrogen and other hormonal therapy), estrogen agonist/antagonist (raloxifene), the receptor activator of nuclear factor kappa-B (RANK) ligand (RANKL) inhibitor (denosumab), and anabolic agents such as parathyroid hormone (PTH), teriparatide, and abaloparatide [1–34]. These agents are summarized in Table 4.6 [9]. Calcitonin does not reduce the risk of fractures but may assist with pain associated with vertebral fracture, and thus it may be utilized accordingly. The FDA-approved treatments have been shown to decrease fracture risk in patients with osteoporosis including those with and without prior fragility fractures [9]. The NOF does not endorse the use of non-FDA-approved therapies to prevent or treat osteoporosis such as calcitriol, sodium fluoride, tibolone, strontium ranelate, and genistein, among others [9]. Genistein is an isoflavone phytoestrogen which is a main ingredient in a prescription "medical food" product Fosteum® and

Table 4.6 Selected FDA-approved treatment for the prevention and treatment of osteoporosis

Agent	Mechanism of action	Dosage
Oral bisphosphonates 1. Alendronate/ Fosamax® 2. Risedronate/ Actonel® 3. Ibandronate/ Boniva®	Antiresorptive Inhibitor of osteoclast-mediated bone resorption	1. Prevention 5 mg daily/35 mg weekly 1. Treatment 10 mg daily/70 mg weekly 2. Prevention and treatment 5 mg daily/35 mg weekly 150 mg monthly 3. Treatment 150 mg monthly
IV bisphosphonate 1. Ibandronate/ Boniva® 2. Zoledronic acid/ Reclast®	Antiresorptive Inhibitor of osteoclast-mediated bone resorption	1. Treatment 3 mg IV every 3 months 2. Prevention 5 mg every 2 years 2. Treatment 5 mg yearly
RANKL/RANKL inhibitor Denosumab/ Prolia®	Antiresorptive Prevents RANKL from activating its receptor, RANK, on the surface of osteoclasts. Prevention of the RANKL/RANK interaction inhibits osteoclast formation, function, and survival, thereby decreasing bone resorption	60 mg SQ every 6 months
SERM Raloxifene/ Evista®	Acts as an estrogen agonist in bone. Decreases bone resorption and bone turnover	Prevention and treatment 60 mg oral daily
PTH (1–34) 1. Teriparatide/ Forteo® 2. Abaloparatide/ Tymlos®	Anabolic Stimulates new bone formation on trabecular and cortical (periosteal and/or endosteal) bone surfaces by preferential stimulation of osteoblastic activity over osteoclastic activity	Treatment 1. 20 mcg SQ daily 2. 80 mcg SQ daily

IV intravenous, *SQ* subcutaneous

may benefit bone health in postmenopausal women; however more data from well-designed randomized-controlled trials are needed to fully understand its effects on bone health and fracture risk [9, 57]. Although there are strong data on the benefits of pharmacologic therapy for patients with osteoporosis with or without prior fractures, the evidence for overall anti-fracture benefit in patients with osteopenia who are not at high risk for fracture is not as compelling [9]. Use of the FRAX tool has helped to identify those patients with osteopenia who are at predictably high risk for fracture who may benefit from treatment; however there are limited data confirming fracture risk reduction with pharmacologic therapy in this group of patients [9]. Each provider must review with each patient the risks and benefits of osteoporosis pharmacotherapies to optimize management and compliance with the goal of risk reduction for vertebral and non-vertebral fractures [9].

Oral Bisphosphonates

Alendronate sodium (Fosamax®, Fosamax Plus D, Binosto™ and generic alendronate), risedronate sodium (Actonel®, Atelvia™), and zoledronic acid (Reclast®) are FDA approved to prevent and treat osteoporosis in postmenopausal women, to increase bone mass in men with osteoporosis, and for the treatment of glucocorticoid-induced osteoporosis (GIOP) in women and men [9, 58–63]. Alendronate, an oral medication, reduces the incidence of hip and vertebral fractures by about 50% over 3 years in patients with osteoporosis as defined by T-score or a prior vertebral fracture and reduces the incidence of vertebral fractures by 50% over 3 years in patients without a previous vertebral fracture [9, 59, 64, 65]. Risedronate sodium (Actonel®, Atelvia™), an oral medication, has been shown to reduce the incidence of non-vertebral fractures by 36% and vertebral fractures by 41–49% over 3 years with significantly reduced risk within 1 year of treatment in patients with a history of a prior vertebral fracture [60, 66]. Ibandronate sodium (Boniva®) is FDA approved for the prevention and treatment of postmenopausal osteoporosis [9]. This medication was shown to reduce the incidence of vertebral fractures by ~ 50% at 3 years, but risk reduction of non-vertebral fractures was not specifically addressed prior to FDA approval of ibandronate [9, 67].

Zoledronic acid (Reclast®), an annual infusion medication, is also indicated for the prevention of new clinical fractures in women and men with a history of a recent hip fragility fracture [9, 68]. This medication reduces the incidence of vertebral fractures by 70% (with significant reduction at 1 year), non-vertebral fractures by 25%, and hip fractures by 41% over 3 years in patients with osteoporosis (defined by BMD in osteoporotic range at the hip and prevalent vertebral fractures) [9, 62]. When receiving zoledronic acid, patients should remain adequately hydrated and may receive premedication with acetaminophen to decrease the risk for an "acute phase reaction" or "flu-like syndrome" (fever, headache, arthralgia, myalgia) which has been reported in up to 32% of patients after the first dose, 7% after the second dose, and 3% after the third dose [9].

All bisphosphonates require adequate renal function prior to administration and have not been studied in patients with an estimated GFR <35 mL/min; zoledronic acid is not advised in patients with GFR <35 mL/min or evidence of acute renal insufficiency. Renal function should be assessed prior to administration of zoledronic acid [9, 69].

Two rare but noteworthy complications that have been reported with bisphosphonate use are osteonecrosis of the jaw (ONJ) and atypical femoral fractures (AFF).

ONJ is a condition in which there is decreased metabolic support to the bony tissue of the mandible and maxilla resulting in bone necrosis and poor healing. ONJ can occur spontaneously or more commonly occurs after invasive dental work such as tooth extractions or dental implants, and thus all patients should be encouraged to have all dental procedures completed prior to starting therapy, as instrumentation appears to heighten the risk for this condition. The FDA has voiced precautions regarding the occurrence of ONJ seen in patients on bisphosphonates, with risks for developing ONJ higher in patients taking the drug intravenously and related to an underlying malignancy [9, 70]. AFF are rare, low trauma fractures that may be associated with long-term (>5 years) use of bisphosphonates and may be preceded by a prodrome of anterior thigh or groin pain which may be unilateral or bilateral [9, 71]. In the presence of a new AFF, bilateral femur x-rays should be obtained. If clinical suspicion remains high even in the presence of negative contralateral plain films, then MRI or radionuclide bone scan should be considered [9, 71]. The risk of atypical femoral fracture, but not osteonecrosis of the jaw, clearly increases with bisphosphonate therapy duration; however the risk of these rare events is outweighed by vertebral fracture risk reduction in high-risk patients [72]. Discontinuation of antiresorptive agents is imperative with the occurrence of ONJ or an AFF.

Rank Ligand Inhibition

Denosumab (Prolia®) is FDA approved for the treatment of osteoporosis in postmenopausal women at high risk for fracture, to increase bone mass in men with osteoporosis, to treat bone loss in women with breast cancer on aromatase inhibitors and men receiving gonadotropin-reducing hormone treatment for prostate cancer who are at high risk for fracture [9]. It is a monoclonal antibody that potently blocks the binding of receptor activator of nuclear factor kappa-B ligand (RANKL) to its osteoclast-derived receptor (RANK), thereby inhibiting osteoclast-mediated bone resorption [73]. It reduces, over 3 years, the incidence of vertebral fractures by~ 68%, non-vertebral fractures by ~ 20%, and hip fractures by ~40% [9, 74]. Denosumab can lead to hypocalcemia and has also rarely been associated with ONJ and AFF. Once treatment with this agent is stopped, bone loss may be rapid, and alternative agents should be considered to maintain BMD.

In addition, recent data suggest discontinuing denosumab may increase the risk of multiple vertebral fractures due to a rebound increase in bone resorption, thus clinicians and patients must be aware of this potential risk [9, 75].

Estrogen Agonist/Antagonist (Formerly Known as SERMs)

Raloxifene (Evista®) is FDA approved for the prevention and treatment of osteoporosis in postmenopausal women. It has been shown to reduce the risk of vertebral fractures by ~ 30% in patients with prior vertebral fracture and by ~ 55% in patients without a prior vertebral fracture over 3 years, though it does not have a demonstrated benefit for non-vertebral fracture risk reduction [76].

Anabolic Agents

Parathyroid hormone (PTH 1–34) teriparatide (Forteo®) is FDA approved for the treatment of postmenopausal women and men at high risk for fracture, and in those with osteoporosis associated with sustained use of systemic glucocorticoid therapy [9, 77]. A similar agent abaloparatide (Tymlos®) (PTH 1–34) is similarly FDA approved for the treatment of postmenopausal women with osteoporosis at high risk for fracture [78]. Teriparatide reduces the risk of vertebral fractures by ~ 65% and non-vertebral fragility fractures by ~ 53% after an average of 18 months of treatment [79]. Abaloparatide (Tymlos) compared with placebo also reduces the risk of new vertebral and non-vertebral fractures and results in higher BMD gains over 18 months [78]. These agents carry a black box warning of osteosarcoma risk, although there has not been an observed increased occurrence in humans clinically. Patients at high risk for osteosarcoma at baseline should not receive these agents such as those with Paget's disease of bone, unexplained increase in alkaline phosphatase, hypercalcemia, history of skeletal malignancy, history of bony metastases, or a history of prior skeletal radiation [9]. Other potential adverse effects from these agents are: leg cramps, dizziness, and orthostatic hypotension. Following treatment with an anabolic agent, an antiresorptive agent should be started to maintain skeletal benefits [9].

Another agent being studied for treatment of osteoporosis is romosozumab, a potent humanized monoclonal antibody that binds to sclerostin, an inhibitor of the Wnt signaling pathway, a major pathway in skeletal development, bone remodeling and adult skeletal homeostasis [80]. Romosozumab is a potent anabolic agent which activates the Wnt signaling pathway and leads to bone formation and an increase in BMD. In the Phase III placebo-controlled FRActure study in postmenopausal woMen with ostEoporosis (FRAME) trial comparing romosozumab to placebo, vertebral fractures were reduced by 73% after 1 year of treatment [80, 81] . Treatment with romosozumab for 1 year, followed by denosumab in the second year, reduced vertebral fractures by 75% compared to the group receiving placebo for 1 year followed by denosumab for 1 year [80, 81].

Treatment for osteoporosis should not be considered indefinite in duration with the realization that all non-bisphosphonate therapies produce temporary effects that fade with stopping the medication, and when these therapies are stopped, the benefits gained will quickly disperse [9]. Bisphosphonates often allow for residual effects even after their discontinuation, and thus it is possible to stop bisphosphonate therapy and retain lingering benefits against fracture for years [9]. Treatment duration must be tailored to individual patients, and after 3–5 years of therapy, a risk assessment should be conducted with assessment of clinical fracture history, BMD testing, new medications and medical illnesses, height loss, and consideration of vertebral imaging [9]. As evidence of efficacy beyond 5 years of treatment is limited, it is reasonable to stop bisphosphonates after 3–5 years in patients with modest risk after the initial treatment timeframe; however in those at high risk for fracture, continued treatment should be considered [9, 82, 83].

The appropriate duration of therapy to treat osteoporosis with medications remains an area of uncertainty and several studies have attempted to clarify this. The Fracture Intervention Trial Long-term Extension (FLEX) evaluated the effects of stopping alendronate/Fosamax® therapy after 5 years versus continuing therapy for 10 years [84]. In this trial, 1099 postmenopausal women who had been randomized to alendronate in FIT (Fracture Intervention Trial), with a mean of 5 years of prior alendronate treatment, were randomized to one of two doses of alendronate or placebo for 5 years [84]. After 5 years, the cumulative risk of non-vertebral fractures (RR, 1.00; 95% CI, 0.76–1.32) was not significantly different between those continuing on (19%) and stopping (18.9%) alendronate. Among those who remained on drug for 10 years, there was a significantly lower risk of clinically recognized vertebral fractures (5.3% for placebo and 2.4% for alendronate; RR, 0.45; 95% CI, 0.24–0.85) but no significant reduction in morphometric vertebral fractures (11.3% for placebo and 9.8% for alendronate; RR, 0.86; 95% CI, 0.60–1.22) [84]. The study concluded that for many postmenopausal women, discontinuation of alendronate after 5 years of therapy does not appear to significantly increase fracture risk but that women at very high risk of vertebral fractures may benefit by remaining on therapy for a total course of 10 years [84]. Based on these data, many authorities recommend therapy with oral bisphosphonates for 5 years followed by consideration for a "drug holiday" while continuing to monitor the patient clinically with DXA scan, assessment of clinical and morphometric fractures, and risk factor assessment.

Another trial, a randomized extension to the HORIZON-Pivotal Fracture Trial (PFT), looked at the effect of 3 years versus 6 years of zoledronic acid treatment for osteoporosis [85]. To investigate the long-term effects of zoledronic acid on BMD and fracture risk, in this extension trial, 1233 postmenopausal women who received zoledronic acid for 3 years in the core study were randomized to 3 additional years of zoledronic acid (Z6, n = 616) versus placebo (Z3P3, n = 617) [85]. They found that new morphometric vertebral fractures were lower in those patients who received 6 years of zoledronic acid compared to those patients receiving zoledronic acid for 3 years followed by placebo infusions for 3 years (odds ratio = 0.51; p = 0.035), but other fractures were not noted to be different [85]. Small differences in bone density and bone turnover markers in those who continued versus those who stopped zoledronic acid suggest residual effects, and it was concluded that after 3 years of annual zoledronic acid infusions, many patients can discontinue therapy for up to 3 years [85]. However, vertebral fracture reductions in this trial suggested that those at high risk of fracture and particularly vertebral fractures may benefit from continued treatment for more than 3 years [85].

Summary

Despite available treatments, many patients are not being given the tools for prevention of osteoporosis and related fractures, and many are not undergoing the testing to diagnose or establish their underlying bone health risk. In addition, many patients who have suffered osteoporotic-related fractures are not receiving any of the very effective FDA-approved pharmacologic therapies for the treatment of osteoporosis [9].

Many of the same principles related to primary prevention, risk assessment, and screening should be implemented once a fracture has occurred to help avoid further fractures.

Primary prevention of osteoporosis includes risk assessment, BMD testing, and pharmacotherapy if indicated. These same principles in patient management apply to those patients who have sustained a fragility fracture (secondary prevention). Many patients who have sustained a fragility fracture do not receive treatment and thus remain at very high risk for subsequent fracture, increased morbidity and mortality. The medical management of osteoporotic fractures is well-supported by data demonstrating medication efficacy. Treatment regimens should be individualized for patient needs including medication selection and duration of therapy. Risk factor assessment, including fall risk, remains an essential part of the management plan.

References

1. Marwick C. Consensus panel considers osteoporosis. JAMA. 2000;283:2093–5.
2. Longo UG, Loppini M, Denaro L, Maffulli N, Denaro V. Osteoporotic vertebral fractures: current concepts of conservative care. Br Med Bull. 2012;102:171–89.
3. Bouxsein M, Genant H. International Osteoporosis Foundation. Vertebral Fracture Audit. www.iofbonehealth.org. 2010.
4. Ballane G, Cauley JA, Luckey MM, El-Hajj Fuleihan G. Worldwide prevalence and incidence of osteoporotic vertebral fractures. Osteoporos Int. 2017;28(5):1531–42.
5. Kanis JA, Odén A, McCloskey EV, Johansson H, Wahl DA, Cooper C, IOF Working Group on Epidemiology and Quality of Life. A systematic review of hip fracture incidence and probability of fracture worldwide. Osteoporos Int. 2012;23(9):2239–56. Epub 2012 Mar 15.
6. Fink HA, Milavetz DL, Palermo L, et al. What proportion of incident radiographic vertebral deformities is clinically diagnosed and vice versa? J Bone Miner Res. 2005;20(7):1216–22.
7. Gehlbach SH, Bigelow C, Heimisdottir M, May S, Walker M, Kirkwood JR. Recognition of vertebral fracture in a clinical setting. Osteoporos Int. 2000;11:577–82.
8. O'Neill TW, Felsenberg D, Varlow J, Cooper C, Kanis JA, Silman AJ, the European Vertebral Osteoporosis Study Group. The prevalence of vertebral deformity in European men and women: the european vertebral osteoporosis study. J Bone Miner Res. 1996;11:1010–8.
9. Cosman F, de Beur SJ, LeBoff MS, Lewiecki EM, Tanner B, Randall S, Lindsay R. Clinician's guide to prevention and treatment of osteoporosis. Position Paper. Osteoporos Int. 2014;25:2359. https://doi.org/10.1007/s00198-014-2794-2.
10. Khosla S, Riggs BL. Pathophysiology of age-related bone loss and osteoporosis. Endocrinol Metab Clin N Am. 2005;34:1015–30.
11. Office of the Surgeon General (US). Bone Health and Osteoporosis: a report of the Surgeon General. Office of the Surgeon General (US), Rockville (MD). Available from https://www.ncbi.nlm.nih.gov/books/NBK45513/. 2004.
12. Day JC. Population projections of the United States by age, sex, race, and hispanic origin: 1995 to 2050. Washington, D.C.: U.S. Government Printing Office; 1996.
13. Burge R, Dawson-Hughes B, Solomon DH, Wong JB, King A, Tosteson A. Incidence and economic burden of osteoporosis-related fractures in the United States, 2005–2025. J Bone Miner Res. 2007;22(3):465–75.
14. The International Society for Clinical Densitometry (ISCD). Official Positions 2015 ISCD Combined (US), Middletown. Available from www.ISCD.org.
15. Kanis JA, on behalf of the World Health Organization Scientific Group. Assessment of osteoporosis at the primary health care level. Technical Report. World Health Organization Collaborating Center for Metabolic Bone Diseases. University of Sheffield, UK. 2007.
16. Lenchik L, Rogers LF, Selmas PD, Genant HK. Diagnosis of osteoporotic vertebral fractures: importance of recognition and description by radiologists. Am J Roentgenol. 2004;183(4):949–58.
17. Ross PD, Davis JW, Epstein RS, Wasnich RD. Pre-existing fractures and bone mass predict vertebral incidence in women. Ann Intern Med. 1991;114(11):919–23.
18. Kanis JA, Johnell O, Oden A, Johansson H, McClaskey EV. FRAX™ and the assessment of fracture probability in men and women for the UK. Osteoporos Int. 2008;19:385–97.
19. Kanis JA, Oden A, Johnell O, et al. The Use of Clinical risk factors enhances the performance of BMD in the prediction of hip and osteoporotic fractures in men and women. Osteoporos Int. 2007;18:1033–46.
20. National Osteoporosis Foundation (NOF) and International Society for Clinical Densitometry (ISCD). Recommendations to DXA manufacturers for FRAX ® Implementation. Available at http://www.nof.org/files/nof/public/content/resource/862/files/392.pdf.
21. Gillespie LD, Gillespie WJ, Robertson MC, et al. Interventions for preventing falls in elderly people. Cochrane Database Syst Rev. 2003;(4):CD000340.
22. Granacher U, Gollhofer A, HortoBágyi T, Kressig RW, Muehlbauer T. The importance of trunk muscle strength for balance, functional performance and fall prevention in seniors: a systematic review. Sports Med. 2013;43(7):627–41.
23. Sherrington C, Whitney JC, Lord SR, Herbert RD, Cumming RG, Close JC. Effective exercise for the prevention of falls: a systematic review and meta-analysis. J Am Geriatr Soc. 2008;56(12):2234–43.
24. Choi M, Hector M. Effectiveness of intervention programs in preventing falls: a systematic review of recent 10 years and meta-analysis. J Am Med Dir Assoc. 2012;13(2):188.e13–21.
25. Berg WP, Alessio HM, Mills EM, et al. Circumstances and consequences of falls in independent community-dwelling older adults. Age Ageing. 1997;26:261–8.
26. Wyman JF, Croghan CF, Nachreiner NM, et al. Effectiveness of education and individualized counseling in reducing environmental hazards in the homes of community-dwelling older women. J Am Geriatr Soc. 2007;55:1548–56.
27. Stevens JA, Baldwin GT, Ballesteros MF, Noonan RK, Sleet DA. An older adult falls research agenda from a public health perspective. Clin Geriatr Med. 2010;26:767–79.
28. Rubenstein LZ, Josephson KR, Robbins AS. Falls in the nursing home. Ann Intern Med. 1994;121:442–51.
29. National Osteoporosis Foundation (NOF). Health Professional's guide to rehabilitation of the patient

with osteoporosis. Washington, D.C.: National Osteoporosis Foundation; 2003.
30. Osteoporosis – Prevention, diagnosis and treatment: a systematic review [Internet]. Swedish Council on Health Technology Assessment. Stockholm: Swedish Council on Health Technology Assessment (SBU); 2003. SBU Yellow Report No. 165/1+2.
31. Waugh EJ, Lam MA, Hawker GA, McGowan J, Papaioannou A, Am C, et al. Risk factors for low bone mass in healthy 40–60 year old women: a systematic review of the literature. Osteoporos Int. 2009; 20:1–21.
32. Maurel DB, Boisseau N, Benhamou CL, Jaffre C. Alcohol and bone: review of dose effects and mechanisms. Osteoporos Int. 2012;23(1):1–16.
33. Larsen ER, Mosekilde L, Foldspang A. Vitamin D and calcium supplementation prevents osteoporotic fractures in elderly community dwelling residents: a pragmatic population-based 3-year intervention study. J Bone Miner Res. 2004;19(3):370–8.
34. Zhao JG, Zeng XT, Wang J, Liu L. Association between calcium or Vitamin D supplementation and fracture incidence in community-dwelling older adults; a systematic review and meta-analysis. JAMA. 2017;318(24):2466–82.
35. Institute of Medicine (US) Committee to review dietary reference intakes for Vitamin D and calcium. In: Ross AC, Taylor CL, Yaktine AL, et al., editors. Dietary reference intakes for calcium and vitamin D. Washington, D.C.: National Academies Press (US); 2011. Available from: http://www.ncbi.nlm.nih.gov/books/NBK56070.
36. Prentice RL, Pettinger MB, Jackson RD, et al. Health risks and benefits from calcium and vitamin D supplementation: Women's Health Initiative clinical trial and cohort study. Osteoporosis Int. 2013;24(2):567–80.
37. Reid IR, Bolland MJ. Calcium supplements: bad for the heart? Heart. 2012;98(12):895–6.
38. Bolland MJ, Grey A, Avenell A, Gamble GD, Reid IR. Calcium supplements with or without vitamin D and risk of cardiovascular events: reanalysis of the Women's Health Initiative limited access dataset and meta-analysis. BMJ. 2011;19, 342
39. Moyer VA, U.S. Preventative Services Task Force. Vitamin D and calcium supplements to prevent fractures in adults: U.S. Preventative Services Task Force recommendation statement. Ann Intern Med. 2013;158(9):691–6.
40. Xiao Q, Murphy RA, Houston DK, Harris TB, Chow WH, Park Y. Dietary and supplemental calcium intake and cardiovascular disease mortality: the National Institutes of Health-AARP diet and health study. JAMA Intern Med. 2013;173(8):639–46.
41. Looker SC, Pfeiffer CM, Lacher DA, Schleicher RL, Picciano MF, Yetley EA. Serum 25-hydroxyvitamin D status of the US population: 1988-1994 compared to 2000-2004. Am J Clin Nutr. 2008;88(6):1519–27.
42. Wortsman J, Matsukoa LY, Chen TC, Lu Z, Holick MF. Decreased bioavailability of vitamin D in obesity. Am J Clin Nutr. 2000;72(3):690–3.
43. Khaw KT, Stewart AW, Waayer D, Lawes CMM, Toop L, Camargo CA Jr, Scragg R. Effect of monthly high-dose vitamin D supplementation on falls and non-vertebral fractures: secondary and post-hoc outcomes from the randomised, double-blind, placebo-controlled ViDA trial. Lancet Diabetes Endocrinol. 2017;5(6):438–47.
44. Sanders KM, Stuart AL, Williamson EJ, Simpson JA, Kotowicz MA, Young D, Nicholson GC. Annual high-dose oral vitamin D and falls and fractures in older women: a randomized controlled trial. JAMA. 2010;303(18):1815–22.
45. Silverman SL. The clinical consequences of vertebral compression fracture. Bone. 1992;13(2):S27–31.
46. Lyles KW. Management of patients with vertebral compression fractures. Pharmacotherapy. 1999;19:21S–4S.
47. Cherasse A, Muller G, Ornetti P. Tolerability of opioids in patients with acute pain due to nonmalignant musculoskeletal disease. A hospital-based observational study. Joint Bone Spine. 2004;71:572–6.
48. Browning R, Jackson JL, O'Malley PG. Cyclobenzaprine and back pain: a meta-analysis. Arch Intern Med. 2001;161:1613–20.
49. Knopp JA, Diner BM, Blitz M. Calcitonin for treating acute back pain of osteoporotic vertebral compression fractures: a systematic review of randomized, controlled trials. Osteoporos Int. 2005;16:1281–90.
50. Prather H, Watson JO, Gilula LA. Nonoperative management of osteoporotic vertebral compression fractures. Injury. 2007;38(S3):S40–8.
51. Kim DH, Vaccaro AR. Osteoporotic compression fractures of the spine; current options and considerations for treatment. Spine J. 2006;6:479–87.
52. Sinaki M, Itoi E, Wahner HW. Stronger back muscles reduce the incidence of vertebral fractures: a prospective 10 year follow-up of postmenopausal women. Bone. 2002;30:836–41.
53. Sinaki M, Lynn SG. Reducing the risk of falls through proprioceptive dynamic posture training in osteoporotic women with kyphotic posturing: a randomized pilot study. Am J Phys Med Rehabil. 2002;81: 241–6.
54. Sinaki M, Brey RH, Hughes CA. Significant reduction in risk of falls and back pain in osteoporotic-kyphotic women through a Spinal Proprioceptive Extension Exercise Dynamic (SPEED) program. Mayo Clin Proc. 2005;80:849–55.
55. Itoi E, Sinaki M. Effect of back-strengthening exercise on posture in healthy women 49 to 65 years of age. Mayo Clin Proc. 1994;69:1054–9.
56. Bennell KL, Matthews B, Greig A. Effects of an exercise and manual therapy program on physical impairments, function and quality-of-life in people with osteoporotic vertebral fracture: a randomized, single-blind controlled pilot trial. BMC Musculoskelet Disord. 2010;11:36.
57. Marini H, Minutoli L, Polito F, Bitto A, Altavilla D, Atteritano M, Gaudio A, Mazzaferro S, Frisina A, Frisina N, et al. Effects of the phytoestrogen genistein

on bone metabolism in osteopenic postmenopausal women: a randomized trial. Ann Intern Med. 2007;146:839–47.

58. Saag KG, Emkey R, Schnitzer TJ, et al. Alendronate for the prevention and treatment of glucocorticoid-induced osteoporosis. Glucocorticoid-Induced Osteoporosis Intervention Study Group. NEJM. 1998;339(5):292–9.
59. Black DM, Cummings SR, Karpf DB, et al. Randomized trial of effect of alendronate on risk of fracture in women with existing vertebral fractures. Fracture Intervention Trial Research Group. Lancet. 1996;348(9041):1535–41.
60. Reginster J, Minne HW, Sorenson OH, et al. Randomized trial of the effects of risedronate on vertebral fractures in women with established postmenopausal osteoporosis. Vertebral Efficacy with Risedronate Therapy (VERT) Study Group. Osteoporos Int. 2000;11(1):83–91.
61. Eastell R, Devogelaer JP, Peel NF, et al. Prevention of bone loss with risedronate in glucocorticoid-treated rheumatoid arthritis patients. Osteoporos Int. 2000;11(4):331–7.
62. Black DM, Delmas PD, Eastell R, Horizon Pivotal Fracture Trial, et al. Once yearly zoledronic acid for treatment of postmenopausal osteoporosis. N Engl J Med. 2007;356(18):189–1822.
63. Buckley L, Guyatt G, Fink HA, Cannon M, Grossman J, Hansen KE, Humphrey MB, Lane NE, Magrey M, Miller M, Morrison L, Rao M, Robinson AB, Saha S, Wolver S, Bannuru E, Osani M, Turgunbaev M, Miller AS, McAlindon T. 2017 American College of Rheumatology Guideline for the prevention and treatment of glucocorticoid-induced osteoporosis. Arthritis Rheumatol. 2017;69(8):1521–37.
64. Black DM, Thompson DE, Bauer DC, et al. Fracture risk reduction with alendronate in women with osteoporosis: the Fracture Intervention Trial. FIT Research Group. J Clin Endocrinol Metab. 2000;85(11):4118–24.
65. Cummings SR, Black DM, Thompson DE, et al. Effect of alendronate on risk of fracture in women with low bone density but without vertebral fractures: results from the Fracture Intervention Trial. JAMA. 1998;280(24):2077–82.
66. Harris ST, Watts NB, Genant HK, et al. Effects of risedronate treatment on vertebral and nonvertebral fractures in women with postmenopausal osteoporosis: a randomized controlled trial. Vertebral Efficacy with Risedronate Therapy (VERT) Study Group. JAMA. 1999;282(14):1344–52.
67. Chestnut CH 3rd, Skag A, Christiansen C, et al. Effects of oral ibandronate administered daily or intermittently on fracture risk in postmenopausal osteoporosis. J Bone Miner Res. 2004;19(18):1241–9.
68. Lyles KW, Colon-Emeric CS, Magaziner JS, et al. Zoledronic acid and clinical fractures and mortality after hip fracture. N Engl J Med. 2007;357(18):1799–809.
69. U.S. Food and Drug Administration. Reclast (zoledronic acid): drug safety communication- new contraindication and updated warning on kidney impairment. Posted 09/01/2011. Available at: http://www.fda.gov/Safety/MedWatch/SafetyInformation/SafetyAlertsforHumanMedicalProducts/ucm270464.htm.
70. Khosla S, Burr D, Abrahmsen B, American Society for Bone and Mineral Research, et al. Bisphosphonate-associated osteonecrosis of the jaw: report of a task force of the American Society for Bone and Mineral Research. J Bone Miner Res. 2007;22(10):1470–91.
71. Shane E, Burr D, Abrahmsen B, American Society for Bone and Mineral Research, et al. Atypical subtrochanteric and diaphyseal femoral fractures: second report of a task force of the American Society for Bone and Mineral Research. J Bone Miner Res. 2014;29(1):1–23.
72. Adler RA, El-Haji FG, Bauer DC, Camacho PM, Clarke BL, Clines GA, Compston JE, Drake MT, Edwards BJ, Favus MJ, Greenspan SL, McKinney R, Pignolo RJ, Sellmeyer DE. Managing osteoporosis in patients on long-term bisphosphonate treatment: report of a Task Force of the American Society for Bone and Mineral Research. J Bone Miner Res. 2016;31(1):16–35.
73. Lacey DL, Timms E, Tan HI, et al. Osteoprotegerin ligand is a cytokine that regulates osteoclast differentiation and activation. Cell. 1998;93:165–76.
74. Cummings SR, San Martin J, McClung MR, et al. Denosumab for prevention of fractures in postmenopausal women with osteoporosis. N Engl J Med. 2009;361(19):1914.
75. Tsourdi E, Langdahl B, Cohen-Solal M, Aubry-Rozier B, Eriksen EF, Guanabens N, Obermayer-Pietsch B, Ralston SH, Eastell R, Zillikens MC. Discontinuation of Denosumab therapy for osteoporosis: a systemic review and position statement by ECTS. Bone. 2017;105:11–7.
76. Ettinger B, Black DM, Mitlak BH, et al. Reduction of vertebral fracture risk in postmenopausal women with osteoporosis treated with raloxifene: results from a 3-year randomized clinical trial. Multiple Outcomes of Raloxifene Evaluation (MORE) Investigators. JAMA. 1999;282(7):637–45. (Erratum in: N Engl J Med 2009;282(22):2124.)
77. Saag K, Shane E, Boonen S, et al. Teriparatide or alendronate in glucocorticoid-induced osteoporosis. N Engl J Med. 2007;357(20):2028–39.
78. Miller PD, Hattersley G, Riis BJ, Williams GC, Lau E, Russo LA, Alexandersen P, Zerbini CA, Hu M-Y, Harris AG, Fitzpatrick LA, Cosman F, Christiansen C, for the ACTIVE Study Investigators. Effect of abaloparatide vs placebo on new vertebral fractures in postmenopausal women with osteoporosis: a randomized clinical trial. JAMA. 2016;316(7):722–33.
79. Neer RM, Arnaud CD, Zanchetta JR, et al. Effect of parathyroid hormone (1-34) on fractures and bone mineral density in postmenopausal women with osteoporosis. N Engl J Med. 2001;344(19):1434–41.

80. Lim SY, Bolster MB. Profile of romosozumab and its potential in the management of osteoporosis. Drug Des Devel Ther. 2017;11:1221–31.
81. Cosman F, Crittenden DB, Adachi JD, et al. Romosozumab treatment in postmenopausal women with osteoporosis. N Engl J Med. 2016;375(16):1532–43.
82. Boonen S, Ferrari S, Miller PD. Postmenopausal osteoporosis treatment with antiresorptives: effects of discontinuation or long-term continuation on bone turnover and fracture risk- a perspective. J Bone Miner Res. 2012;27(5):963–74.
83. Black DM, Bauer DC, Schwartz AV, Cummings SR, Rosen CJ. Continuing bisphosphonate treatment for osteoporosis- for whom and for how long? N Engl J Med. 2012;366(22):2051–3.
84. Black DM, Schwartz AV, Ensrud KE, Cauley JA, Levis S, Quandt SA, Satterfield S, Wallace RB, Bauer DC, Palermo L, Wehren LE, Lombardi A, Santora AC, Cummings SR, FLEX Research Group. Effects of continuing or stopping alendronate after 5 years of treatment: the Fracture Intervention Trial Long-term Extension (FLEX): a randomized trial. JAMA. 2006;296(24):2927–38.
85. Black DM, Reid IR, Boonen S, Bucci-Rechtweg C, Cauley JA, Cosman F, Cummings SR, Hue TF, Lippuner K, Lakatos P, Leung PC, Man Z, Martinez RL, Tan M, Ruzycky ME, Su G, Eastell R. The effect of 3 versus 6 years of zoledronic acid treatment of osteoporosis: a randomized extension to the HORIZON-Pivotal Fracture Trial (PFT). J Bone Miner Res. 2012;27(2):243–54.

Biomechanics of Vertebral Compression Fractures

5

Peter J. Ostergaard and Thomas D. Cha

Microstructure of the Vertebral Body

The vertebral body is composed of superior and inferior endplates, with a thin cortical shell surrounding a network of trabecular bone. The endplate is in fact a bilayer of cartilage and bone [5–7]. The cartilage is composed of chondrocytes within an extracellular matrix composed of proteoglycans, water, and type I and III collagen fibers that, in contrast to articular cartilage, are arranged parallel to the ends of the vertebral body [5, 6]. The bony portion of the endplate is composed of thickened trabecular bone. This endplate is thinnest in the central portions of the vertebral bodies and becomes progressively thicker as it moves toward the periphery [7–9]. The cranial endplate is consistently thinner than the more caudal endplate on histologic examination, which in large part explains why the cranial endplate has been shown to fracture first in VCFs [8, 10].

The structure of the trabecular bone can be described in terms of vertical columns, as well as horizontal struts that interconnect the columns [11, 12]. The density of the horizontal connections changes depending on the location within the vertebral body, with more horizontal struts existing closer to the endplates [12]. Changes in trabecular bone orientation can directly affect the mechanical properties and corresponding loads to failure, without changing the overall bone density of the trabecular bone itself [11]. Variation in structure also exists within the vertebral body itself. The anterior vertebral body is preferentially affected by disease processes such as osteoporosis and is structurally weaker than the more central or posterior vertebral body [8, 13–16]. This is due in part to stress shielding as under normal axial loading, the posterior elements of the spinal column tend to see anywhere between 60% and 80% of the forces applied in compression (Fig. 5.1) [15, 17]. In osteoporosis, the trabecular bone is preferentially affected, causing a decrease in overall bone mass [18]. This bone loss seems to be regionally specific as well, affecting the anterior vertebral bodies more heavily.

P. J. Ostergaard · T. D. Cha (✉)
Department of Orthopaedic Surgery, Massachusetts General Hospital, Harvard Medical School, Boston, MA, USA
e-mail: postergaard@partners.org; tcha@mgh.harvard.edu

A. E. Razi, S. H. Hershman (eds.), *Vertebral Compression Fractures in Osteoporotic and Pathologic Bone*, https://doi.org/10.1007/978-3-030-33861-9_5

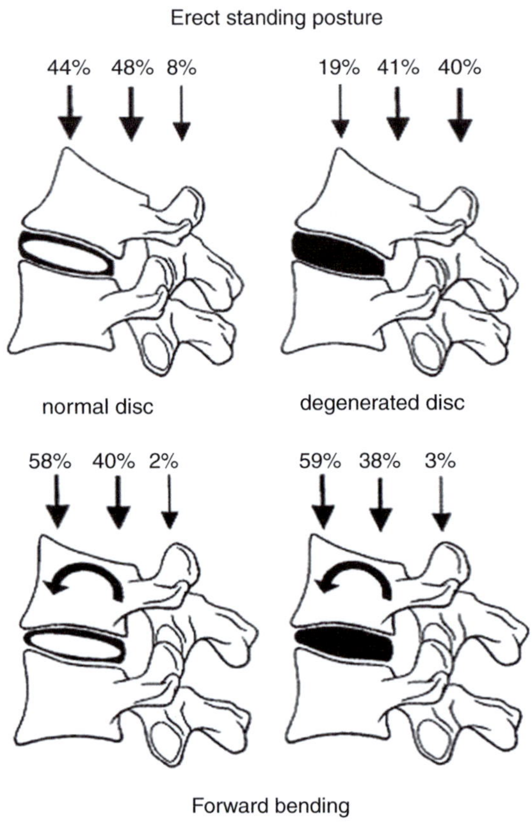

Fig. 5.1 Distribution of forces in erect and flexed positioning of the vertebral column. The left side shows normal force distribution in a non-diseased disc; the right shows the distribution of force in a patient with disc degeneration. (Reproduced from Pollintine et al. [17], with permission from s, Inc.)

Microstructure of the Intervertebral Disc

The intervertebral disc is made up of the inner nucleus pulposus and outer annulus fibrosus. The nucleus pulposus is comprised of type II collagen, proteoglycans, and water. It possesses a characteristic low collagen to high proteoglycan ratio, with a resulting high water content which gives it the ability to resist compressive forces. With aging, the ratio of proteoglycan to collagen decreases within the nucleus pulposus, leading to decreased water content and loss of the normal compressive properties [19–23]. The annulus fibrosus is composed of obliquely oriented type I collagen, as well as both proteoglycans and water. In contrast to the nucleus pulposus, the annulus has a high collagen to proteoglycan ratio, making it a more rigid structure with high tensile strength.

Creep Deformity and Fatigue Failure

As noted earlier, many patients present with VCFs without recall of a specific time of injury and frequently these injuries are noted incidentally on imaging for other injuries or medical conditions [1–4]. This is thought in large part to be due to the idea of "creep" deformity. This is defined as the slow, progressive deformation of the vertebral bodies that occurs with repetitive physiologic cyclic loading. Over time, this repetitive stress can cause microfractures and irreversible deformities of the vertebral endplates [24–26]. The idea of progressive "creep" can also explain the mechanism by which a biconcavity fracture type can progress to a crush-type, as is discussed later in this chapter.

Fracture Patterns

Vertebral compression fractures occur in several major patterns, depending mostly on the forces that caused the initial deformity. Many classification systems of compression fractures have been described, some purely based off of radiographic description, while others have included factors such as chronicity and dynamic stability [14, 27–31]. When describing the morphology of compression fractures, three subtypes are described: anterior wedge, biconcave, and crush (Fig. 5.2) [14, 27, 29, 32].

Anterior wedge fractures are the most common type of compression fracture in osteoporotic patients, making up just over 50% of all VCFs [33]. This is thought to be due to the stress shielding effect that occurs in the degenerative spine [17]. When the adult degenerative spine is subjected to cyclic daily activities, the posterior elements of the spinal column bear anywhere between 60% and 80% of the compressive forces, leaving the anterior endplates and trabecular bone relatively shielded from daily compressive

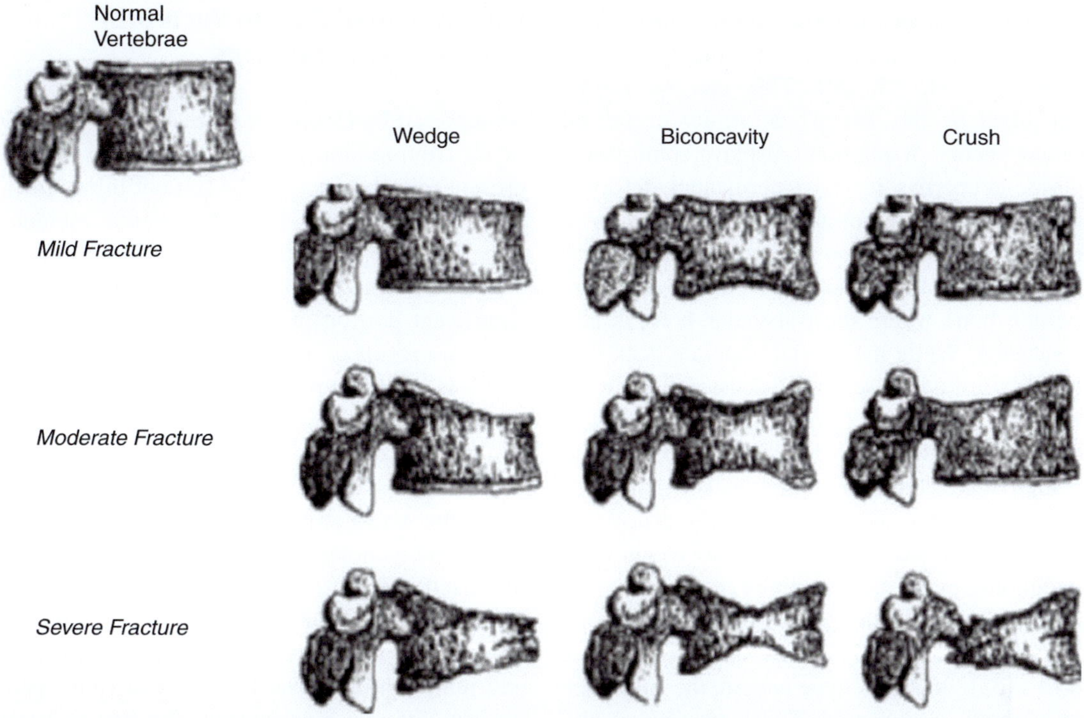

Fig. 5.2 Classification system for vertebral compression fractures: Pattern types include anterior wedge, biconcave, and crush. (Reproduced from Genant et al. [32] with permission from John Wiley and Sons)

forces, hence weakening the bone [8, 15, 17, 20, 34, 35]. However, in the setting of sudden forced flexion, the anterior vertebral bodies see an abrupt increase in compressive forces. This results in higher than normal physiologic forces acting on an already weakened portion of the vertebral body, causing the characteristic anterior wedge fracture deformity. Landham et al. suggest that the anterior wedge compression fracture occurs in a two-stage process, whereby the endplate undergoes a sentinel injury, causing a shift in load bearing onto the anterior vertebral cortex and away from the adjacent intervertebral disc and central endplate [36]. With repetitive flexion and further cyclic loading, the relatively weak anterior cortex and trabecular bone continue to collapse, leading to a progressive anterior wedge deformity. As discussed previously, the idea of fatigue failure and gradual creep deformity can also contribute to a resulting anterior wedge VCF. The less-dense anterior trabecular bone in osteoporosis is gradually compressed under normal physiologic loads, causing a preferential deformity of the anterior vertebral body [37]. This is likely the reason that a high percentage of patients with anterior wedge VCFs do not recall a specific overt injury. Of note, anterior wedge fractures tend to occur in the thoracic or thoracolumbar spine most commonly, followed by the lumbar spine [28, 30, 33].

Biconcave fracture patterns are the second most common morphological presentation, comprising roughly 17% of VCFs [33]. The mechanism by which biconcave fracture patterns occur is largely explained by the anatomy of the cranial and caudal vertebral endplates discussed previously. With physiologic aging, the intervertebral disc, particularly the nucleus pulposus, changes in regard to the relative proteoglycan and water content [19–23]. Decreasing proteoglycan and water content preferentially affects the outer nucleus pulposus, leaving the central portion as the only remaining compression-resisting element of the disc [19, 20]. The central portion of the endplates also happens to be the thinnest and most porous area as well, likely in order to supply metabolites to the otherwise avascular intervertebral discs [38]. Hence, the compressive forces of the central nucleus pulposus on the thin central endplates can cause a deformation of the endplate [23, 34, 35, 39]. This can be further explained by the "creep" deformity or fatigue failure theory. While bone displays some viscoelastic properties to resist permanent deformation, repetitive microtrauma or compression of the nucleus pulposus on the central endplate can eventually result in fracture, especially in osteoporotic bone where the trabecular bone is also weakened. While the cranial endplate does tend to fracture first for reasons discussed earlier, the eventual progressive fracture of both the cranial and caudal endplate in their central-most regions results in the characteristic biconcave pattern [8, 10]. Unlike the anterior wedge or crush-type fractures, biconcave VCFs tend to occur more commonly in the lumbar spine [28, 30, 33].

Crush-type fracture patterns are the least common, comprising only an estimated 13% of all VCFs [33]. In a crush-type pattern, the entire vertebral body is collapsed. There are several proposed mechanisms by which crush-type fractures can occur. The first is an extension of a concept discussed earlier, stating that with disc degeneration, more forces are transmitted through the outer annulus due to decreased compression resistance from the nucleus pulposus [14, 19, 20]. This in turn increases the amount of force exerted on the relatively weak vertebral cortices [14, 19, 20, 40]. When the proper amount of flexion to disengage the posterior elements of the vertebral column occurs, combined with axial loading, the fracture then occurs through the vertebral cortices, causing a crush-type fracture. The second theory is one in which a biconcave VCF becomes a crush-type injury with progressive creep. The two mechanisms differ in that the vertebral endplates will be relatively flat in the first theory in which adjacent disc degeneration is the culprit for collapse, versus a more concave appearance in the second model [14]. An extension of the crush-type pattern is a burst fracture, which has a similar mechanism of injury to the crush-type but with more energy transmitted, causing greater displacement of the cortices. As in anterior wedge-type VCFs, crush-type fractures occur most commonly in the thoracic or thoracolumbar junction [28, 30, 33].

Mechanism of Pain in Vertebral Compression Fractures

As reported by Cooper et al. in 1992, over 60% of all compression fractures that occur do not present to a physician at the time of injury [41]. These fractures are later discovered incidentally, especially with the advent of three-dimensional CT imaging. Nonetheless, there is a significant portion of patients who suffer from pain as a result of a VCF. Pain that arises from VCFs is multifactorial and can be broken down into acute pain that occurs at the time of injury and chronic pain that occurs for months or even years after the initial insult [42].

In the timeframe immediately following a VCF, pain is thought to be mediated by the fracture itself and subsequent inflammation [42–46]. The sensation of pain itself originates from the nociceptors, which dwell within the periosteum and joint capsules. The fracture can cause pain via two different mechanisms. The first is direct structural damage or compression from damaged tissues, while the second is chemically mediated by release of inflammatory substances that activate nociceptive nerve endings [44, 46]. Often, patients suffering from this intense, acute pain have significant collapse seen on initial imaging but will typically not have recurrences of pain or prolonged symptoms [42].

In contrast to the group of patients who suffer from acute pain are those who have a more chronic and cyclic-type pain associated with VCFs. Lyritis et al. defined this group as those who have minimal collapsed seen on initial imaging but progressively worsen over a timeframe of months to years [42]. The chronic pain associated with VCFs is thought to be multifactorial and a result of a more gradual biomechanical disturbance than from the initial insult of the fracture itself. The final amount of deformity seen on imaging can in fact correspond to the severity and distribution of pain the patient describes [47]. With increased kyphosis from wedge-type deformities, for instance, it is not hard to imagine that this would alter the articulation between adjacent zygapophyseal joints, which are rich in nociceptive nerve endings [43, 47]. This in turn can lead to long-term facet joint arthrosis and neural irritation [30, 43]. Progressive kyphosis may also result in more chronic paraspinous muscle fatigue from both the kyphosis itself, as well as from the forward shift of the upper trunk [30]. With the severe kyphosis that is often associated with multilevel VCFs, chronic pain can result from impingement of the rib cage on the pelvic rim [30, 46]. Not surprisingly, multilevel VCFs are a predictor for chronic pain, largely in part to the degree of increased kyphosis [48].

Vertebral augmentation (i.e., kyphoplasty and vertebroplasty) is a commonly accepted though somewhat controversial method of treating persistent pain from VCFs. Multiple studies have shown that vertebroplasty is as effective or even superior to non-operative management in the treatment of persistent pain from VCFs (Figs. 5.3 and 5.4) [30, 49–51]. The mechanism of pain relief from vertebral augmentation is thought to be due to decreased micromotion and increased stabilization at the fracture site [52]. Vertebral augmentation may also prevent further collapse and increased resistance to compressive forces in VCFs, which may also lead to less deformity and resulting pain [52].

In order to understand VCFs properly, it is essential to have a baseline understanding of the relevant anatomy and physiologic forces that act upon the non-pathologic vertebral bodies. The ability to conceptualize the morphologic classification system in terms of these forces is what allows clinicians to better assess and treat patients with VCFs. In classifying VCFs biomechanically, it allows the clinician the ability to understand the deforming forces that act upon the osteoporotic spine and predict further deformity. Similarly, knowledge of the mechanism by which VCFs cause pain and deformity allows for the advancement of future therapeutic measures.

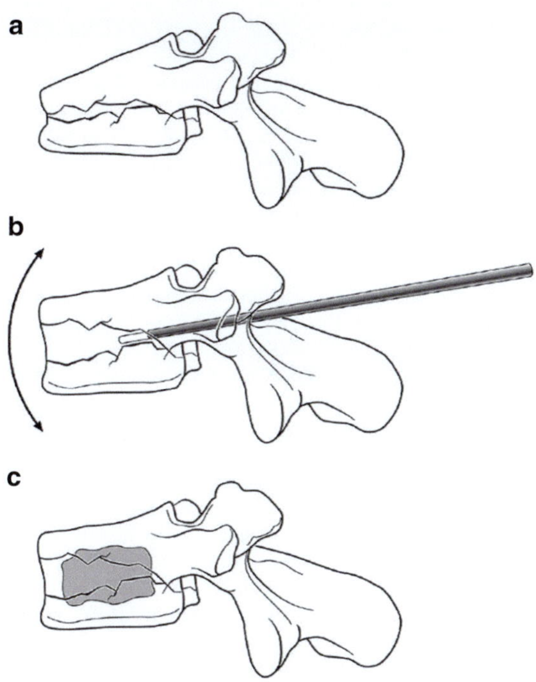

Fig. 5.3 Mechanism of vertebroplasty in the augmentation of VCFs. (**a**) Compression fracture demonstrating loss in vertebral body height (**b**) Trochar is inserted through pedicle posteriorly into the collapsed vertebral body (**c**) Balloon is inserted into the vertebral body in an attempt to restore vertebral body height. (Reproduced from Rao and Singrakhia [30], with permission from Wolters Kluwer Health, Inc.)

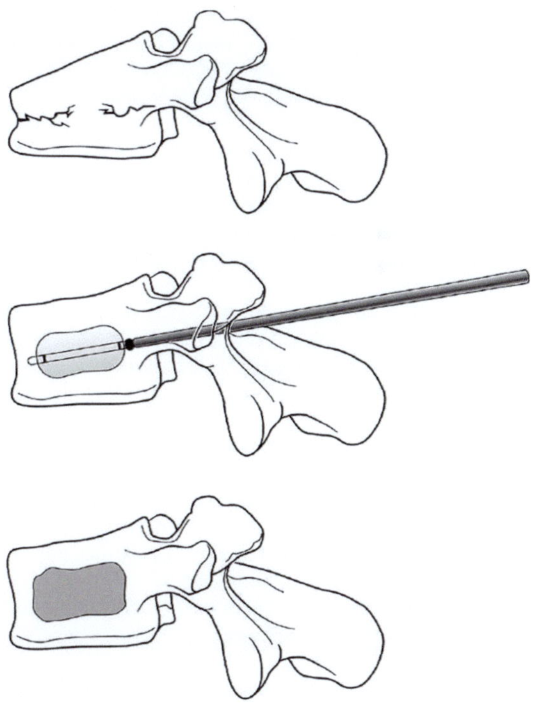

Fig. 5.4 Mechanism of kyphoplasty in the augmentation of VCFs. (Reproduced from Rao and Singrakhia [30], with permission from Wolters Kluwer Health, Inc.)

References

1. Ensrud KE, Schousboe JT. Vertebral fractures. N Engl J Med. 2011;364(17):1634–42. https://doi.org/10.1056/nejmcp1009697.
2. Riggs Bl, Melton Lj. The worldwide problem of osteoporosis: insights afforded by epidemiology. Bone. 1995;17(5):S505. https://doi.org/10.1016/8756-3282(95)00258-4.
3. Fink HA, et al. What proportion of incident radiographic vertebral deformities is clinically diagnosed and vice versa? J Bone Miner Res. 2005;20(7):1216–22. https://doi.org/10.1359/jbmr.050314.
4. Melton LJ, et al. Epidemiology of vertebral fractures in women. Am J Epidemiol. 1989;129(5):1000–11. https://doi.org/10.1093/oxfordjournals.aje.a115204.
5. Antoniou J, et al. The human lumbar endplate. Spine. 1996;21(10):1153–61. https://doi.org/10.1097/00007632-199605150-00006.
6. Aspden RM, et al. Determination of collagen fibril orientation in the cartilage of vertebral end plate. Connect Tissue Res. 1981;9(2):83–7. https://doi.org/10.3109/03008208109160244.
7. Lotz JC, et al. The role of the vertebral end plate in low back pain. Global Spine J. 2013;3(3):153–63. https://doi.org/10.1055/s-0033-1347298.
8. Hou Y, Luo Z. A study on the structural properties of the lumbar endplate. Spine. 2009;34(12):E427. https://doi.org/10.1097/brs.0b013e3181a2ea0a.
9. Zhao F-D, et al. Vertebral fractures usually affect the cranial endplate because it is thinner and supported by less-dense trabecular bone. Bone. 2009;44(2):372–9. https://doi.org/10.1016/j.bone.2008.10.048.
10. Jiang G, et al. Vertebral fractures in the elderly may not always be osteoporotic. Bone. 2010;47(1):111–6. https://doi.org/10.1016/j.bone.2010.03.019.
11. Jensen Ks, et al. A model of vertebral trabecular bone architecture and its mechanical properties. Bone. 1990;11(6):417–23. https://doi.org/10.1016/8756-3282(90)90137-n.
12. Smit TH, et al. Structure and function of vertebral trabecular bone. Spine. 1997;22(24):2823–33. https://doi.org/10.1097/00007632-199712150-00005.
13. Hulme Pa, et al. Regional variation in vertebral bone morphology and its contribution to vertebral fracture strength. Bone. 2007;41(6):946–57. https://doi.org/10.1016/j.bone.2007.08.019.
14. Adams MA, Dolan P. Biomechanics of vertebral compression fractures and clinical application. Arch Orthop Trauma Surg. 2011;131(12):1703–10. https://doi.org/10.1007/s00402-011-1355-9.
15. Pollintine P, et al. Neural arch load-bearing in old and degenerated spines. J Biomech. 2004;37(2):197–204. https://doi.org/10.1016/s0021-9290(03)00308-7.
16. Hordon Ld, et al. Trabecular architecture in women and men of similar bone mass with and without vertebral fracture: I. two-dimensional histology. Bone. 2000;27(2):271–6. https://doi.org/10.1016/s8756-3282(00)00329-x.
17. Pollintine P, et al. Intervertebral disc degeneration can lead to stress-shielding of the anterior vertebral body. Spine. 2004;29(7):774–82. https://doi.org/10.1097/01.brs.0000119401.23006.d2.
18. Mosekilde L. Sex differences in age-related loss of vertebral trabecular bone mass and structure – biomechanical consequences. Bone. 1989;10(6):425–32. https://doi.org/10.1007/978-1-4612-3450-0_4.
19. Adams MA, et al. Stress distributions inside intervertebral discs. J Bone Joint Surg. 1996;78-B(6):965–72. https://doi.org/10.1302/0301-620x.78b6.0780965.
20. Adams MA, et al. Intervertebral disc degeneration can predispose to anterior vertebral fractures in the thoracolumbar spine. J Bone Miner Res. 2006;21(9):1409–16. https://doi.org/10.1359/jbmr.060609.
21. Humzah MD, Soames RW. Human intervertebral disc: structure and function. Anat Rec. 1988;220(4):337–56. https://doi.org/10.1002/ar.1092200402.
22. Roughley PJ. Biology of intervertebral disc aging and degeneration. Spine. 2004;29(23):2691–9. https://doi.org/10.1097/01.brs.0000146101.53784.b1.
23. Twomey L, Taylor J. Age changes in lumbar intervertebral discs. Acta Orthop Scand. 1985;56(6):496–9. https://doi.org/10.3109/17453678508993043.
24. Hansson TH, et al. Mechanical behavior of the human lumbar spine. II. Fatigue strength during dynamic compressive loading. J Orthop Res. 1987;5(4):479–87. https://doi.org/10.1002/jor.1100050403.
25. Keller TS, et al. Mechanical behavior of the human lumbar spine. I. Creep analysis during static compressive loading. J Orthop Res. 1987;5(4):467–78. https://doi.org/10.1002/jor.1100050402.
26. Zioupos P, et al. Microcracking damage and the fracture process in relation to strain rate in human cortical bone tensile failure. J Biomech. 2008;41(14):2932–9. https://doi.org/10.1016/j.jbiomech.2008.07.025.
27. Eastell R, et al. Classification of vertebral fractures. J Bone Miner Res. 2009;6(3):207–15. https://doi.org/10.1002/jbmr.5650060302.
28. Ismail AA, et al. Number and type of vertebral deformities: epidemiological characteristics and relation to back pain and height loss. Osteoporos Int. 1999;9(3):206–13. https://doi.org/10.1007/s001980050138.
29. Faciszewski T, Mckiernan F. Calling all vertebral fractures classification of vertebral compression fractures: a consensus for comparison of treatment and outcome. J Bone Miner Res. 2002;17(2):185–91. https://doi.org/10.1359/jbmr.2002.17.2.185.
30. Rao RD, Singrakhia MD. Painful osteoporotic vertebral fracture. J Bone Joint SurgAm. 2003;85(10):2010–22. https://doi.org/10.2106/00004623-200310000-00024.
31. Smith-Bindman R, et al. A comparison of morphometric definitions of vertebral fracture. J Bone Miner Res. 2009;6(1):25–34. https://doi.org/10.1002/jbmr.5650060106.
32. Genant HK, et al. Vertebral fracture assessment using a semiquantitative technique. J Bone Miner Res. 1993;8(9):1137–48. https://doi.org/10.1002/jbmr.5650080915.

33. Black DM, et al. Prevalent vertebral deformities predict hip fractures and new vertebral deformities but not wrist fractures. J Bone Miner Res. 1999;14(5):821–8. https://doi.org/10.1359/jbmr.1999.14.5.821.
34. Holmes Ad, Hukins Dwl. Fatigue failure at the disc-vertebra interface during cyclic axial compression of cadaveric specimens. Clin Biomech. 1994;9(2):133–4. https://doi.org/10.1016/0268-0033(94)90037-x.
35. Holmes AD, et al. End-plate displacement during compression of lumbar vertebra-disc-vertebra segments and the mechanism of failure. Spine. 1993;18(1):128–35. https://doi.org/10.1097/00007632-199301000-00019.
36. Landham PR, et al. Pathogenesis of vertebral anterior wedge deformity. Spine. 2015;40(12):902–8. https://doi.org/10.1097/brs.0000000000000905.
37. Pollintine P, et al. Bone creep can cause progressive vertebral deformity. Bone. 2009;45(3):466–72. https://doi.org/10.1016/j.bone.2009.05.015.
38. Roberts S, et al. Biochemical and structural properties of the cartilage end-plate and its relation to the intervertebral disc. Spine. 1989;14(2):166–74. https://doi.org/10.1097/00007632-198902000-00005.
39. Brinckmann P, et al. Deformation of the vertebral end-plate under axial loading of the spine. Spine. 1983;8(8):851–6. https://doi.org/10.1097/00007632-198311000-00007.
40. Rockoff SD, et al. The relative contribution of trabecular and cortical bone to the strength of human lumbar vertebrae. Calcif Tissue Res. 1969;3(1):163–75. https://doi.org/10.1007/bf02058659.
41. Cooper C, et al. Incidence of clinically diagnosed vertebral fractures: a population-based study in Rochester, Minnesota, 1985–1989. J Bone Miner Res. 1992;7(2):221–7. https://doi.org/10.1002/jbmr.5650070214.
42. Lyritis GP, et al. Analgesic effect of Salmon calcitonin suppositories in patients with acute pain due to recent osteoporotic vertebral crush fractures: a prospective double-blind, randomized, placebo-controlled clinical study. Clin J Pain. 1999;15(4):284–9. https://doi.org/10.1097/00002508-199912000-00004.
43. Bogduk N, et al. The pain of vertebral compression fractures can arise in the posterior elements. Pain Med. 2010;11(11):1666–73. https://doi.org/10.1111/j.1526-4637.2010.00963.x.
44. Gennari C, et al. Use of calcitonin in the treatment of bone pain associated with osteoporosis. Calcif Tissue Int. 1991;49(S2):S9. https://doi.org/10.1007/bf02561370.
45. Knopp JA, et al. Calcitonin for treating acute pain of osteoporotic vertebral compression fractures: a systematic review of randomized, controlled trials. Osteoporos Int. 2004;16(10):1281–90. https://doi.org/10.1007/s00198-004-1798-8.
46. Silverman S. The clinical consequences of vertebral compression fracture. Bone. 1992;13:S27. https://doi.org/10.1016/8756-3282(92)90193-z.
47. Doo T-H, et al. Clinical relevance of pain patterns in osteoporotic vertebral compression fractures. J Korean Med Sci. 2008;23(6):1005. https://doi.org/10.3346/jkms.2008.23.6.1005.
48. Huang C. Vertebral fracture and other predictors of physical impairment and health care utilization. Arch Intern Med. 1996;156(21):2469–75. https://doi.org/10.1001/archinte.156.21.2469.
49. Klazen CA, Lohle PN, De Vries J, et al. Vertebroplasty versus conservative treatment in acute osteoporotic vertebral compression fractures (Vertos II): an Open-Label Randomised Trial. Lancet. 2010;376(9746):1085–92. Epub 2010 Aug 9." *The Spine Journal*, vol. 11, no. 1, 2011, pp. 88–88. https://doi.org/10.1016/j.spinee.2010.11.011.
50. Blasco J, et al. Effect of vertebroplasty on pain relief, quality of life, and the incidence of new vertebral fractures: a 12-month randomized follow-up, controlled trial. J Bone Miner Res. 2012;27(5):1159–66. https://doi.org/10.1002/jbmr.1564.
51. Lieberman I. Vertebral augmentation for osteoporotic and osteolytic vertebral compression fractures: vertebroplasty and kyphoplasty. *Advances in Spinal Stabilization.* Prog Neurol Surg. 2003:240–50. https://doi.org/10.1159/000072646.
52. Bostrom MPG, Lane JM. Future directions: augmentation of osteoporotic vertebral bodies. Spine. 1997;22(Supplement):38S. https://doi.org/10.1097/00007632-199712151-00007.

6 Osteoporotic Vertebral Compression Fractures

Ahmed Saleh and Michael Collins

Osteoporotic vertebral compression fractures (OVCFs) are frequently encountered in clinical practice. As the population continues to age and the number of people living past the age of 65 continues to increase, osteoporotic compression fractures will continue to be a significant concern to the medical provider. These fractures often require multidisciplinary care, including primary care physicians, radiologists, endocrinologists, spinal surgeons, and nursing.

Osteoporosis and osteopenia are major public health concerns in the United States and are estimated to effect 54 million Americans or approximately 55% of the people over the age of 50. By the year 2020, it is estimated that there will be 121 million people in the United States over the age of 50, with an estimated 14 million having osteoporosis [1, 2]. Currently, the cost of osteoporotic fractures is nearly $19 billion annually, and this number expected to increase to $25 billion by the year 2025 [1].

It is important to note that there are different types of osteoporosis. Type I, also known as postmenopausal osteoporosis, is found in the trabecular bone of women and hypogonadal men less than 60 years of age. Type II, or senile osteoporosis, is seen in both men and women over the age of 65 and is found in the cortical bone. Type III is osteoporosis secondary to any other underlying pathology – this form is a result of medications and various disease states. One may find elevated endogenous or exogenous cortisol in this form of osteoporosis.

Osteoporotic vertebral compression fractures are extremely common; they occur at a rate ten times higher than that of femoral fractures in Japan, and many occur without a fall or antecedent trauma [3, 4]. Racial, ethnic, and dietary differences play a role in the incidence and prevalence of vertebral compression fractures. Studies have demonstrated that Japanese women have both a higher prevalence of vertebral fractures and a higher likelihood of sustaining two or more vertebral compression fractures than American women [4]. Additionally, people in Japan develop vertebral compression fractures at nearly twice the rate of their European counterparts [3, 4].

Different parts of the world exhibit different rates of osteoporotic vertebral compression fractures. Eastern Europe has a rate of 18%, while Scandinavia has a rate of 26%. North America has a rate of 20–24% with Caucasian women having a higher rate than African-American women, the ratio between the two being approximately 1.6. Latin America has a rate of 11–19%.

Osteoporosis is more common in women. One in every two women and one in every four men over the age of 50 in the United States will break

A. Saleh (✉) · M. Collins
Department of Orthopaedic Surgery, Maimonides Medical Center, Brooklyn, NY, USA
e-mail: Asaleh@maimonidesmed.org; MIcollins@maimonidesmed.org

A. E. Razi, S. H. Hershman (eds.), *Vertebral Compression Fractures in Osteoporotic and Pathologic Bone*, https://doi.org/10.1007/978-3-030-33861-9_6

a bone secondary to osteoporosis [1]. In the United States, a woman older than 50 has a 40% chance of developing an osteoporotic compression fracture in her lifetime. Radiographic studies show that 8–13% of women in their 60s and 30–40% of women in their 70s are found to have evidence of vertebral compression fractures on plain radiographs in epidemiological studies [3].

OVCFs are diagnosed radiographically by having a loss of more than 4 mm or 20% of the vertebral body height on plain films [5]. Back pain is the primary symptom; however the severity can vary greatly among individuals who sustain fractures. In fact, a large portion of fractures remain asymptomatic. Symptomatic back pain is found in only 25–33% of patients with vertebral compression fractures [6, 7].

A decrease in bone mineral density is a risk factor for OVCF. However, a decrease in bone mineral density does not necessarily predict who will eventually fracture. Risk factors identified by the World Health Organization (WHO) include age, personal and family history of fracture, heavy alcohol use, chronic steroid use, rheumatoid arthritis, and smoking [3, 8]. The United States Preventative Services Task Force (USPSTF) recommends screening for osteoporosis in women aged 65 years and older and in younger women whose fracture risk is equal to or greater than that of a 65-year-old white woman with no additional risk factors [9]. Screening is also recommended for men age 70 and older as well as men younger than the age of 70 with risk factors for low bone mass such as prior fracture, high-risk medication consumption, low body weight, or conditions associated with bone loss.

DEXA scores come into play when evaluating bone mineral density on scans. The two numbers given are the T-score and the Z-score. The T-score compares the bone density of the patient to that of normal young adult female bone. The T-score represents how many standard deviations away from the mean a patient's bone density is, assuming a Gaussian distribution. The Z-score compares the bone density of the patient with that of age-matched controls. A T-score greater than or equal to −1.0 is considered normal. T-scores between −1.0 and −2.5 indicate low bone mass or osteopenia. While other factors may also confer a diagnosis of osteoporosis, a patient meets WHO criteria for a diagnosis of osteoporosis with a T-score that is less than −2.5.

Frailty is defined as the accumulation of age-related deficits in different physiological systems leading to greater risks of adverse health outcomes, such as falls, fractures, hospitalizations, loss of independence, and death [10]; OVCFs have been implicated to be a marker of frailty. Low-trauma fractures related to osteoporosis have been shown to increase frailty. There are gender differences present in the development of frailty. Hip fractures and vertebral compression fractures both have significant and similar influence on the progression of frailty in women. When the same two fractures were looked at in men, first-time hip fractures had an impact on the progression of frailty, but initial vertebral compression fractures did not.

Other than aging, gender, and racial factors, medication can also play a role in the development of osteoporotic compression fractures. Systemic corticosteroid use has been shown to decrease bone mineral density [11]. Chronic oral glucocorticoid therapy is the most common form of secondary osteoporosis, leading to increased risk for osteoporotic fractures [12]. Chronic glucocorticoid therapy significantly influences lumbar bone density T-scores and bone mineral density (BMD). Studies show that bone loss and alterations of bone occur at higher doses irrespective of the method of administration [12]. Oral glucocorticoids are associated specifically with a higher incidence of vertebral compression fractures [12, 13].

Epidural steroid injections can also lead to an increased risk for vertebral compression fractures in those individuals at risk for osteoporotic fractures [10]. This should be taken in consideration when administering such injections and should be used with caution in those with an increased risk of sustaining these fractures.

Although these fractures are primarily associated with pain and an overall decline in function, osteoporotic vertebral compression fractures can also be associated with neurologic compromise [12, 14]. A study examined 28 patients with osteoporotic vertebral compression fractures that required surgery due to neurologic compromise. These patients had significant neurologic compromise including the inability to ambulate, the ability to ambulate only with significant assistance, and sphincter disturbances. It is important to keep in mind that these neurological manifestations are often delayed in the setting of vertebral compression fractures. OVCFs with neurologic symptoms were associated with retropulsion caused by an average canal compromise of 36.5% in the aforementioned study [14].

Vertebral compression fractures often go undiagnosed [12]. Some fractures may cause minimal symptoms or be asymptomatic altogether, leading to many fractures being discovered incidentally. These asymptomatic and undiagnosed vertebral compression fractures still have a high association and an increased risk of additional osteoporotic fractures at the same site or different sites of the body [12].

Different tools are used in assessing risk for vertebral compression fractures. Commonly, used measurements are femoral and lumbar T-scores. Capozzi et al. showed a correlation between age and femoral T-scores but did not find a correlation between lumbar spine T-scores and a patient's age [12]. One thought is that the lumbar bone density reading can be affected by arthrosis, osteoarthritis, or calcification, while the femoral T-score is less affected by this.

Body mass index (BMI) has also been shown to have a significant correlation with femoral T-scores and bone mineral density. Fat tissues have a positive effect on bone preservation by converting androgens to estrogens peripherally, therefore resulting in a protective effect on bone density [12]. Other risk factors include smoking, a family history of fractures, alcohol consumption, and other causes of secondary osteoporosis [12].

Percutaneous vertebroplasty is somewhat controversial but has been shown to be an effective minimally invasive treatment option for symptomatic vertebral compression fractures. This technique involves injecting polymethyl methacrylate into the fractured vertebral body providing fracture stability and pain relief. There are advantages and disadvantages associated with this and other cement augmentation techniques; however, this topic is outside the scope of this chapter and will be discussed thoroughly elsewhere in this book.

Lumbar degenerative disc disease and lumbar spinal stenosis are very common problems that spinal surgeons are faced with treating. These conditions are much more prevalent in patients over 55 years of age, which is also the group of people in whom osteoporosis is more common [15]; a significant portion of stenosis patients who are symptomatic will require surgery. Two broad categories of operative treatment include decompression alone and decompression with fusion [15]. One study investigated the association with lumbar decompression surgery and subsequent vertebral body compression fractures [15]. They found that lumbar decompression alone without fusion did not place patients at a higher risk for sustaining vertebral compression fractures in the future. However, they found that instrumenting the spine in addition to the decompression was associated with a higher rate of vertebral body compression fractures within one or two vertebral segments of the instrumentation [15]. Patients were at a higher risk of sustaining a subsequent vertebral body fracture regardless of the implant [15, 16]. Even a one-level interspinous stabilization device was associated with a higher rate of sustaining a subsequent fracture [16].

Low bone mass is widely accepted as a risk factor for vertebral compression fractures and osteoporosis [17]. It is a condition which is often asymptomatic until one suffers sequelae such as a vertebral body fracture or hip fracture [17, 18]. An individual's peak bone mass is typically found between the ages of 20 and 30. Individuals who reach lower peak bone mass compared to their peers are at higher risk for fracture later in their lifetime [19, 20]. Increased risk is largely due to genetic factors [21]. Additionally, being female has a large role in one's susceptibility to osteoporosis. These factors are non-modifiable but should be considered when treating and screening patients [22].

Patients and providers should also be aware of modifiable risk factors. Influences to consider include physical activity, body composition, and dietary intake of nutrients such as calcium and vitamin D. Although there is not a clear conclusion on what the proper amount of calcium intake is among males, females, races, or age groups, low calcium intake has been shown to be a significant risk factor for the development of osteoporosis, and it should be addressed with supplementation in at risk patients [19]. Additionally, individuals with metabolic deficits of calcium absorption such as a past history of bariatric surgery should not be ignored [17].

Vitamin D deficiency is another risk factor for the development of osteoporosis that can be modified. Vitamin D helps in the absorption of calcium in the intestine and thus can help decrease the risk for osteoporosis. Additionally, Vitamin D has positive effects on calcium metabolism and bone strength [17]. Similar to calcium, the best way to screen for vitamin D deficiency is not clear, nor are the values for determining the threshold for deficiency [22]. Although vitamin D deficiency may be recognized, the appropriate amount of supplementation for those needing it remains unanswered [23]. Adequate intake of protein and fruit can help to decrease the risk of fracture by having a benefit on bone mass in young adults [19]. Milk consumption has been shown to have a positive effect on bones in adolescent girls as well [32]. Like calcium and vitamin D, however, the ideal intake is unknown.

Alcohol consumption and tobacco smoking are factors that can increase the risk of osteoporosis and, thus, vertebral compression fractures [24, 25]. Both have been shown to have direct negative effects on bone as well as other organs and organ systems. This is particularly important to consider in growing individuals as it can hinder reaching one's optimal peak bone mass during young adulthood [24, 25]. Consumption of greater than four alcoholic beverages a day has been shown to have a negative effect on bone; even consumption of more than two alcoholic beverages daily increases one's risk of sustaining an osteoporotic fracture secondary to both the direct effect on bone itself and the decreased coordination leading to fall risk [24, 33]. Smoking has a direct negative effect on osteoblasts, upregulation of receptor activator of nuclear factor-kB (RANKL), alterations in calciotropic hormones, and decreased intestinal calcium absorption [34]. Additionally, there is a large group of smokers who are physically inactive and have lower body weights, both of which increase fracture risk [17].

Physical activity may decrease the risk of OVCF; people have developed a more sedentary lifestyle in the modern day, and this lack of activity leads to an increased risk of lower bone density and lower peak bone mass [26]. Specifics on the duration and intensity of physical activity remain unanswered, but physical activity has been shown to have favorable results on BMD and peak bone mass [27].

As touched on before, patients with a lower T-score are at an increased risk for osteoporotic fractures [28]. It is important to recognize that there are many fractures that occur in patients that have a decreased T-score but who do not meet the T-score criteria for a diagnosis of osteoporosis [29].

FRAX, another assessment tool in fracture risk, is a computer-based algorithm that gives a patient's 10-year probability of a major fracture (defined as forearm, proximal humerus, or vertebral compression fracture) [30]. This is another useful tool to help recognize patients at increased risk for sustaining osteoporotic vertebral compression fractures and osteoporotic fractures overall. Several factors are considered in FRAX such as prior fractures, BMI, age, smoking history, alcohol consumption, chronic use of glucocorticoids, rheumatoid arthritis, parental history of hip fracture, and other secondary causes of osteoporosis [17].

Another modifiable factor is the use of anti-osteoporotic drugs. Although medications are widely available, it has been observed that a large number of patients who are at risk for osteoporotic fractures and could benefit from treatment with such medications are not being treated [31, 32]. It has been shown in Europe that even in its best-performing country, the gap between diagnosis and treatment was 25%. Most countries in Europe showed a treatment gap of 40–95% with an overall average of 50% across countries in the European Union which tend to have adequate resources [31, 32]. Minimizing this gap could lead to a decrease in overall osteoporotic fracture risk. Despite the possibility of side effects from the medications, the benefit of decreasing fracture risk is reported to be between 30% and 70%.

Several factors can influence the risk of developing osteoporotic vertebral compression fractures, some are modifiable, and others are not. Healthcare providers should be knowledgeable about both in order to spread awareness to others in healthcare as well as to patients. An attempt to address modifiable factors should be performed in order to help reduce the incidence of these otherwise preventable injuries.

References

1. National Osteoporosis Foundation. nof.org. Accessed May 2018.
2. O'Neill TW, et al. J Bone Miner Res. 1996;11:1010–8.
3. Tsuda T. Epidemiology of fragility fractures and fall prevention in the elderly: a systematic review of the literature. Curr Orthop Pract. 2017;28(6):580–5. https://doi.org/10.1097/BCO.0000000000000563.
4. Orimo H, Yaegashi Y, Onoda T, et al. Hip fracture incidence in Japan: estimates of new patients in 2007 and 20-year trends. Arch Osteoporos. 2009;4:71–7.
5. Consensus development conference: prophylaxis and treatment of osteoporosis. Am J Med. 1991;90:107–10.
6. Sakuma M, Endo N, Oinuma T, et al. Incidence and outcome of osteoporotic fractures in 2004 in Sado City, Niigata Prefecture, Japan. J Bone Miner Metab. 2008;26:373–8.
7. Black DM, Cummings SR, Karpf DB, et al. Randomized trial of effect of alendronate on risk of fracture in women with existing vertebral fractures. Lancet. 1996;348:1535–41.
8. WHO Scientific Group. Prevention and management of osteoporosis. WHO Technical Report Series, World Health Organ Tech Rep Ser. 2003;921:1–164.
9. United States Preventive Services Task Force. https://www.uspreventiveservicestaskforce.org. Accessed May 2018.
10. Gajic-Veljanoski O, Papaioannou A, Kennedy C, et al. Osteoporotic fractures and obesity affect frailty progression: a longitudinal analysis of the Canadian multicentre osteoporosis study. BMC Geriatr. 2018;18(1):4. Published 2018 Jan 5. https://doi.org/10.1186/s12877-017-0692-0.
11. Kanis JA, Johansson H, Oden A, et al. A meta-analysis of prior corticosteroid use and fracture risk. J Bone Miner Res. 2004;19:893–9.
12. Capozzi A, et al. Clinical management of osteoporotic vertebral fracture treated with percutaneous vertebroplasty. Clin Cases Miner Bone Metab. 2017;14(2):161–6.
13. Amiche MA, Albaum JM, Tadrous M, et al. Fracture risk in oral glucocorticoid users: a Bayesian meta-regression leveraging control arms of osteoporosis clinical trials. Osteoporos Int. 2016; 27(5):1709–18. https://doi.org/10.1007/s00198-015-3455-9. Epub 2015
14. Yeung YK, Ho ST. Delayed neurological deficits after osteoporotic vertebral fractures: clinical outcomes after surgery. Asian Spine J. 2017;11(6):981–8.
15. Granville M, Berti A, Jacobson RE. Vertebral compression fractures after lumbar instrumentation. Cureus. 2017;9:0.
16. Lems WF, Raterman HG. Critical issues and current challenges in osteoporosis and fracture prevention. An overview of unmet needs. Ther Adv Musculoskelet Dis. 2017;9(12):299–316. https://doi.org/10.1177/1759720X17732562.
17. Kilbanski A, Adams-Campbell L, Bassford T, et al. Osteoporosis prevention, diagnosis, and therapy. JAMA. 2001;285:785–95.
18. Weaver CM, Gordon CM, Janz KF, et al. The National Osteoporosis Foundation's position statement on peak bone mass development and lifestyle factors: a systematic review and implementation recommendations. Osteoporos Int. 2016;27:1281–386.
19. Berger C, Goltzman D, Langsetmo L, et al. Peak bone mass from longitudinal data: implications for the prevalence, pathophysiology, and diagnosis of osteoporosis. J Bone Miner Res. 2010;25:1948–57.
20. Eisman JA. Genetics of osteoporosis. Endocr Rev. 1999;20:788–0.
21. Gilsanz V, Kovanlikaya A, Costin G, et al. Differential effect of gender on the sizes of the bones in the axial and appendicular skeletons. J Clin Endocrinol Metab. 1997;82:1603–7.
22. Cameron MA, Paton LM, Nowson CA, et al. The effect of calcium supplementation on bone density in premenarcheal females: a co-twin approach. J Clin Endocrinol Metab. 2004;89:4916–22.
23. Manson JE, Brannon PM, Rosen CJ, et al. Vitamin D deficiency–is there really a pandemic? N Engl J Med. 2016;375:1817–20.
24. Kanis JA, Johansson H, Johnell O, et al. Alcohol intake as a risk factor for fracture. Osteoporos Int. 2005;16:737–42.
25. Herrmann D, Buck C, Sioen I, et al. Impact of physical activity, sedentary behaviour and muscle strength on bone stiffness in 2–10-year-old children—cross-sectional results from the IDEFICS study. Int J Behav Nutr Phys Act 2015; 12: 112.
26. Pasqualini L, Leli C, Ministrini S, et al. Relationships between global physical activity and bone mineral density in a group of male and female students. J Sports Med Phys Fitness. 2017;57:238–43.
27. Marshall D, Johnell O, Wedel H. Meta-analysis of how well measures of bone mineral density pre-

dict occurrence of osteoporotic fractures. BMJ. 1996;312:1254–9.
28. Siris ES, Chen YT, Abbott TA, et al. Bone mineral density thresholds for pharmacological intervention to prevent fractures. Arch Intern Med. 2004;164:1108–12.
29. Kanis JA, Hans D, Cooper C, et al. Interpretation and use of FRAX in clinical practice. Osteoporos Int. 2011;22:2395–411.
30. Diez-Perez A, Hooven FH, Adachi JD, et al. Regional differences in treatment for osteoporosis. The Global Longitudinal Study of Osteoporosis in Women (GLOW). Bone. 2011;49:493–8.
31. Cadogan J, Eastell R, Jones N, et al. Milk intake and bone mineral acquisition in adolescent girls: randomised, controlled intervention trial. BMJ. 1997;315:1255–60.
32. Rasch LA, de van der Schueren MA, van Tuyl LH, et al. Content validity of a short calcium intake list to estimate daily dietary calcium intake of patients with osteoporosis. Calcif Tissue Int. 2017;100:271–7.
33. Kanis JA, Johnell O, Oden A, et al. Smoking and fracture risk: a meta-analysis. Osteoporos Int. 2005;16:155–62.
34. Lewiecki EM. Risk communication and shared decision making in the care of patients with osteoporosis. J Clin Densitom. 2010;13:335–45.

Pathologic Vertebral Compression Fractures: Diagnosis and Management

7

Daniel G. Tobert and Joseph H. Schwab

Introduction

Vertebral compression fractures (VCF) are common and can cause significant morbidity and utilization of healthcare resources. Approximately one quarter of all postmenopausal women in the United States will sustain a VCF at some point. Osteoporotic bone is the most common culprit for these injuries, which typically occur by disproportionately low-energy mechanisms. The term *pathologic* vertebral compression fracture (pVCF) historically excludes osteoporosis in its definition. Etiologies for pVCF include primary spine tumors, metastatic disease to the axial skeleton, infection, and dysregulations in bone metabolism, such as Paget's disease.

The diagnosis of VCF is made with a combination of history and imaging modalities. However, differentiation between VCF and pVCF can be difficult radiographically, especially if the finding prompts the initial suspicion for a pathologic state. The goal of management in pVCF is pain control, preservation of mobility and neurologic function, and avoidance of symptomatic deformity. Currently, the clinician is afforded an array of nonsurgical, minimally invasive, and open surgical techniques to treat patients with VCF. A consideration of the underlying pathology and baseline patient function is critical when choosing management for patients with pVCF. The scope of this chapter will focus on pVCF caused by metastatic disease and is intended to review the diagnosis and management of pVCF caused by metastatic disease.

Metastatic Disease in the Spine

There are an estimated 8.2 million cancer deaths worldwide each year; approximately 600,000 of those deaths occur in the United States [1]. After the liver and lungs, the skeletal system is the third most common site of metastatic disease. One study estimated 280,000 people in the United States live with bone metastases [2]. The mechanism of bone metastasis has been elucidated through a large body of research – a tumor's affinity for bone includes its vascularity, a molecular attraction to marrow stromal cells, and the depot of growth factors available in the bone [3, 4]. The spine is the most commonly observed location for metastatic disease within the skeletal system; this was first described by Batson who postulated and reported a redundant, valveless venous plexus as the reason for this observation [5].

D. G. Tobert · J. H. Schwab (✉)
Department of Orthopaedic Surgery, Massachusetts General Hospital, Harvard Medical School, Boston, MA, USA
e-mail: jhschwab@partners.org

A. E. Razi, S. H. Hershman (eds.), *Vertebral Compression Fractures in Osteoporotic and Pathologic Bone*, https://doi.org/10.1007/978-3-030-33861-9_7

The thoracic and thoracolumbar spine are the most common sites of metastatic involvement, with less than 10% of spinal metastases occurring in the cervical spine [6]. However, metastases to the thoracic and cervical spine are the most likely to cause neurologic impairment due to the relative size of the spinal canal and neuroforamina. The relentless advance of metastatic disease in the spine leads to a spectrum of worsening symptoms and sequelae. The initial seeding of metastatic disease within the spine is often asymptomatic and, depending on the location within the vertebra, may have little initial implications on the structural stability on the vertebral column. Similar to fractures in other locations, vertebral compression fractures occur after metastatic spine disease has progressed to the point that physiologic loads are no longer tolerated by the vertebral structure. In the absence of a retropulsed bony fragment (pathologic burst fracture) or epidural tumor burden, a pVCF rarely causes spinal cord dysfunction. However, radicular pain is frequently present due to foraminal stenosis.

Diagnosis of Pathologic Vertebral Compression Fractures

History

The patient's clinical scenario and history help form the foundation to an accurate diagnosis of pVCF. Traumatic compression fractures typically occur in the thoracolumbar junction and are most often caused by axial load forces. In healthy patients with normal bone density, it can require considerable energy to cause a VCF; identification of a VCF in a young patient most commonly occurs after high-energy blunt trauma. Although blunt trauma can precede a diagnosis of pVCF, pathologic fractures frequently occur with physiologic loading. The mechanism of injury is an important component of the history as it can alert the clinician to an incompetent vertebral column.

The hallmark of pVCF due to metastatic disease is pain (usually atraumatic onset or after low-energy trauma), often at night, and exacerbated by movement [7]. The prevalence of low back pain in the general population can make it difficult to discriminate mechanical/arthritic pain from pathologic pain in patients with a history of cancer. Clinicians must be aware of the "red flag" symptoms, such as night pain, progressively worsening pain, or pain out of proportion to injury. This is especially true for patients without a history of cancer as spinal metastasis are the initial finding in up to 20% of cancer diagnoses [8].

Further imaging should be obtained if a patient has low back pain and a prior oncologic history. Premkumar et al. showed that there is a 10% chance of spinal malignancy if both an oncologic history and low back pain are present [9]. Imaging is also warranted if a patient has a history of spinal metastases and presents with new or worsening back or neck pain. Pain at a different segment of the spine could indicate a non-contiguous pVCF, and significantly worsening pain could result from a contiguous pVCF or progression of the known metastases.

Physical Examination

A comprehensive, documented physical exam is necessary to establish the diagnosis, inform clinical decisions, and provide longitudinal care. Inspection of the patient's gait upon arrival to the examination room can clue the examiner to the degree of functional impairment that the patient is experiencing. The clinical posture in the sagittal plane can illustrate how much kyphosis may be present during ambulation.

Spinal palpation is notoriously unreliable and has poor interrater reliability. However, a comprehensive systematic review by Seffinger et al. found that pain provocation maneuvers are more reliable [10]. In that same study, landmark palpation had intermediate reliability, and paraspinal soft-tissue pain was found to be the least reliable. It is the authors' opinion that pain with spinous process palpation is useful for correlation to imaging studies; therefore, a non-tender spinous process plays little role in the evaluation of a patient with back pain. The physical exam should thoroughly interrogate the nerve root's motor and sensory function. Patellar reflexes, Babinski's maneuver, and ankle clonus should be performed to discriminate upper and lower motor neuron involvement.

Imaging

The major categories of imaging available to screen for pVCF include plain film radiography (XR), multi-detector computer tomography (MD-CT), and magnetic resonance imaging (MRI). Plain films are helpful to understand the spinal alignment in the sagittal and coronal planes under physiologic loading. While cost-effective, plain films are not sensitive or specific enough to detect metastatic disease of the spine. By the time the pathologic process is apparent on plain films, up to half of the trabecular bone has been replaced with tumor [11]. The classic "winking owl" finding of pediculosis on the anterior-posterior view usually indicates a prolonged involvement of metastatic disease in that vertebra.

If history and physical exam raise concern for a pVCF due to metastatic disease, MRI is the screening modality of choice. Although MD-CT provides a better understanding of the osseous structures, MD-CT has an unfavorable sensitivity of 66% [8]. MRI better delineates the soft-tissue structures and the relationship of the tumor with respect to the sensitive neural elements. The authors recognize the recommendation for MRI as a screening tool carries a potential for overuse; however, a careful history and comprehensive physical exam can establish an appropriate pretest probability helping to determine where MRI can be usefully employed as a screening tool.

Differentiating between benign (osteoporotic or traumatic) and pathologic VCF can be difficult on MRI (Table 7.1). This is especially true for acute compression fractures, where the short-tau inversion recovery (STIR) sequences show high-intensity signal, similar to pVCF. However, studies using early MRI technology (1.5T) noticed a more homogenous appearance and complete absence of marrow signal on STIR in pVCF [12]. In another study using a 1.5T magnet, Jung et al. found the following characteristics in metastatic pVCF: (1) convex posterior border of the vertebral body, (2) abnormal signal intensity of the pedicle or posterior elements, and (3) epidural mass (Fig. 7.1) [13]. In contrast, acute osteoporotic compression fractures had areas of spared bone marrow signal, a low signal intensity band on T1 and T2 sequences, and a

Table 7.1 Characteristics on magnetic resonance imaging (MRI) used to discriminate between traumatic/osteoporotic vertebral compression fractures and pathologic compression fractures due to metastatic disease

Pathologic VCF	Acute/subacute VCF
Homogenous marrow signal intensity	Nonhomogenous marrow signal intensity
Convex posterior vertebral body border	Retropulsion of posterior bony elements (burst component)
Epidural mass extension	Low signal intensity band on T1 and T2 sequences

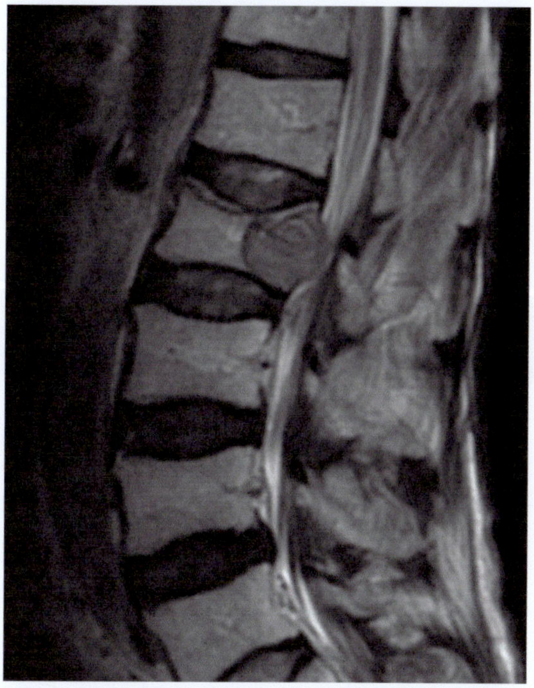

Fig. 7.1 Sagittal T2 sequence magnetic resonance image (MRI) of a 69-year-old man with a history of hepatocellular carcinoma in remission who presented with low back pain found to have a L3 pathologic vertebral compression fracture. A homogenous marrow appearance and extension of the mass into the epidural space are noted

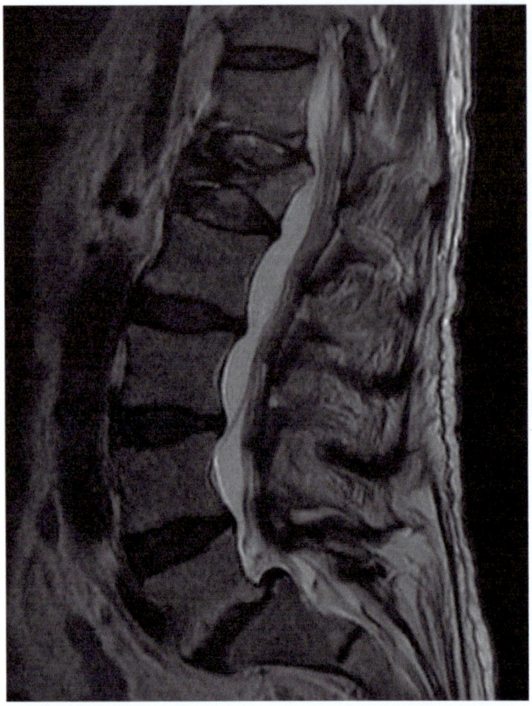

Fig. 7.2 Sagittal T2 sequence magnetic resonance image (MRI) of a 71-year-old woman with osteoporosis who presented with a subacute L1 osteoporotic vertebral compression fracture. Nonhomogenous marrow intensity and a retropulsion component are noted

component of retropulsion of the posterior elements (Fig. 7.2). If the conventional MRI sequences are equivocal, a dynamic contrast-enhanced MRI has been shown to help differentiate between benign acute and pathologic compression fractures [14].

If imaging demonstrates concern for metastatic pVCF, the oncologic status of the patient would influence the subsequent clinical decisions. Patients with evidence of spinal metastases on imaging but without a previous cancer diagnosis should undergo local and remote staging including MRI of the entire spine to look for noncontiguous metastases; MD-CT of the chest, abdomen, and pelvis to screen for a source tumor; and laboratory tests including complete blood counts; creatinine, serum, and urine electrophoresis; and a thyroid panel. For patients with a known cancer history but without metastasis, a tissue sample is necessary to confirm the source of spinal metastasis. The authors recommend close collaboration with radiology as open biopsy is often unnecessary and can be supplanted by image-guided (CT or fluoroscopic) core-needle biopsy. A new finding of spinal metastasis in a patient with known spinal metastasis can be presumed to originate from the known source and treated accordingly.

Management of Pathologic Vertebral Compression Fractures

The goal of management in pVCF is to safely minimize pain and restore function while recognizing the high potential morbidity of this disease state. A treatment plan should consider treatment of the fracture and any sequelae (deformity or stenosis) alongside treatment of the metastatic tumor. These two considerations overlap substantially because successful fracture union requires eradication of the pathologic tissue in the vertebral body. The most important initial consideration in the treatment of pVCF is the degree of spinal canal involvement by the tumor. In a landmark study by Patchell et al., a clear functional benefit was shown for patients with current or impending spinal cord compression treated with surgical decompression and stabilization (unless the tumor was exquisitely radiosensitive) [15]. Patients in this scenario should be educated about the relative morbidity of surgical treatment and adjuvant radiotherapy in context with the expected functional benefits.

Although there is high-quality data to support treatment decisions for patients with pVCF and neurologic instability, there is less robust data available to define and prognosticate biomechanical instability conferred by pVCF. For example, the revised Tokuhashi scoring system incorporates tumor histology, overall function, and the number and site of metastases to create a prognostic score but does not consider morphologic characteristics of the spine [16]. The Spinal Instability in Neoplastic Score (SINS) considers several biomechanical factors, including the alignment of the spine, degree of vertebral body collapse, posterior vertebral element involvement, and location of the metastatic disease within the spine [17]. The calculated score provides a more objective measure of biomechanical instability for the clinician. A pVCF that receives a SINS of "indeterminate" or "unstable" (more than 6 points) warrants consultation from a spine surgeon to determine whether surgical stabilization is necessary prior to treatment of the spinal metastasis.

If the metastatic disease responsible for a pVCF does not portend imminent neurologic or biomechanical instability risk, more measured options are available for treatment. In this scenario, radiotherapy is the mainstay of treatment. Radiotherapy successfully treats the pain from bone metastasis in approximately 75% of patients [18]. The success of radiotherapy is directly related to the radiosensitivity of the tumor. Lymphoma and multiple myeloma have the most robust response to radiotherapy, whereas metastases from solid-organ malignancy typically respond less favorably to radiotherapy. Chemotherapy is not commonly used as the primary treatment of spinal metastasis except when the tumor histology has demonstrated a dramatic response to chemotherapeutic agents, such as germ-cell tumors and neuroblastoma.

Following treatment for metastatic disease in the spine, the patient should be reevaluated to determine the degree of dysfunction and pain from the remaining fractured vertebra. The authors recommend bracing as a therapeutic modality for comfort only; however it should be noted that there is no high-quality data suggesting bracing will prevent the kyphotic sequela of pVCF. If pain from the pVCF is a persistent limitation, kyphoplasty or vertebroplasty may ameliorate some of the symptoms and improve function. Berenson et al. performed a randomized controlled trial comparing percutaneous vertebral augmentation with non-operative management for patients with cancer and VCF [19]. They reported an improvement in patient-reported disability and quality of life for those who received cement augmentation and few adverse events. It is important to recognize certain contraindications to kyphoplasty or vertebroplasty, including a vertebral height that limits safe transpedicular access to the vertebral body, multiple contiguous levels, and posterior cortex disruption as these increase the risk of the procedure.

Conclusion

Metastatic disease of the spine resulting in pVCF is relatively common. This condition most often occurs in the thoracic or thoracolumbar spine, and the predilection of spine involvement is likely due to a combination of vascularity and availability of growth factors within the vertebral trabecular bone. Any patient presenting with weight loss, night pain, atraumatic back pain, or a disproportionate degree of pain without a history of malignancy should receive further work-up as spinal metastasis is often the initial finding in malignancy diagnoses. Patients with a history of malignancy who present with back pain should have a neurologic exam documented and an MRI to screen for metastatic disease.

MRI is the most sensitive modality to confirm the diagnosis of pVCF. As discussed earlier, homogenous marrow involvement and a convex posterior vertebral body border help discriminate a metastatic pVCF from acute or subacute traumatic/osteoporotic VCF. The treatment of pVCF is dependent on the degree of neurologic and biomechanical instability. High-quality evidence demonstrates that patients with pVCF and spinal cord compression have better functional outcomes after surgical treatment and adjuvant radiotherapy. The SINS is a helpful tool to objectively determine the degree of biomechanical instability. Patients without neurologic or biomechanical instability should undergo treatment directed at eradicating the spinal metastatic disease that caused pVCF; most commonly, this is accomplished with radiotherapy. Following successful treatment of the metastatic spinal tumor, patients with continued pain from pVCF can undergo percutaneous vertebral cement augmentation which has been shown to have a high likelihood of benefit with relatively low risk.

References

1. American Cancer Society. Cancer facts & figure 2018. Atlanta: American Cancer Society.
2. Arneson TJ, Shuling L, Yi P, et al. Estimated number of prevalent cases of metastatic bone disease in the US adult population. Clin Epidemiol. 2012;4:87–93.
3. Roodman GD. Mechanisms of bone metastasis. N Engl J Med. 2004;350(16):1655–64.
4. Poste G, Fidler IJ. The pathogenesis of cancer metastasis. Nature. 1980;283(5743):139–46.
5. Batson OV. The function of the vertebral veins and their role in the spread of metastases. Ann Surg. 1940;112(1):138–49.
6. Brihaye J, Ectors P, Lemort M, Van Houtte P. The management of spinal epidural metastases. Adv Tech Stand Neurosurg. 1988;16:121–76.
7. Boland PJ, Lane JM, Sundaresan N. Metastatic disease of the spine. Clin Orthop Relat Res. 1982;(169):95–102.
8. Buhmann Kirchhoff S, Becker C, Duerr HR, Reiser M, Baur-Melnyk A. Detection of osseous metastases of the spine: comparison of high resolution multi-detector-CT with MRI. Eur J Radiol. 2009;69(3):567–73.
9. Premkumar A, Godfrey W, Gottschalk MB, Boden SD. Red flags for low back pain are not always really red: a prospective evaluation of the clinical utility of commonly used screening questions for low back pain. J Bone Joint Surg Am. 2018;100(5):368–74.
10. Seffinger MA, Najm WI, Mishra SI, et al. Reliability of spinal palpation for diagnosis of back and neck pain: a systematic review of the literature. Spine. 2004;29(19):E413–25.
11. Edelstyn GA, Gillespie PJ, Grebbell FS. The radiological demonstration of osseous metastases. Experimental observations. Clin Radiol. 1967;18(2):158–62.
12. Baker LL, Goodman SB, Perkash I, Lane B, Enzmann DR. Benign versus pathologic compression fractures of vertebral bodies: assessment with conventional spin-echo, chemical-shift, and STIR MR imaging. Radiology. 1990;174(2):495–502.
13. Jung H-S, Jee W-H, McCauley TR, Ha K-Y, Choi K-H. Discrimination of metastatic from acute osteoporotic compression spinal fractures with MR imaging. Radiogr Rev Publ. 2003;23(1):179–87.
14. Arevalo-Perez J, Peck KK, Lyo JK, Holodny AI, Lis E, Karimi S. Differentiating benign from malignant vertebral fractures using T1 -weighted dynamic contrast-enhanced MRI. J Magn Reson Imaging. 2015;42(4):1039–47.
15. Patchell RA, Tibbs PA, Regine WF, et al. Direct decompressive surgical resection in the treatment of spinal cord compression caused by metastatic cancer: a randomised trial. Lancet Lond Engl. 2005;366(9486):643–8.
16. Tokuhashi Y, Matsuzaki H, Oda H, Oshima M, Ryu J. A revised scoring system for preoperative evaluation of metastatic spine tumor prognosis. Spine. 2005;30(19):2186–91.
17. Fisher CG, DiPaola CP, Ryken TC, et al. A novel classification system for spinal instability in neoplastic disease: an evidence-based approach and expert consensus from the Spine Oncology Study Group. Spine. 2010;35(22):E1221–9.
18. Foro Arnalot P, Fontanals AV, Galcerán JC, et al. Randomized clinical trial with two palliative radiotherapy regimens in painful bone metastases: 30 Gy in 10 fractions compared with 8 Gy in single fraction. Radiother Oncol. 2008;89(2):150–5.
19. Berenson J, Pflugmacher R, Jarzem P, et al. Balloon kyphoplasty versus non-surgical fracture management for treatment of painful vertebral body compression fractures in patients with cancer: a multicentre, randomised controlled trial. Lancet Oncol. 2011;12(3):225–35.

8 History, Physical Exam, and Differential Diagnosis of Vertebral Compression Fracture

Michael Dinizo and Aaron Buckland

Introduction

Osteoporotic vertebral compression fractures (VCFs) are associated with pain, physical deformity, worsening social function, decreased self-esteem, impaired quality of life, and increased morbidity and mortality [1]. VCFs are a warning of subsequent osteoporotic fracture because they occur both earlier and more frequently than other fragility fractures. Patients with a single VCF have a fivefold increase of future vertebral fracture and a threefold increased risk of sustaining a hip fracture [2, 3].

VCF treatment varies widely from non-operative symptomatic management to vertebral augmentation procedures and surgical intervention. Treatment decisions are based on the symptoms, etiology, and chronicity of the VCF, making a timely and accurate diagnostic evaluation critical for treatment success. In addition, patients with a VCF often require interdisciplinary and multimodal treatment that necessitates proper clinical assessment, imaging, laboratory testing, and subspecialist referral. As patients with a VCF often seek the care of an orthopedic or spine surgeon, these practitioners are in a unique position to identify patients who are at high risk for further fragility fractures and, therefore, can initiate the workup to diagnose, treat, and prevent future fractures. Unfortunately, when presented with these patients, physicians are not always acquainted with the appropriate course of action. In a study of patients with a low-energy VCF initially presenting to a spine surgeon, only 60% of surgeons ordered a DEXA scan, only 39% initiated a metabolic laboratory evaluation, and only 63% referred the patient to a primary care physician or endocrinologist for further treatment [4].

Despite the critical importance of detecting VCFs, these fractures remain under diagnosed [5]. The differential diagnosis of a patient presenting to his/her doctor with back pain, deformity, and/or limited range of motion is vast. Many older, osteoporotic patients have these symptoms chronically, making it difficult to distinguish chronic mechanical back pain from a vertebral insufficiency fracture without the proper clinical suspicion [4]. As such, only one in four VCFs is detected clinically, often because symptoms do not correlate well with the underlying fracture [5]. Once a VCF is suspected, the physician should investigate secondary causes of osteoporosis, metabolic bone disease, malignancy, osteomalacia, hyperthyroidism, hyperparathyroidism, and renal failure. Treatment

M. Dinizo (✉) · A. Buckland
Department of Orthopedic Surgery, NYU Langone Orthopedic Hospital, NYU Langone Medical Center, New York, NY, USA
e-mail: Michael.Dinizo@nyulangone.org; aaron.buckland@nyulangone.org

A. E. Razi, S. H. Hershman (eds.), *Vertebral Compression Fractures in Osteoporotic and Pathologic Bone*, https://doi.org/10.1007/978-3-030-33861-9_8

should be initiated after ordering the appropriate imaging tests and laboratory studies and initiating the proper referrals, without a delay in care or diagnosis.

Accurate diagnostic evaluation of VCFs will enhance patient outcomes and allow clinicians to target therapeutic intervention to those patients who would benefit most thereby preventing additional fragility fractures. In this chapter we describe the clinical presentation, differential diagnosis, and laboratory evaluation for patients presenting with a VCF. In osteopenic patients presenting with back pain, the history and physical exam remain the cornerstone of diagnosis. The role of radiographs, CT, MRI, and DEXA is discussed in further detail in other chapters. In patients with "red flag symptoms," such as a history of infection, cancer, or neurologic involvement, or those with constitutional symptoms such as fever, chills, weight loss, or night pain, the indications for additional imaging and testing are reviewed.

Clinical Presentation

History

The most common etiology of VCF is osteoporosis, although trauma, infection, and neoplasm can also lead to a VCF. A thorough diagnostic evaluation of patients with a VCF is required to determine treatment, prevent further VCFs, begin treatment for a secondary cause of osteoporosis, and rule out or initiate a malignancy workup. In patients with known or suspected VCFs, obtaining a detailed history of a patient's onset of symptoms, pain pattern, chronicity, and medical history is critical. Understanding the chronicity of the patient's symptoms is especially crucial as both acute and chronic fractures have a different natural history and sequelae that may aid the physician when counseling the patient.

Studies have suggested that having one VCF increases the risk of future VCFs. Irrespective of bone density, having one or more VCFs leads to an increase in a patient's risk of developing another vertebral fracture [3]. When an osteoporotic VCF is suspected, inquiring about the onset of menopause, prior bone density studies, and the presence of modifiable risk factors can help narrow the differential diagnosis and may alter treatment. Risk factors include alcohol and/or tobacco use, estrogen deficiency, early menopause, premenopausal amenorrhea, corticosteroid use, insufficient physical activity, low body weight, and dietary calcium and vitamin D deficiency. Generally, patients will give a history of some trauma or inciting event with each compression fracture. In some cases of osteoporosis, the cause of fracture may be negligible such as lifting a household object, a low-energy fall, or even normal activities of daily living. Interestingly, up to 30% of compression fractures in patients with osteoporosis occur while the patient is in bed [6].

Differentiating VCF from muscular or spondylotic pain is often difficult. The pain associated with a VCF can be severe and has significant overlap with other causes of back pain, which includes difficulty with bending, lifting, descending stairs, and impairment with activities of daily living. Discogenic or spondylotic pain are classically exacerbated by activities that load the disc, such as sitting, arising from a seated position, awaking in the morning, lumbar flexion, lifting, coughing, laughing, and a Valsalva maneuver. Patients with musculoskeletal low-back pain may indicate a regional rather than localized pain, often being unable to localize the pain. In many cases VCF pain can be more localized to a specific segment of the back by a patient.

When obtaining the history of a patient with a VCF, it is important to keep in mind that VCF may also cause referred pain and that low-back pain is not always the only presenting symptom. Gibson et al. looked at 288 patients with one or more compression fractures and found that non-midline pain was present in 68%. The typical pain pattern was referred to the ribs, hip, groin, or buttocks [7]. In some cases, the main symptom can be radicular pain rather than axial pain, mimicking foraminal stenosis or disc herniation. This often happens in the case of osteoporotic VCF combined with preexisting stenosis of the intervertebral foramen, thus resulting in root compression when the vertebral height decreases due to fracture [8]. The incidence of acute radiculopathy after lumbar compression fracture is uncommon but rises when VCF occurs at lower lumbar spinal levels [9].

Although pain may prompt a patient to seek treatment, many compression fractures are painless and are detected incidentally. Often, a patient will present with symptoms of progressive scoliosis, kyphosis, or mechanical lower-back pain, and it is not until after routine radiographs that the vertebral compression deformity is diagnosed. Patients with multiple compression deformities and progressive loss of vertebral body height are at the highest risk of developing excessive thoracic kyphosis and lumbar lordosis; every 4 cm loss of vertebral height leads to ~15 degrees of kyphosis [10]. Excessive kyphosis may lead to constipation, bowel obstruction, prolonged inactivity, deep vein thrombosis, progressive muscle weakness, decreased height, and respiratory disturbances [11].

In addition to treating the initial presenting symptoms, physicians that diagnose a VCF are in a unique position to initiate the proper medical and malignancy workup when the cause of the VCF is not clear. A review of systems should include constitutional symptoms as well as a thorough medical history, especially whether there is a history of cancer. Systemic disease or symptoms may increase susceptibility to infection, which can lead to vertebral osteomyelitis; vertebral osteomyelitis may mimic or cause a VCF. Typically, the most common organisms in a chronic infection are staphylococci or streptococci. A history of night pain, fever, drug use, depression, or symptoms suggestive of metabolic disease can aid diagnosis and guide subsequent workup and treatment. Obtaining a travel history as well as history of prior infections can help narrow the diagnosis because tuberculosis (Pott's disease) can occur in the spine and mimic VCF.

Compression fractures are often the presenting manifestation leading to the diagnosis of malignancy. Up to 10% of patients with cancer will ultimately have spinal metastasis [12], and metastasis is the most common malignancy leading to spinal fractures. The most common malignancies that metastasize to the spine are renal, prostate, breast, and lung. The two most common primary spinal malignancies are multiple myeloma and lymphoma [13]. If malignancy is suspected, additional lab work and imaging should be guided by the suspected malignancy.

Physical Exam

A well-performed, well-documented, and consistent physical examination during the initial and follow-up visits can yield accurate and consistent clinical information that can guide the diagnostic evaluation. Physical examination findings should always be put into the context of the reported symptoms and diagnostic test results. Physical examination should always include an accurate measurement of height. Midline back pain is the most common symptom of a VCF, and the pain is often axial and aching and may range from mild to severe. However, pain may also be referred to the ribs, hip, groin, or buttocks [14]. Upon inspection of the spine, a patient with a VCF may have a new onset kyphotic posture that cannot be corrected caused by the anterior wedging of the fractured vertebra. Clinical measures of kyphosis can be used and include parameters such as the distance from a patient's occiput to the wall (normally 0 cm). Additional features of advanced vertebral deformity may also be used such as cervical hyperextension and abdominal protuberance.

Examining a patient's gate may yield additional clues to diagnosis. Patients may walk with their hips flexed and hunched forward. This may be caused by hip flexor contractures due to iliopsoas shortening secondary to vertebral height loss and compensation for increased kyphosis. When examining a patient with a suspected VCF, close attention should be paid to the thoracolumbar junction. This is a transitional zone between the more rigid thoracic vertebral column and the relatively mobile lumbar vertebral column, making the junction more prone to fractures. This location is the site for approximately 60% of all VCFs [15].

Simple palpation will often reveal moderate tenderness at the level of the fracture. Extreme pain and warmth elicited with superficial palpation should raise the suspicion of an infectious process. Paraspinal tenderness is commonly due to continuous contraction of the paraspinal musculature in order to maintain posture in the context of altered spinal mechanics due to fracture.

A detailed neurologic examination is essential in VCF patients as it is in all patients presenting with back pain, spinal deformity, or trauma. The patient should be assessed for sensory deficits, motor weakness, and upper motor neuron signs. Neurologic abnormalities may indicate retropulsion of a bone fragment into the spinal canal or foraminal stenosis that may require surgical intervention. Examination should always attempt to distinguish between neuropathy, peripheral nerve injury, nerve root problems, and myelopathy, which is one of the common causes of fall secondary to imbalance.

Differential Diagnosis

There are many potential causes of back pain which mimic a vertebral compression fracture. These may include but are not limited to bony metastasis, osteomyelitis, Pott's disease, and other lesions. Chronic degenerative spine pathology which could mimic a VCF includes spondylolisthesis, degenerative disc disease, and facet arthropathy. A thorough history, exam, and proper imaging can help distinguish these pathologies from an osteoporotic vertebral compression fracture. The etiology of a VCF is varied and includes osteomalacia, excessive glucocorticoid intake, hyperparathyroidism, chronic kidney disease, trauma, and malignancy. After a thorough history and exam, the radiograph should be carefully assessed for features that favor a pathologic fracture which would necessitate further diagnostic workup with advanced imaging. Signs that can be used to differentiate osteoporotic fractures from non-osteoporotic include accentuated secondary or vertical trabeculae which give a striated appearance and sharply outlined cortical endplates [16]. Further details on the radiologic characteristics of VCFs are available in other chapters throughout this text.

There are various normal variants, congenital abnormalities, degenerative changes, and other pathologies that can change the shape of vertebrae and be easily confused with VCF [17]. For example, in osteochondritis there is anterior wedging of multiple adjacent vertebrae, endplate irregularities, and kyphosis. This can be differentiated by the changes in multiple adjacent vertebrae, rather than at a single spinal level. Other characteristics to look for on plain radiographs include endplate erosion which should raise the suspicion of an infectious process and spondylosis characterized by endplate sclerosis, marginal osteophytes, and decreased intervertebral disc spaces along with anterior wedging [18].

Difficultly arises when differentiating acute or subacute osteoporotic fractures from neoplastic fracture. The spine is the most common site of skeletal metastases as well as osteoporotic fracture, and both occur in a similar patient population. Any cortical destruction or the presence of lesions in the fractured or surrounding vertebrae should immediately trigger a malignancy workup and further investigation. However, clinicians should be aware that up to 1/3 of vertebral fractures in patients with known malignancies are due to osteoporosis and not metastasis [19].

Blood Work

Laboratory evaluation in osteoporotic vertebral compression fractures is used mainly to exclude malignancy and infection and evaluate any causes of secondary osteoporosis. Screening lab studies in elderly patients with osteoporotic fractures should be individualized to each patient based on history, exam, and imaging findings.

Endocrine organs that are important to bone metabolism include the skin, parathyroid glands, liver, kidneys, gonads, adrenals, and thyroid. Pituitary and hypothalamic function also affects bone physiology. Endocrine abnormalities can lead to a failure of maintaining normal serum calcium levels – secondary osteoporosis can be caused by renal or liver disease, hyperthyroidism, hyperparathyroidism, Cushing's syndrome, hypogonadism, and nutritional deficiencies, metabolic disorders, and many other causes.

Failure to identify underlying disorders of bone and mineral metabolism can result in inappropriate or inadequate treatment. The most efficient and cost-effective laboratory screening strategy to unmask underlying disorders remains unknown. The National Osteoporosis Foundation (NOF) guidelines recommend that patients with a newly diagnosed fragility fracture undergo a rigorous battery of laboratory tests, including serum calcium, phosphate, creatinine, alkaline phosphatase, liver function, 25(OH) vitamin D, total testosterone, complete blood count, 24-hour urinary calcium, serum magnesium, thyroid-stimulating hormone, parathyroid hormone, and bone turnover markers [20]. A study by Johnson et al. recommends that initially, screening blood tests should only include 25(OH) vitamin D, calcium, PTH, creatinine/eGFR, and serum testosterone in men. Serum testosterone helps detect a sex hormone deficiency as a secondary cause of osteoporosis. This limited laboratory evaluation strategy has both reasonable diagnostic yield and may substantially reduce cost [21].

In women without a history of disease or medication use known to adversely affect bone, 32% were found to have disorders of calcium metabolism. By including the measurement of 24-hour urine calcium, serum calcium, and PTH, the accuracy of diagnosing the underlying causes in this group was improved by 85% [22]. In patients who are receiving thyroid hormone supplementation, determination of the TSH level is useful to be certain that thyroid replacement is not excessive. In patients at high risk for subsequent fracture, more specialized tests should also be considered based on clinical suspicion, including serum and urine protein electrophoresis to detect multiple myeloma and a 24-hour urinary free cortisol or an overnight dexamethasone suppression test to exclude Cushing's syndrome, which, although uncommon, can lead to rapidly progressive osteoporosis [23].

Markers of bone turnover, including various collagen breakdown products, may also serve to distinguish between high and low turnover bone loss. Bone turnover is characterized by bone formation and bone resorption. Biochemical bone turnover markers (BTMs) have been developed to capture measurements of these two activities. International expert groups in the fields of clinical chemistry and osteoporosis have come to a consensus that the amino-terminal propeptide of type I procollagen (PINP) and the carboxy-terminal telopeptide of type I collagen (CTX-I) should be the markers for bone formation and bone resorption, respectively [24].

If malignancy is suspected, serum and urine protein electrophoresis as well as PSA in men should be included. A normal protein electrophoresis pattern excludes the presence of multiple myeloma or a related lymphoproliferative disorder in 90% of patients [25]. Any febrile patient in whom infection is suspected should also have C-reactive protein and blood cultures drawn to evaluate for infection. Bone biopsy is not routinely performed in the setting of fracture and currently has little practical value in dictating treatment but can be obtained when a hematologic disorder is suspected [26].

Conclusion

A VCF may be the initial sign of a patient's subsequent downhill spiral if the underlying etiology of the fracture is not properly diagnosed and addressed. The presentation of a patient with a VCF is often generalized low-back pain which may be poorly localized and without a known etiology or direct traumatic event, making the diagnosis difficult. Neurologic symptoms are rare. Comprehensive evaluation of these patients should include a detailed history and examination, radiographic studies, and laboratory evaluation. Osteoporotic patients with a VCF may have a progressive spinal deformity that affects functional levels and mortality. These patients are at an increased risk of additional VCFs and fragility fractures. It is important to rule out a metastatic process and infection. Advanced radiographic imaging may be helpful to determine the etiology and chronicity of a VCF. Improved and accurate diagnostic evaluation of vertebral compression fractures may improve the ability to target appropriate therapeutic intervention to those patients who would benefit most.

References

1. Ross PD. Clinical consequences of vertebral fractures. Am J Med. 1997;103:30–42.
2. Black DM, Arden NK, Palermo L, Pearson J, Cummings SR. Prevalent vertebral deformities predict hip fractures and new vertebral deformities but not wrist fractures. Study of Osteoporotic Fractures Research Group. J Bone Miner Res. 1999;14(5):821–8.
3. Lindsay R, Silverman SL, Cooper C, Hanley DA, Barton I, Broy SB, et al. Risk of new vertebral fracture in the year following a fracture. JAMA. 2001;285(3):320–3.
4. C Dipaola JB, Biswas D, Dipaoloa M, Grauer J, Rechtine G. Survey of spine surgeons on attitudes regarding osteoporosis and osteomalacia screening and treatment for fractures, fusion surgery and pseudarthrosis. Spine. 2009;9(7):537–44.
5. Fink HAMD, Palermo L, Nevitt MC, Cauley JA, Genant HK. What proportion of incident radiographic vertebral deformities is clinically diagnosed and vice versa? J Bone Miner Res. 2005;20:1216–22.
6. Garfin SR, Yuan HA, Reiley MA. New technologies in spine: kyphoplasty and vertebroplasty for the treatment of painful osteoporotic compression fractures. Spine (Phila Pa 1976). 2001;26(14):1511–5.
7. Gibson JE, Pilgram TK, Gilula LA. Response of nonmidline pain to percutaneous vertebroplasty. AJR Am J Roentgenol. 2006;187(4):869–72.
8. Chung SK, Lee SH, Kim DY, Lee HY. Treatment of lower lumbar radiculopathy caused by osteoporotic compression fracture: the role of vertebroplasty. J Spinal Disord Tech. 2002;15(6):461–8.
9. Kim DE, Kim HS, Kim SW, Kim HS. Clinical analysis of acute radiculopathy after osteoporotic lumbar compression fracture. J Korean Neurosurg Soc. 2015;57(1):32–5.
10. Katzman WB, Huang MH, Lane NE, Ensrud KE, Kado DM. Kyphosis and decline in physical function over 15 years in older community-dwelling women: the Study of Osteoporotic Fractures. J Gerontol A Biol Sci Med Sci. 2013;68(8):976–83.
11. Theodorou DJ, Theodorou SJ, Duncan TD, Garfin SR, Wong WH. Percutaneous balloon kyphoplasty for the correction of spinal deformity in painful vertebral body compression fractures. Clin Imaging. 2002;26(1):1–5.
12. Godersky JC, Smoker WR, Knutzon R. Use of magnetic resonance imaging in the evaluation of metastatic spinal disease. Neurosurgery. 1987;21(5):676–80.
13. Hansen EJM, Simony A, Carreon L, Andersen MO. Rate of unsuspected malignancy in patients with vertebral compression fracture undergoing percutaneous vertebroplasty. Spine. 2016;41(6):549–52.
14. Kim DE, KH, Kim SW, Kim HS. Clinical analysis of acute radiculopathy after osteoporotic lumbar compression fracture. J Korean Neurosurg Soc. 2015;57(1):32–5.
15. Cooper C, Atkinson EJ, O'Fallon WM, Melton LJ III. Incidence of clinically diagnosed vertebral fractures: a population-based study in Rochester, Minnesota, 1985–1989. J Bone Miner Res. 1992;7:221–7.
16. Guglielmi G, Muscarella S, Leone A, Peh WC. Imaging of metabolic bone diseases. Radiol Clin N Am. 2008;46(4):735–54.. vi
17. Kim DH, Vaccaro AR. Osteoporotic compression fractures of the spine; current options and considerations for treatment. Spine J. 2006;6(5):479–87.
18. Ferrar L, Jiang G, Schousboe JT, DeBold CR, Eastell R. Algorithm-based qualitative and semiquantitative identification of prevalent vertebral fracture: agreement between different readers, imaging modalities, and diagnostic approaches. J Bone Miner Res. 2008;23(3):417–24.
19. Fornasier VL, Czitrom AA. Collapsed vertebrae: a review of 659 autopsies. Clin Orthop Relat Res. 1978;131:261–5.
20. Cosman F, de Beur SJ, LeBoff MS, Lewiecki EM, Tanner B, Randall S, et al. Clinician's guide to prevention and treatment of osteoporosis. Osteoporos Int. 2014;25(10):2359–81.
21. Johnson K, Suriyaarachchi P, Kakkat M, Boersma D, Gunawardene P, Demontiero O, et al. Yield and cost-effectiveness of laboratory testing to identify metabolic contributors to falls and fractures in older persons. Arch Osteoporos. 2015;10(1):21.
22. Tannenbaum C, Clark J, Schwartzman K, Wallenstein S, Lapinski R, Meier D, et al. Yield of laboratory testing to identify secondary contributors to osteoporosis in otherwise healthy women. J Clin Endocrinol Metab. 2002;87(10):4431–7.
23. Parreira PCS, Maher CG, Megale RZ, March L, Ferreira ML. An overview of clinical guidelines for the management of vertebral compression fracture: a systematic review. Spine J. 2017;17(12):1932–8.
24. Gaitanis IN, Hadjipavlou AG, Katonis PG, Tzermiadianos MN, Pasku DS, Patwardhan AG. Balloon kyphoplasty for the treatment of pathological vertebral compressive fractures. Eur Spine J. 2005;14(3):250–60.
25. Cannada LK, Hill BW. Osteoporotic hip and spine fractures: a current review. Geriatr Orthop Surg Rehabil. 2014;5(4):207–12.
26. Pignolo RJ. Evaluation of bone fragility and fracture prevention. In: Pignolo RJ, Keenan MA, Hebela NM, editors. Fractures in the elderly: a guide to practical management. Totowa: Humana Press; 2011. p. 309–28.

9 Radiographic Diagnosis of Patients with Vertebral Compression Fractures

R. Aaron Marshall and Mohammad Samim

Abbreviations

18F FDG PET/CT	18F-fluorodeoxyglucose positron emission tomography/computed tomography
ADC	Apparent diffusion coefficient
CSI	Chemical shift imaging
DCI	Dynamic contrast-enhanced imaging
DWI	Diffusion-weighted imaging
MDCT	Multidetector computed tomography
MRI	Magnetic resonance imaging
SPECT	Single-photon emission computed tomography
STIR	Short tau inversion recovery
Tc 99m-MDP	Technetium 99m-methyl diphosphonate
Tc-99m HMDP	Technetium 99m hydroxy-methylene diphosphonate
VCF	Vertebral compression fracture

Key Points

1. In a patient with suspicion for vertebral compression fracture with low risk for spinal cord injury, conventional radiography with lateral and anteroposterior views is the most appropriate initial imaging study. In the setting of known vertebral compression deformities detected on radiograph or CT, MRI is of particular use in evaluating the chronicity of vertebral fractures, for differentiation of benign versus malignant compression deformities, and for the evaluation of associated extra- and intradural soft tissue pathologies.
2. MRI is the cornerstone of vertebral fracture characterization, and a multitude of qualitative and quantitative features have been studied for better differentiation of benign and pathologic VCFs, including morphometric criteria (vertebral body contour, cortex, trabecula, and cleft signs), signal intensity criteria (edema/inflammation, and contrast enhancement patterns), and extravertebral soft tissue abnormalities. Newer techniques for fracture characterization include diffusion-weighted imaging,

R. A. Marshall · M. Samim (✉)
Department of Radiology, NYU Langone Orthopedic Hospital, NYU Langone Medical Center, New York, NY, USA
e-mail: Mohammad.samim@nyulangone.org

A. E. Razi, S. H. Hershman (eds.), *Vertebral Compression Fractures in Osteoporotic and Pathologic Bone*, https://doi.org/10.1007/978-3-030-33861-9_9

chemical shift imaging, and dynamic contrast-enhanced imaging.

3. In patients with contraindications to MRI, positron emission tomography (PET)/CT or SPECT/CT may be useful for discrimination of benign and malignant VCF etiologies using a combination of metabolic and morphologic criteria; however, the gold standard for definitive characterization in patients with contraindication to MRI and concern for malignant compression fracture remains tissue diagnosis with percutaneous or open biopsy.

Initial Radiologic Evaluation

A multitude of imaging modalities are available to the clinician for the evaluation for suspected vertebral injury, with the most appropriate modality depending on both the clinical presentation and the location of the suspected injury. For patients with low-back pain and low risk for spinal cord injury, conventional radiography with lateral and anteroposterior radiographs is the most appropriate initial imaging study, particularly when vertebral compression fracture (VCF) is in the differential. Patients who may meet a low-risk profile for spinal cord injury include those with acute, subacute, or chronic uncomplicated low-back pain with a history of low-velocity trauma (e.g., fall from a height), osteoporosis, advanced age, or steroid use [1, 2]. In these populations, cross-sectional imaging with CT and MRI may be useful to identify fractures which are occult on conventional radiography and for further characterization of complicated fractures, particularly when there is concern for canal compromise or fracture extension into the posterior elements of the spine [3]. CT and MRI are appropriate first-line imaging studies in patients with high risk for spinal injury, which may include trauma patients with neurologic signs and symptoms, certain high impact mechanisms of injury (e.g., high-speed motor vehicle accidents), or other injuries associated with possible cervical spine injury (e.g., significant closed head injury or multiple pelvic or extremity fractures) [4–6].

MRI is indicated as the first-line imaging test in the setting of low-back pain when there is concern that symptoms may be a result of an underlying life or limb-threatening condition such as malignancy, infection, aortic aneurysm, dissection, or complicated fracture. In a patient with vertebral compression deformities detected on radiograph or CT, MRI is of particular use in evaluating the chronicity of vertebral fractures, for differentiation of benign versus malignant compression deformities, and for the evaluation of associated extra- and intradural soft tissue pathologies.

When a VCF is identified, imaging of the entirety of the spine with conventional radiographs or scintigraphy is suggested, since additional fractures are identified in up to 30% of patients at the time of initial diagnosis [7]. These additional fractures may be in vertebra directly adjacent to the compressed vertebra, or in distant vertebra, most commonly in the lower thoracic and lumbar spine where axial loading forces are greatest [8].

Imaging Definition of Vertebral Compression Fracture

VCFs are characterized by the location of endplate depression within the anteroposterior dimension of the vertebral body (anterior third, wedge fracture; middle third, biconcave fracture; posterior third, crush fracture) [9]. Fractures with compression of the entirety of the anteroposterior dimension of the vertebral body are likewise denoted as crush fractures or alternatively as "complete" fractures [10, 11]. Most commonly, compression fractures are wedge- or biconcave-type fractures, resulting from physiologic axial loading and kyphotic flexion forces on the anterior and middle aspect of the vertebra [12, 13].

In the clinical setting, vertebral compression fractures are diagnosed based on a qualitative or semiquantitative imaging assessment of the vertebral body height. A 20% reduction in anterior, middle, or posterior vertebral body height relative to the unaffected portions of the vertebral body defines the minimum threshold for compression fracture with conventional radiography [9, 14]. While 4 mm has traditionally been considered the minimum height loss to define compression on radiography, since normal vertebra demonstrates a 1–3 mm difference in anterior and posterior height [15, 16], however, modern high-resolution multidetector computed tomography (MDCT) and MRI allow detection of more subtle compression deformities. The percentage of vertebral body height loss incrementally aids in grading the severity of the compression deformity, with under 25% defining mild compression (Grade I), 25–40% defining moderate compression (Grade II), and >40% defining severe compression (Grade III) [9].

Vertebral Compression Fracture Chronicity

The chronicity of a vertebral compression deformity is of clinical significance both for diagnosis and for appropriate patient management and follow-up. At initial presentation, characterizing VCF chronicity aids the treating physician in establishing a probable cause for patients presenting symptoms (i.e., back pain), since acute and subacute fractures are more likely to present with pain than chronic (healed) fractures. Additionally, fracture chronicity plays a role in differentiating a multitude of etiologies for the VCF, since only benign, osteoporotic VCFs are expected to fully heal without appropriate intervention. Finally, chronicity is integral in determining the optimal management and follow-up. Fractures in the acute or subacute phase of healing, best marked by marrow edema on MRI or the early phases of increased metabolic activity on scintigraphy, are more likely to benefit from invasive management such as cement augmentation as compared to chronic fractures [17, 18].

Although conventional radiography and CT may play a role in establishing chronicity, these modalities are often insufficient for definitive characterization. This is particularly true in an elderly population with severe osteoporosis, where diminished bone density may obscure features of the healing process typically seen in the subacute or chronic phases of VCF evolution [19]. The primary role of conventional radiography in establishing chronicity is for comparison to prior imaging to determine a timeframe in which a fracture has occurred. In the absence of priors, radiography is typically insufficient for definitive characterization. CT with multiplanar reformatting – specifically in the sagittal plane – may suggest an acute fracture when there is endplate disruption, trabecular impaction, or intra-trabecular gas (the "vacuum cleft" sign) [20]. Findings on CT which may suggest a chronic fracture include a well-corticated compression deformity and bone mineral density similar to unaffected adjacent vertebra [21]. In the absence of these features, the chronicity of a compression fracture is indeterminate with CT, and other advanced imaging techniques are required for definitive characterization.

MRI is a preferred modality for establishing chronicity and fully characterizing vertebral compression fractures. On conventional MRI sequences including T1 and fluid-sensitive sequences such as short tau inversion recovery (STIR) or fat-suppressed T2-weighted sequences, findings of an acute osteoporotic VCF include a distinct fracture line and secondary marrow edema. The fracture line will be hypointense on T1 and T2 and may either parallel or extend obliquely along the endplate with or without disruption of the compressed endplate (Fig. 9.1) [22]. Edema, hemorrhage, and inflammatory changes accompanying the acute fracture result in increased trabecular fluid signal in a band-like pattern paralleling the acutely fractured endplate [23]. This acute intra-spongious edema is hypointense on T1-weighted imaging and hyperintense on STIR or fat-suppressed

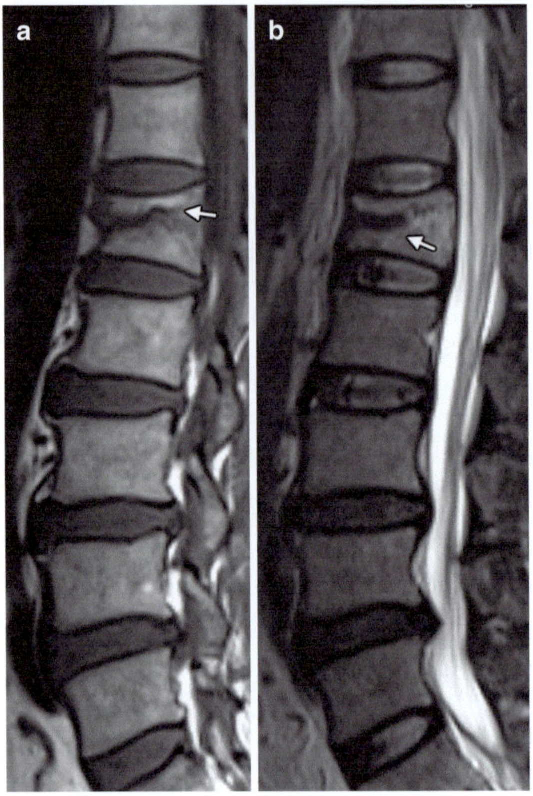

Fig. 9.1 A 65-year-old male with low-back pain and no history of malignancy. Sagittal (**a**) T1 pre-contrast and (**b**) T2 images demonstrate a hypointense fracture line paralleling the endplates (arrow), extending >50% of the vertebral body AP dimension to the anterior cortex suggesting this is an acute benign osteoporotic VCF

T2-weighted images [20, 24]. Edema will persist from the time of the injury for an average of 1–4 months and up to 6 months in up to 18% of patients, after which signal abnormalities should return to normal [18, 23, 25–28]. These transient marrow signal abnormalities are thought to accompany the acute healing process in benign osteoporotic VCFs and have been associated with a favorable clinical response to cement augmentation [17].

Scintigraphy with technetium 99m-methyl diphosphonate (Tc 99m-MDP) is an alternative study for characterization of VCF chronicity. Radiotracer is concentrated at sites of osteoblastic activity, which occurs as a result of the physiologic healing cascade at the site of a compression fracture [29]. Increased scintigraphic uptake may be encountered during the acute, subacute, and, in some cases, early chronic phases of fracture healing. In fact, studies have demonstrated residual activity in 10% of fractures 2 years after the injury and 3% of fractures 3 years after the injury [30]. Scintigraphy plays a role in determining which group of patients may benefit from procedural management. Metabolic activity on bone scan has been shown to be correlated with a favorable clinical response to cement augmentation [18, 31]. Scintigraphy may be of particular benefit compared to MRI in patients with chronic pain related to a compression deformity. In these patients, a fracture may be characterized as healed on MRI when the marrow signal returns to normal approximately 1–4 months post injury, while scintigraphy may detect the ongoing metabolic reparative processes which have been associated with clinical benefit following cement augmentation (Fig. 9.2) [18, 31, 32]. Other better established roles for bone scan, especially for patients unable to have MRI, include the exclusion of occult fractures when conventional radiography or CT is negative and VCF is suspected, and for screening the spine for VCFs at other levels when a single compression deformity is initially identified.

Bone scan imaging in the initial and acute setting has several limitations. First, in the initial setting, a fracture may be falsely negative on bone scan before the body is able to mount the inflammatory response and initiate the healing cascade. Studies have demonstrated this "lag period" for clinically significant metabolic activity to last for up to 1 week in an average patient and even longer in patients with osteoporosis or otherwise deficient osteoblastic activity [30, 33]. Additionally, when fractures are present at multiple levels with different chronicity, the "lag period" for the acute fractures combined with the prolonged uptake duration in the setting of more chronic fractures may confound the acutely painful/injured level and may result in treatment of pain free levels [19, 34]. Studies have indeed confirmed a decreasing specificity of bone scan for identifying the acutely symptomatic level as the number of hypermetabolic vertebrae increases, with only 50% specificity for new

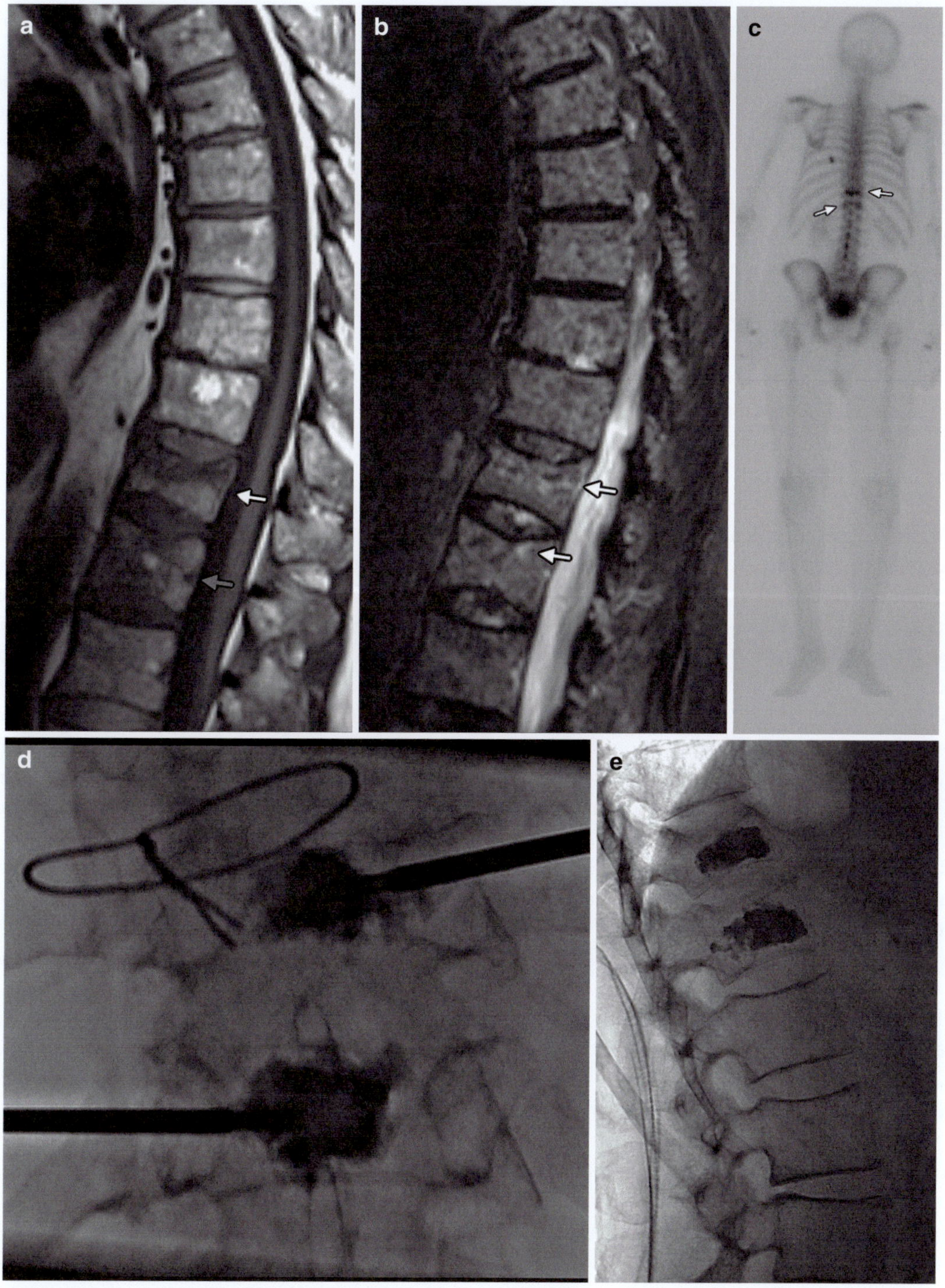

Fig. 9.2 A 93-year-old male with 3 months of low-back pain and no history of malignancy. (**a**) Sagittal T1 MRI demonstrates a wedge-shaped VCF at T11 (white arrow) and biconcave VCF at T12 (gray arrow), both of which demonstrate fracturing of the superior endplate and band-like low T1 signal with preserved remainder of the marrow fat signal suggestive of benign VCF. (**b**) Sagittal STIR MRI demonstrates only mild residual T2 hyperintensity at the fractured endplates (arrows) suggesting that the fracture is subacute to chronic in age. (**c**) Subsequent bone scan demonstrated linear uptake along the endplates of T11 and T12 (arrows), consistent with ongoing metabolic processes at the fracture sites. Therefore (**d** and **e**) vertebroplasty was performed, which resulted in improvement in the patients' symptoms

fractures when two vertebrae demonstrate uptake and 36% specificity when three or more demonstrate uptake [20, 35]. Finally, although increased metabolic activity in bone scan is considered highly sensitive for fracture, it is relatively nonspecific and can be seen in other conditions such as infections, neoplasms, and degenerative changes. Thus, given the limitations of bone scan in the setting of acute trauma and the fact that it is a lengthy exam, MRI is generally preferred for fully characterizing and establishing chronicity of vertebral compression fractures.

Early studies indicate promise for dual-energy CT for the accurate dating of a vertebral compression fracture [36–38]. Dual-energy CT scanners image the patient at two separate energy levels (conventionally 80 kV and 140 kV) and use differences in attenuation values (based on the photoelectric effect) to characterize the composition of tissues. This technology has proven sensitive and specific for detection of bone marrow edema in acute vertebral fractures. In fact, a recent study demonstrated a sensitivity of 92% and a specificity of 82% for the presence of marrow edema using a third-generation dual-energy scanner at 90 kV and 150 kV with a cutoff value of −42 Hounsfield units [38]. The study authors concluded that dual-energy CT could serve as an alternate imaging modality for establishing the chronicity of a vertebral fracture when contraindications to MRI are present [38].

Differentiating Benign Versus Pathologic Fractures

Introduction and Imaging Techniques

Vertebral compression fractures may occur with any process that undermines the structural integrity of a vertebral body, including most commonly osteoporosis and malignancy. Acute fractures present a diagnostic dilemma since the acute healing process, edema, and inflammation may confound the differentiation of benign versus malignant or infectious etiologies. On the other hand, a spontaneously healed chronic fracture can be confidently diagnosed as a benign osteoporotic fracture, since infectious and pathologic VCFs typically will not completely heal without appropriate treatment. Chronic osteoporotic VCFs are readily diagnosed on MRI when there is normalization of marrow signal and resolution of enhancement.

Conventional radiography and scintigraphy, while useful to initially diagnose VCF and collapse, are relatively nonspecific for differentiation of benign and malignant etiologies [39]. CT is likewise relatively nonspecific; however, several morphologic features seen together may suggest a specific etiology.

MRI is the cornerstone of vertebral compression fracture characterization, and a multitude of qualitative and quantitative features have been studied for better differentiation of benign and pathologic VCFs (Table 9.1). Traditionally, MRI protocols for spine imaging include conventional or fast spin echo T1- and T2-weighted images, fat-suppressed T2-weighted or STIR images, and gadolinium-enhanced T1-weighted images. Multiplanar images are acquired in the axial and the sagittal planes. Qualitative features assessed on conventional sequences include vertebral body morphology, marrow signal intensity and enhancement characteristics, as well as associated extravertebral features. A quantitative evaluation is performed with specialized sequences including diffusion-weighted imaging, perfusion imaging, and chemical shift imaging.

In patients with contraindication to MRI, positron emission tomography (PET)/CT may be useful for discrimination of benign and malignant VCF etiologies using a combination of metabolic and morphologic criteria. The gold standard for definitive characterization remains tissue diagnosis with percutaneous or open biopsy [40].

Morphology

Evaluation of the morphology of the acutely compressed vertebral body can yield important clues toward the etiology of a compression deformity. Morphologic features have conventionally been assessed with high-resolution multidetector CT imaging with multiplanar reformatting in the

Table 9.1 Imaging features favoring benign and pathologic vertebral compression fractures

Benign osteoporotic fracture	Pathologic fracture
Morphologic features	
Wedge or biconcave VCF	Crush VCF
Posterior wall: Normal, concave, or angulated	Posterior wall: smooth convex
Retropulsed “burst” fragment	No retropulsed fragments
Perpendicular fracture line extending to anterolateral or posterior cortex	No fracture line
No cortical erosion	Cortical erosion
Trabecular impaction/sclerotic fracture line paralleling endplate	Eroded rather than impacted trabecula
Vacuum cleft/fluid sign	No vacuum cleft
Marrow signal features	
Band-like T2 hyperintense signal (edema) paralleling fractured endplate	T2 hyperintense edema throughout vertebra
Sparing of normal fatty T1 marrow signal within portions of the vertebra	Infiltrative tumor (T1 hypointense to paraspinal muscle and intervertebral disk) throughout vertebra
T1 or T2 signal abnormality in vertebral body only	T1 or T2 signal abnormality extends to pedicles
Extravertebral features	
Thin, poorly marginated signal abnormality circumferentially about vertebra	Focal, nodular, enhancing soft tissue mass with extension into the epidural space
Healed benign VCFs at other levels	Metastases elsewhere in spine
Quantitative features	
DWI: increased diffusivity (high ADC, low SI on DWI)	DWI: restricted diffusivity (low ADC, high SI on DWI)
CSI: signal suppression on opposed phase imaging	CSI: maintained signal on opposed phase imaging
DCE: mild alteration in blood flow kinetics	DCE: marked alteration in blood flow kinetics
PET/CT	
Band-like linear FDG uptake	Round FDG uptake Uptake extending to posterior elements

axial and sagittal plane; however, it is important to note that the majority of these CT imaging features are readily assessed in modern, high-resolution thin slice MR images. Conventional radiography lacks the sensitivity for morphologic evaluation of the vertebra due to overlapping bony structures.

The most commonly described morphologic features for discrimination of benign from malignant osteoporotic vertebral compression fractures include:

- Vertebral Body Contour
  - Benign VCFs most commonly demonstrate anterior or middle vertebral body height loss, resulting in the classical “wedge” shaped or “biconcave” compression deformities. This is the result of a combination of repeated physiologic axial loading and kyphotic flexion forces on abnormally weakened osteoporotic bone [12, 13]. Malignant VCFs, on the other hand, are more likely to present with balanced anteroposterior “complete” crush-type height loss, since pathologic collapse typically only occurs once the majority of the AP dimension of the vertebra is infiltrated with tumor and eroded [12, 13, 28]. Compression deformity of the posterior aspect of the vertebral body is more likely to suggest pathologic fracture, which may relate to preferential blood flow and seeding of the posterior elements of the spine [41].
  - The contour of the anterior and posterior vertebral body walls in benign osteoporotic VCFs is most commonly of normal physiologic contour or increasingly concave compared to a normal vertebra. Less commonly, when the fracture extends to the anterior or posterior cortex, the contour may be convex outward with angulation at

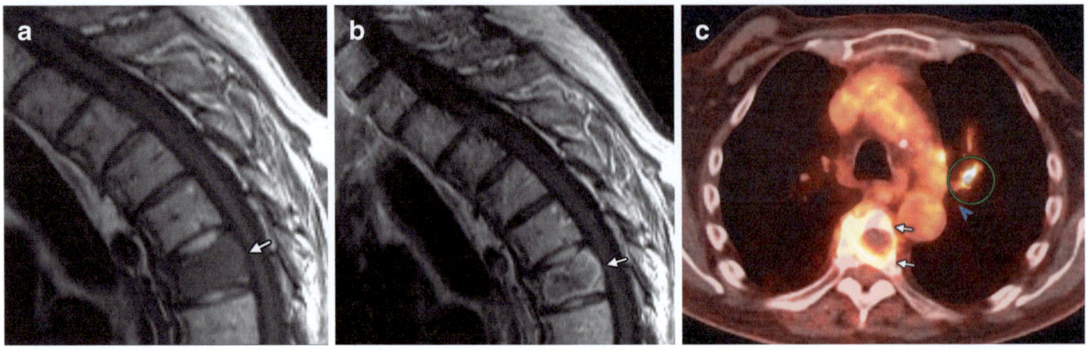

Fig. 9.3 An 88-year-old male with metastatic lung cancer and back pain. Sagittal T1 (**a**) pre-contrast and (**b**) post-contrast images demonstrate a crush-type VCF of T7 (arrow). The marrow is diffusely infiltrated (hypointense to the disk and skeletal muscle), and the posterior cortex of the vertebra is smoothly convex "bulging" outward, suggesting malignancy. (**c**) PET/CT confirms malignant VCF (white arrows) with high FDG uptake (SUVmax 5.4) at the site of the fracture. Lung mass is partially seen (green circle)

the acute fracture line. When the posterior wall is fractured, a retropulsed fragment may be present, which has also been associated with a benign process [22, 23, 25]. In malignancy, due to diffuse tumor infiltration, the posterior wall will be smoothly convex outward (Fig. 9.3). The smooth outward convexity represents an outward bulging of the minimally compressible malignant tissue [23, 25].

- Cortex
  - In the sagittal plane, the presence of a distinct fracture line paralleling the fractured endplate and extending to the anterolateral or posterior cortex of the vertebra is specific for benign fractures [22, 42]. Accuracy for benign fractures is increased when the fracture extends greater than 50% of the AP dimension of the vertebral body or extends to include both the anterolateral and posterior cortices (Fig. 9.1) [22, 42]. Reactive bone formation may be identified where the fracture extends to the endplate or cortex [22, 42]. In the axial plane, the benign fracture fragments may appear as closely opposed and nondisplaced with irregular shapes. This appearance has been termed the "puzzle sign," since the nondisplaced fragments may fit together like a puzzle [22]. Burst fractures arising from high-impact trauma are more highly comminuted than osteoporotic fractures, and the bone fragments are more disordered and distracted [28]. Malignant fractures are less likely than osteoporotic fractures to demonstrate any fracture line in pre-treatment imaging [42]. Additionally, malignant VCFs often demonstrate erosion of the cortices of the vertebral body and/or pedicles [42]. Cortical erosion typically occurs with metastases rather than primary marrow malignancies such as multiple myeloma, which are more likely to erode the trabecula while sparing the cortex [22, 42].
- Trabecula
  - In a benign fracture, the horizontal fracture line may be associated with a dense band of compressed cancellous bone paralleling the endplate. This dense band of trabecular bone may result from a combination of chronically accumulated microtrabecular compression deformities in the structurally weakened osteoporotic bone as well as sclerosis/callous formation resulting from the healing cascade [28, 41, 43]. In burst fractures, increased axial forces result in the outward displacement of fragments, rather than the gradual in-line impaction seen in low-energy osteoporotic fractures. Malignancies are more likely to erode rather than impact the trabecula prior to compression fracture [22, 42].

- Vacuum Cleft/Fluid Sign
  - A final morphologic sign of an acute benign osteoporotic compression fracture is the "vacuum cleft" sign on CT, which is analogous to the "fluid sign" on MR. These signs describe a gas or fluid-filled horizontally oriented cavity paralleling the compressed trabecula and vertebral fracture (Fig. 9.4). The cavity fills with gas when the patient is upright and gradually fills with fluid when the patient is supine [44]. Thus, on a rapid acquisition multidetector CT, one may encounter a gas filled "vacuum cleft." On MR, one may encounter a cleft with signal void (representing gas), or T2 hyperintense signal (representing fluid), depending on the duration the patient has been supine (Fig. 9.4) [43, 45, 46]. The presence of the vacuum cleft or fluid sign has likewise been associated with fracture severity, possibly suggesting a larger quantity of necrotic bone [45, 46].

Marrow Signal Intensity

- Marrow Edema and Inflammation
  - In benign osteoporotic VCFs, T2 hyperintense and T1 hypointense marrow edema may be distributed in a band-like pattern paralleling the horizontal fracture line and the impacted trabecula. There is a gradual transition from the band-like edema to normal fatty marrow signal extending toward the non-fractured endplate (Fig. 9.5) [25, 28, 41]. Thus, normal marrow signal, which appears slightly hyperintense to paraspinal muscle and the intervertebral disk, is commonly preserved in a portion of the vertebral body in a benign osteoporotic fracture (Fig. 9.5) [25, 47]. With malignancy, near-complete marrow replacement and trabecular erosion by tumor are generally required to weaken a vertebra sufficiently for a compression fracture to occur. Therefore, malignant VCFs commonly demonstrate abnormal marrow signal

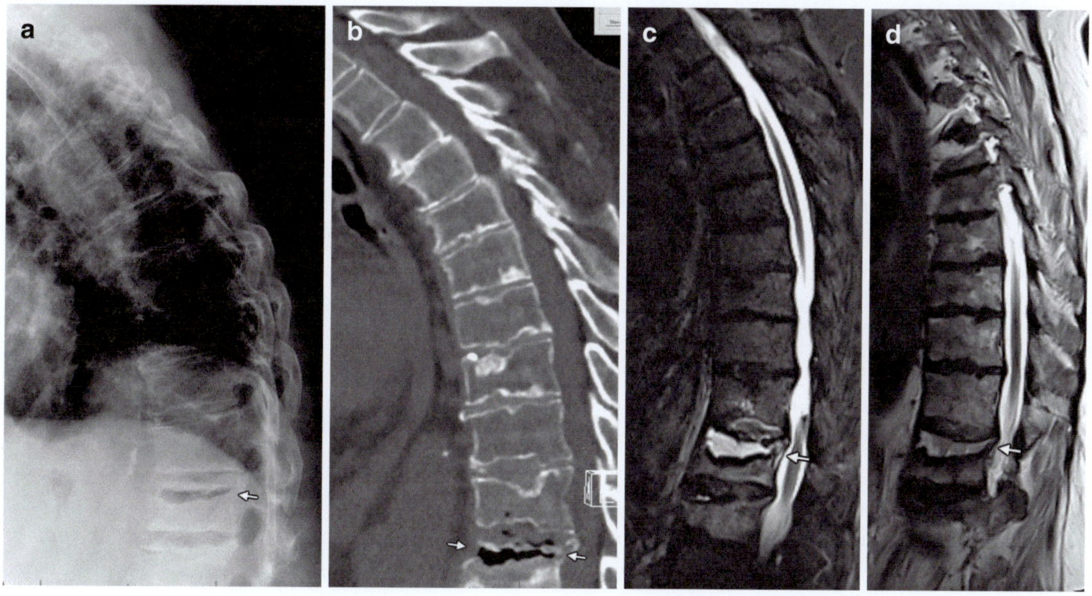

Fig. 9.4 A 67-year-old female with atraumatic low-back pain and new benign osteoporotic VCF of T12. (**a**) Lateral radiograph and (**b**) sagittal CT images demonstrate a linear gas-filled cleft which parallels the fractured T12 endplate ("vacuum cleft sign") (arrow). Subsequent (**c**) sagittal STIR MR image demonstrates filling of the cleft (arrow) with fluid ("fluid sign") while supine in the MRI scanner. (**d**) T2-weighted image demonstrates fluid-fluid levels (arrow) within the fluid cleft, suggesting a mixture of acute blood products and edema within the cleft

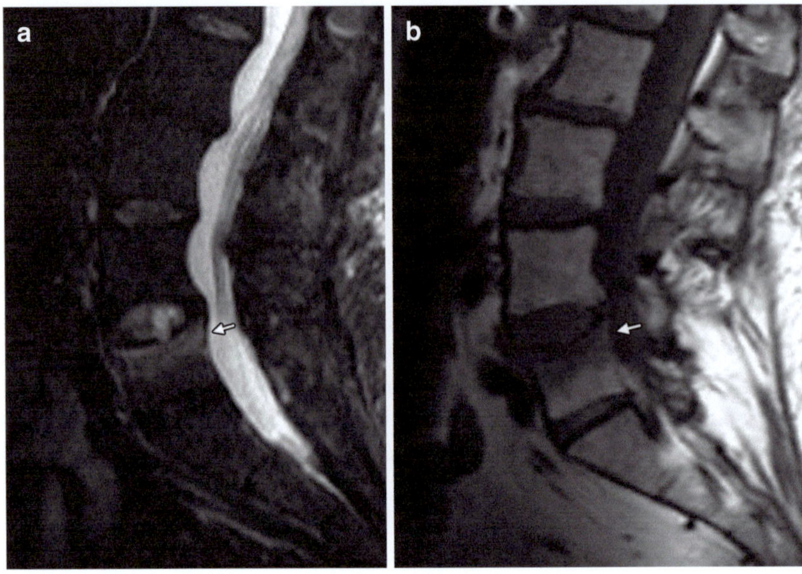

Fig. 9.5 An 85-year-old male with new onset low-back pain and no history of malignancy. Sagittal (**a**) STIR and (**b**) T1 pre-contrast images demonstrate band-like signal abnormality paralleling the fractured superior endplate of L5 (arrow). There is gradual transition to spared normal fatty marrow signal toward the inferior endplate of L5

throughout nearly the entirety of the vertebral body resulting from a combination of marrow edema (T2 hyperintense) and infiltrative tumor (T1 hypointense to paraspinal muscle and the intervertebral disk) (Fig. 9.6) [22, 23, 25]. Alternatively, though less likely, edema may be circular or spherically radiating outward from a rounded tumor deposit [25]. Finally, abnormal T2 or T1 marrow signal extending from the compressed vertebral body into to the pedicles and bony neural arch is suggestive of a metastatic VCF (Fig. 9.6); however, in rare cases, this can be seen in osteoporotic fractures when the fracture extends to the posterior column [22, 25, 28, 48, 49].

- Contrast Enhancement
  - Contrast enhancement in the setting of VCFs is best assessed with fat-suppressed T1-weighted sequences. Since contrast material and normal fatty marrow may have similar signal intensity, fat suppression is necessary to discriminate a boundary between abnormal enhancement and normal background fatty marrow. A benign fracture is suggested when contrast enhancement mimics the band-like trabecular impaction and reactive edema seen on T2 and pre-contrast T1-weighted sequences. In the majority of VCFs, however, contrast enhancement patterns are heterogeneous and insufficient for accurate discrimination between benign and malignant etiologies [23, 49, 50].

Extravertebral Features

- Paraspinal Soft Tissue
  - Both benign and malignant VCFs commonly present with extravertebral signal abnormalities. In benign VCFs, paravertebral signal abnormality is caused by edema and hemorrhage and typically presents as a thin (<10 mm), poorly marginated, T2-weighted signal abnormality circumferentially about the vertebral body [22, 42]. It is typically most pronounced anterolaterally and virtually always spares the epidural space [22]. In malignant VCFs, a paraspinal soft tissue mass will typically have a nodular contour and well-defined margin which characteristically enhances following contrast administration. The enhancing soft tissue mass will frequently protrude focally from the diffusely infiltrated vertebral body (Fig. 9.6) [25]. An enhancing paravertebral soft tissue mass

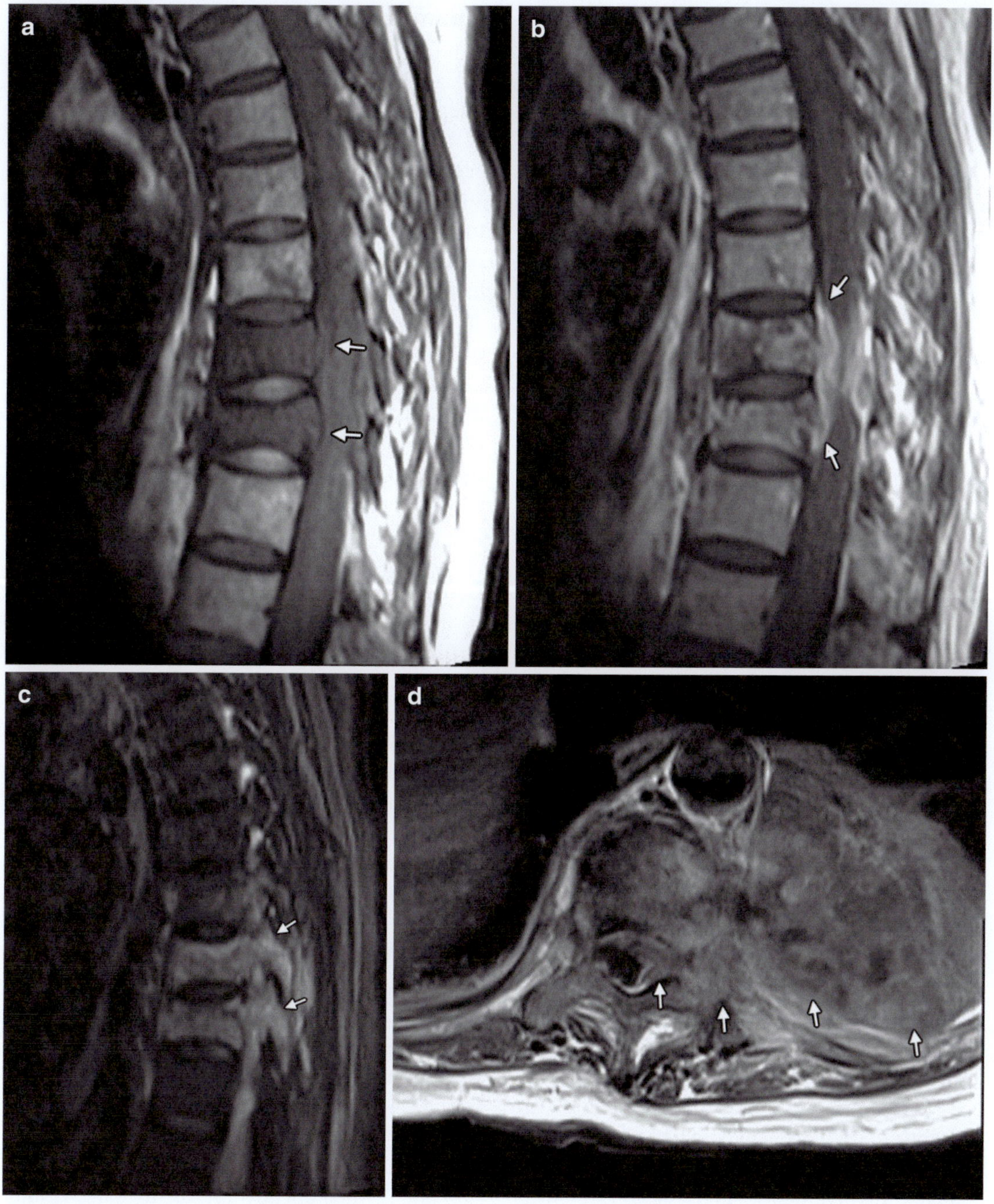

Fig. 9.6 A 67-year-old female with history of lung cancer and new pathologic VCF. (**a**) Sagittal T1 pre-contrast image demonstrates complete malignant infiltration of the marrow of T11 and T12 (arrows), which is hypointense to the paraspinal skeletal muscle and the intervertebral disk. (**b**) The post-contrast sagittal T1 images demonstrate heterogeneous enhancement of the disk and an enhancing epidural mass (arrow), a finding which is virtually pathognomonic for malignancy. (**c**) Sagittal STIR image demonstrates extension of the T2 hyperintense marrow edema to the pedicles (arrow), which is more commonly seen in malignancy. (**d**) Axial T1 post-contrast images demonstrate a focal nodular enhancing mass extending from the left lateral aspect of the vertebra which is contiguous with the dominant left lower lobe lung adenocarcinoma (arrow)

extending into the epidural space is virtually pathognomonic for malignancy (Fig. 9.6) [22, 28].

- Distant Osseous Findings
  - The presence of healed compression deformities at adjacent levels or distant levels can be suggestive of benign, osteoporotic VCF. This suggests that abnormally weakened bone is a result of a diffuse process, such as osteoporosis, rather than a focal abnormality such as a metastasis [22, 28]. On the other hand, the majority of malignant VCFs are associated with focal metastases in distant vertebra, particularly to the posterior elements of the spine, or in the ribs [25].

Conventional MR: Combined Evaluation of Features

Though morphologic features may suggest benign or malignant etiologies for VCFs, no single feature, in isolation, is sufficiently accurate for reliable discrimination. Recent studies have therefore examined the use of combinations of morphologic features to improve accuracy. One group created a scoring system of morphologic features and correctly characterized 99 of 100 fractures as benign or malignant based on the combination of the following features: pedicle or posterior element involvement (MRI), paravertebral extension (MRI), normal marrow signal preservation (MRI), intact posterior vertebral body cortex (MRI), osteolytic destruction (CT), and distinct fracture lines (CT) [51]. A second group demonstrated 99.3% probability of malignancy when three malignant features (diffuse posterior wall protrusion, pedicle involvement, and posterior wall involvement) were present, and the benign feature of a band-like edema pattern was absent [52]. When only two of the listed malignant features were present, probability of malignancy was 75–87% [52].

Quantitative Evaluation

A combined qualitative evaluation of signal intensity and morphologic features using CT and MRI is typically sufficiently accurate for discrimination between benign and malignant VCFs; however, at times, due to significant feature heterogeneity and overlap, diagnosis can remain challenging. Quantitative MRI techniques have been studied for characterization of VCFs in an attempt to improve diagnostic accuracy, simplify characterization, and reduce inter-reader variability in interpretation of often nonspecific qualitative features. The most well-studied quantitative techniques include diffusion-weighted imaging (DWI), chemical shift imaging (CSI), and dynamic contrast-enhanced imaging (DCI).

Diffusion-Weighted Imaging

Diffusion-weighted imaging is used to quantify the diffusivity of water molecules within a voxel of tissue. In the setting of acute osteoporotic VCFs, diffusivity is expected to be increased (high apparent diffusion coefficient (ADC), low signal intensity on DWI) as a result of interstitial fluid space expansion related to the acute inflammatory response and marrow edema (Fig. 9.7). On the contrary, in malignant VCFs, diffusivity is expected to decrease (low ADC and high signal intensity on DWI) as a result of interstitial fluid displacement and diffusivity restriction due to the infiltrating hypercellular tumor (Fig. 9.7) [53, 54]. Exceptions to this rule include both sclerotic metastases and previously treated metastases, which may appear hypointense on DWI and therefore cannot reliably be discriminated from benign fractures with DWI [55, 56].

Though theoretically useful, to date, results have been mixed regarding the utility of DWI to discriminate benign from malignant VCFs. Variability in outcomes are likely multifactorial relating to sequence acquisition variability (fat saturation, pulse sequences, and diffusion

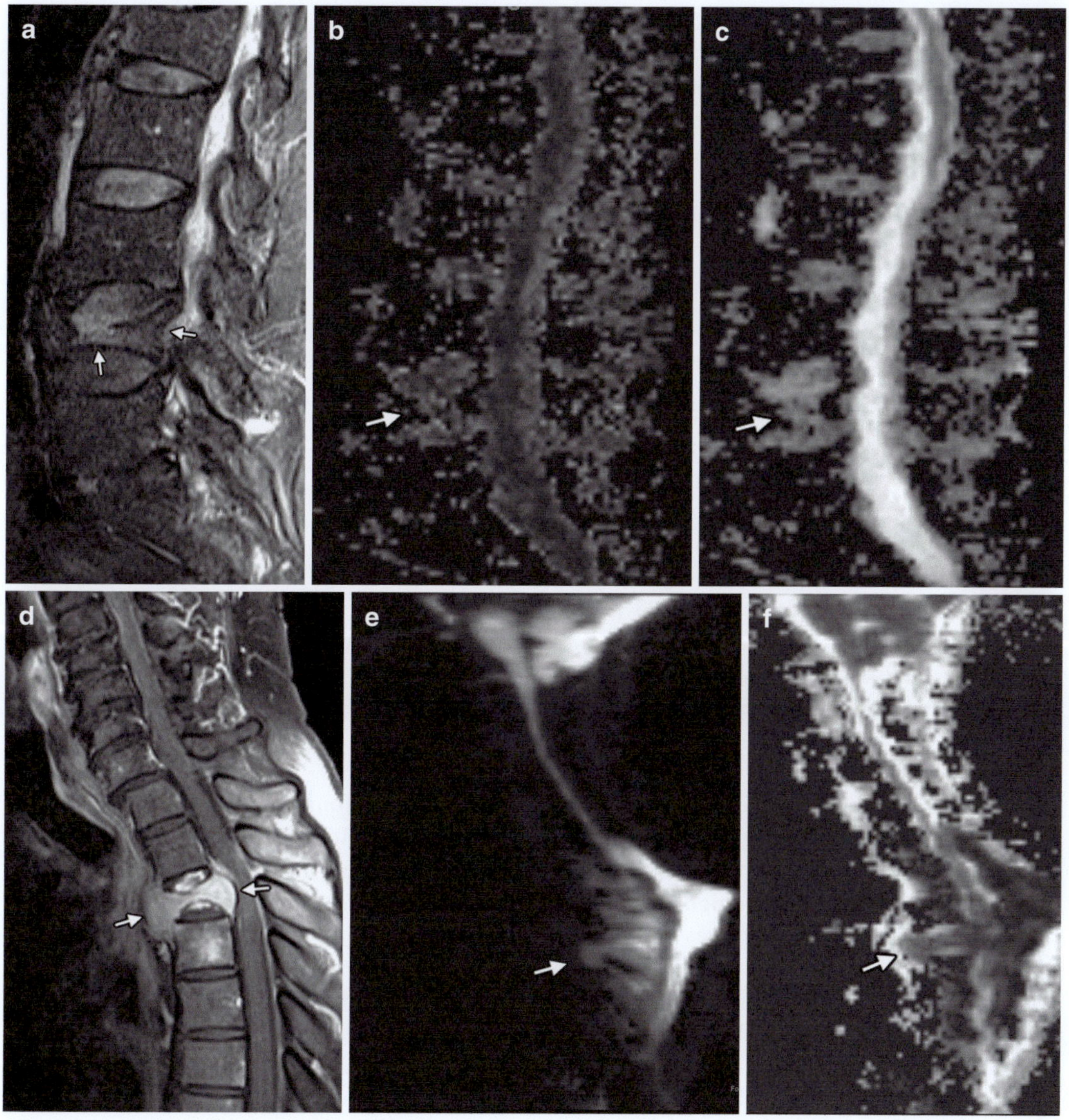

Fig. 9.7 A 63-year-old male with a benign osteoporotic VCF of L4. (**a**) Sagittal STIR images demonstrate a severe compression fracture of T4 with mild edema (arrow). (**b**) DWI images demonstrate isointensity to mild hyperintensity at the fracture site (arrow), but there is no loss of signal on (**c**) ADC image suggesting that the fracture is benign. (**d**) T1 post-contrast, (**e**) DWI, and (**f**) ADC images in a 74-year-old male with lymphoma demonstrate an enhancing compression deformity at T3 which is hyperintense on DWI and hypointense on ADC (arrows) consistent with a pathologic VCF

weighting/b-values), interpretation variability (qualitative assessment versus quantitative using ADC, as well as region of interest selection) [55–63], and possibly tumor inclusion characteristics (lytic, sclerotic, and/or treated metastases). These discrepancies may explain the wide ranges of ADC values demonstrated in benign and malignant fractures across studies available in the literature (benign, 0.32 to 2.23 × 10^{-3} mm^2/s, and malignant, 0.19 to 1.04 × 10^{-3} mm^2/s) [64]. In light of the significant variability in acquisition techniques, analysis, and cutoffs recommended, the optimal use for DWI may be in combination with signal intensity and morphologic features characterized on conventional MRI sequences in patients without sclerotic metastases or prior therapy [55, 56, 63]. In fact, recent studies have demonstrated that the inclusion of axial DWI with ADC measurements to conventional MR imaging features can improve the accuracy to discriminate benign from malignant fractures from 92% to 98% [63].

Chemical Shift Imaging

Chemical shift imaging provides a semiquantitative characterization of the relative fat and water content of a tissue on a voxel-by-voxel basis. When the relative quantity of fat and water is balanced in a tissue, such as in normal marrow or benign VCFs, the MRI signal of that tissue will be suppressed on "opposed phase" imaging. In contrast, when the fat content is diminished relative to the water content, such as when fatty marrow is replaced with infiltrative malignancy, the signal will be relatively maintained or will not suppress as much on opposed phase imaging. Therefore, the percentage drop in signal intensity on the opposed phase imaging compared to the signal on inphase imaging is expected to be greater in benign fractures as compared to malignant fractures (Fig. 9.8). Recent studies using dual-echo chemical shift-encoded imaging have demonstrated signal intensity drop cutoffs of 20–35% to accurately discriminate benign from malignant fractures [65–67]. A recent study using a 20% drop in signal as a cutoff value demonstrated a sensitivity of 91.7%, a specificity of 73.3%, and a diagnostic accuracy of 82.5% for chemical shift imaging to discriminate benign from malignant VCFs [68]. Another study performed using a T2∗-corrected six-echo Dixon method for chemical shift quantification of tissue fat content demonstrated a fat fraction of 5.26% to be 96% sensitive and 95% specific for discrimination of benign and malignant fractures [69]. As with DWI, significant feature overlap has been demonstrated in the acute phase of fracture healing,

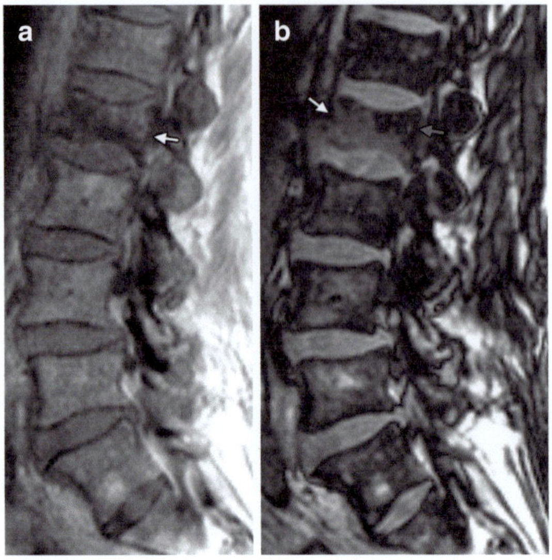

Fig. 9.8 An 89-year-old female with new onset back pain and no history of malignancy. Sagittal T1 (**a**) in phase and (**b**) opposed phase images demonstrate a wedge-shaped compression deformity of L1 (white arrow). Regions of signal drop on the opposed phase images are suggestive of normal fatty marrow sparing in a benign osteoporotic VCF (gray arrow)

which may confound results when evaluated in isolation. Therefore, evaluation in concert with conventional imaging parameters remains recommended [59].

Dynamic Contrast-Enhanced Imaging

Dynamic contrast-enhanced MRI is used to evaluate qualitative and quantitative hemodynamic characteristics of tissues by measuring relative signal intensity changes over time after the administration of gadolinium. Both benign osteoporotic VCFs and malignant VCFs are expected to have altered contrast enhancement kinetics compared to normal marrow. Expected differences in contrast enhancement kinetics include more rapid initial contrast uptake, increased peak maximal enhancement, and more rapid contrast washout [70–73]. Altered blood flow kinetics are expected to be mild in benign VCFs due to the acute inflammatory cascade and more marked in malignant VCFs due to tumor neovascularity; however, significant overlap is observed between these etiologies. Results have been mixed for the discrimination of benign and malignant VCFs using dynamic contrast enhancement MRI [70–73]. This may be due to the overlapping kinetics, variability of injection protocols, fracture age, and patient features including patient age, spinal level, and fat/water content in bone marrow [70–73]. Recent studies have demonstrated accurate discrimination of benign and malignant fractures in the acute phase when quantitative perfusion parameters including plasma volume and vessel permeability are evaluated; however, more research is required in this area for validation [74].

Evaluation When MRI Is Contraindicated

In patients who cannot receive MRI, morphologic imaging alone with CT or combination morphologic and functional imaging with 18F fluorodeoxyglucose (FDG) PET/CT or single-photon emission computed tomography (SPECT)/CT can be performed.

Though not as well studied as MRI, 18F FDG PET/CT has proven useful for discrimination of benign and malignant VCFs, based on the principle that metabolically active tumor cells should metabolize glucose at an increased rate compared to normal marrow. Although osteoporotic VCFs can demonstrate FDG uptake in acute and subacute injuries for up to 3 months, it typically occurs at a lower uptake level than malignant VCFs [75–78]. There is however significant overlap in ranges of FDG uptake between malignant VCFs and acute benign VCFs [75–78]. Analogous to metabolic imaging with bone scintigraphy, absent uptake in a VCF is diagnostic of a healed VCF [78]. If uptake is present, diagnosis can be suggested based on both the pattern of uptake and the maximum tracer uptake. Rounded tracer uptake or uptake involving the vertebral body and the posterior elements/pedicles contiguously is suggestive of malignancy (Fig. 9.9) [79]. Linear tracer uptake paralleling the disk space or at a facet joint is suggestive of a benign process (Fig. 9.10) [79]. Studies have demonstrated a maximum standardized uptake value (SUVmax) of greater than 3.0 to be suggestive of a pathologic fracture, with optimal accuracy when SUVmax of 4.25 is exceeded, yielding a sensitivity of 85% and a specificity of 71% [77, 80, 81]. In a comparison study, PET/CT at optimal SUVmax of 4.25 was demonstrated to be more sensitive (85% versus 64%) but slightly less specific (71% versus 82%) than an MRI combined evaluation of three conventional features (cortical bulge, epidural mass, and pedicle enhancement) for discrimination of benign from malignant VCFs [78]. Studies have concluded that the optimal role of PET/CT is in patients with contraindications for MRI and in patients with equivocal or nondiagnostic MRI findings, rather than as a primary screening test [77, 78].

SPECT with technetium 99m hydroxymethylene diphosphonate (Tc-99m HMDP) has also been evaluated in comparison with MRI with morphologic criteria for discrimination of benign and pathologic VCFs. A study by Tokuda et al. demonstrated superior sensitivity and specificity of MRI compared to SPECT in compression fractures with partial replacement of the fatty marrow on T1-weighted images [82]. Sensitivity and specificity, however, were comparable between SPECT and MRI when there was complete replacement of the fatty marrow on T1-weighted imaging (sensitivity up to 87.1 for SPECT and 89.5% for MRI; specificity up to 89.5% for SPECT and 89.5% for MRI) [82].

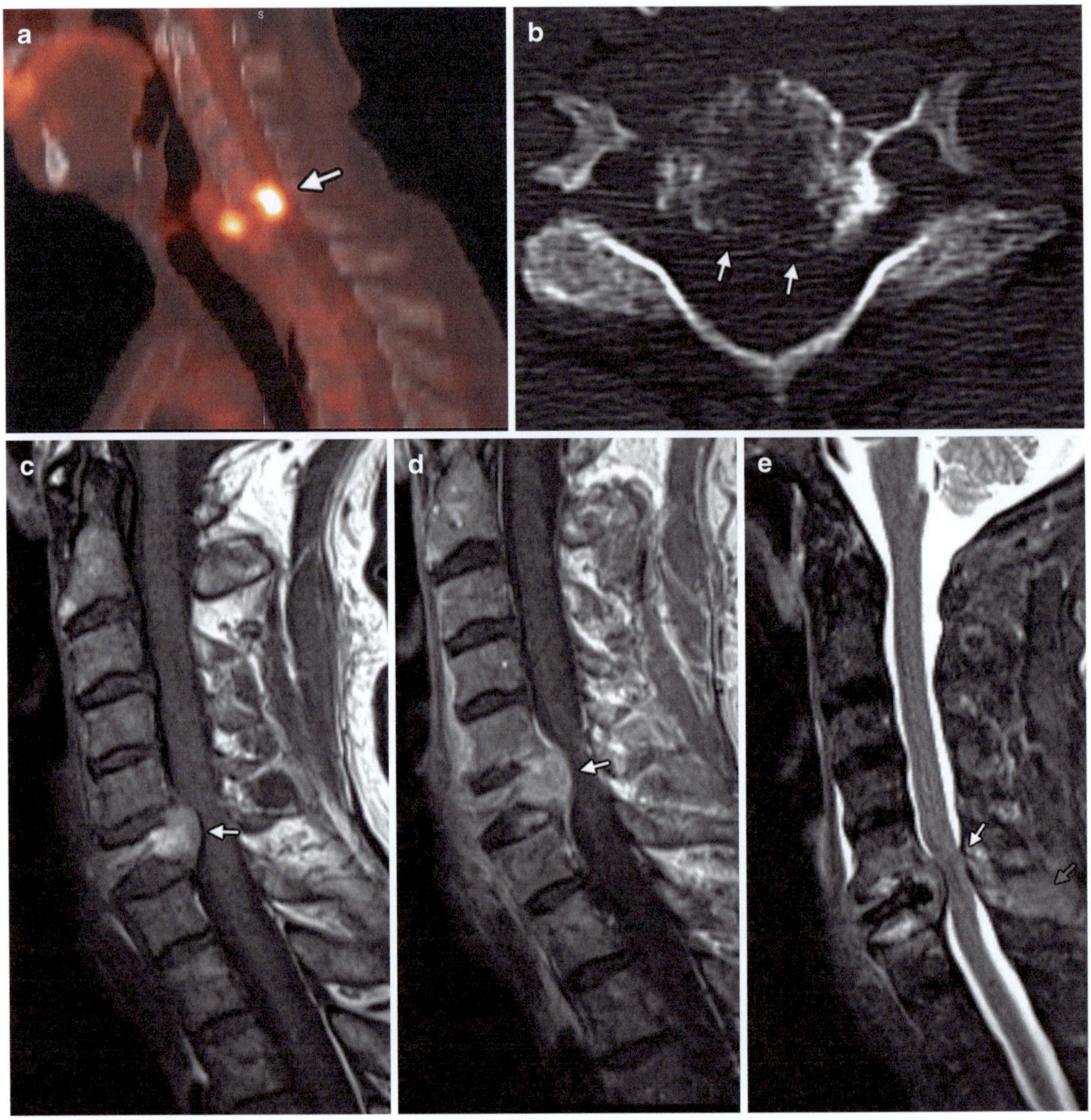

Fig. 9.9 A 70-year-old male with back pain and pathologic VCF. (**a**) Sagittal PET/CT demonstrates rounded FDG uptake at the site of VCF (with high SUVmax of 10.1) (arrow). (**b**) Simultaneously performed axial CT demonstrates erosion of the posterolateral cortex of T5 (arrow). Sagittal T1 (**c**) pre-contrast and (**d**) post-contrast images demonstrate an inherently T1 hyperintense enhancing mass with near-complete infiltration of the T5 vertebra with epidural extension (arrow). (**e**) Sagittal STIR image demonstrates signal abnormality extension into the posterior elements (white arrow) and adjacent posterior soft tissues (gray arrow), which are likewise suggestive of a malignant VCF

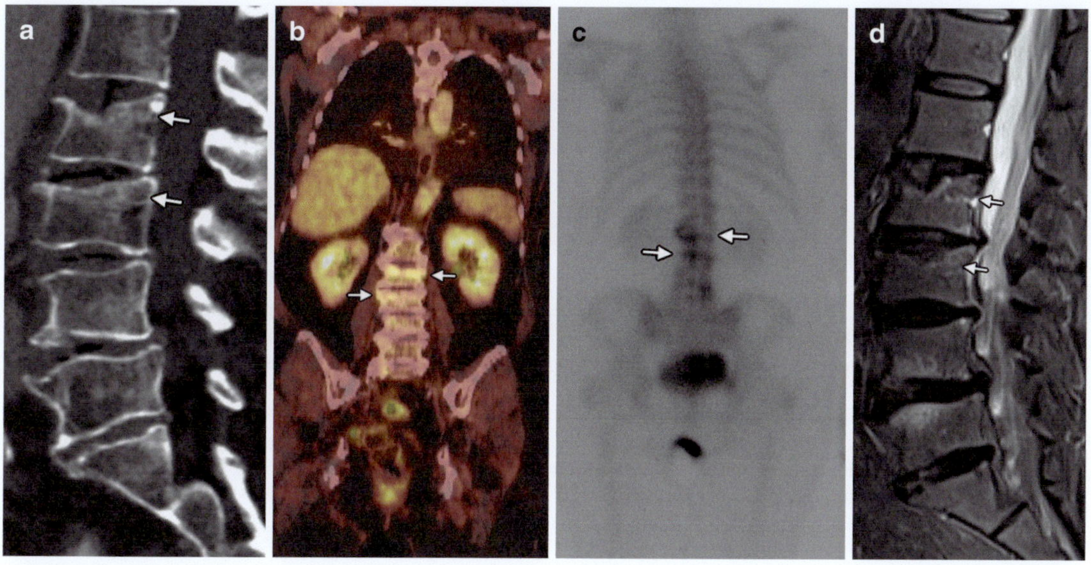

Fig. 9.10 An 80-year-old man with history of colon cancer status post colectomy with new benign VCF. (**a**) Sagittal CT images demonstrate wedge-type VCFs of L2 and L3, with linear trabecular impaction/sclerosis paralleling the fractured superior endplates (arrows). (**b**) PET/CT and (**c**) bone scan demonstrate linear uptake (SUVmax of 4.1) (arrows) which also parallels the endplates, suggesting a benign etiology for the fractures. Sagittal (**d**) STIR image demonstrates mild band-like T2 signal paralleling the endplate (arrows), transitioning to normal fatty marrow signal in the remainder of the vertebra

References

1. Patel ND BD, Burns J, et al. ACR appropriateness criteria: low back pain. Available at https://acsearch.acr.org/docs/69483/Narrative/. American College of Radiology; [8/6/2017].
2. Daffner RH WB, Wippold FJ, et al. ACR appropriateness criteria: suspected spine trauma. Available at https://acsearch.acr.org/docs/69359/Narrative/. American College of Radiology; [8/6/2017].
3. Williams AL, Gornet MF, Burkus JK. CT evaluation of lumbar interbody fusion: current concepts. AJNR Am J Neuroradiol. 2005;26(8):2057–66.
4. Hoffman JR, Mower WR, Wolfson AB, Todd KH, Zucker MI. Validity of a set of clinical criteria to rule out injury to the cervical spine in patients with blunt trauma. National Emergency X-Radiography Utilization Study Group. N Engl J Med. 2000;343(2):94–9.
5. Stiell IG, Wells GA, Vandemheen KL, Clement CM, Lesiuk H, De Maio VJ, et al. The Canadian C-spine rule for radiography in alert and stable trauma patients. JAMA. 2001;286(15):1841–8.
6. Hanson JA, Blackmore CC, Mann FA, Wilson AJ. Cervical spine injury: a clinical decision rule to identify high-risk patients for helical CT screening. AJR Am J Roentgenol. 2000;174(3):713–7.
7. Old JL, Calvert M. Vertebral compression fractures in the elderly. Am Fam Physician. 2004;69(1):111–6.
8. Patel U, Skingle S, Campbell GA, Crisp AJ, Boyle IT. Clinical profile of acute vertebral compression fractures in osteoporosis. Br J Rheumatol. 1991;30(6):418–21.
9. Genant HK, Wu CY, van Kuijk C, Nevitt MC. Vertebral fracture assessment using a semiquantitative technique. J Bone Miner Res. 1993;8(9):1137–48.
10. Cummings SR, Kelsey JL, Nevitt MC, O'Dowd KJ. Epidemiology of osteoporosis and osteoporotic fractures. Epidemiol Rev. 1985;7:178–208.
11. Alexandru D, So W. Evaluation and management of vertebral compression fractures. Perm J. 2012 Fall;16(4):46–51.
12. Ismail AA, Cooper C, Felsenberg D, Varlow J, Kanis JA, Silman AJ, et al. Number and type of vertebral deformities: epidemiological characteristics and relation to back pain and height loss. European Vertebral Osteoporosis Study Group. Osteoporos Int. 1999;9(3):206–13.
13. Buckley JM, Kuo CC, Cheng LC, Loo K, Motherway J, Slyfield C, et al. Relative strength of thoracic vertebrae in axial compression versus flexion. Spine J. 2009;9(6):478–85.
14. Nevitt MC, Ettinger B, Black DM, Stone K, Jamal SA, Ensrud K, et al. The association of radiographically detected vertebral fractures with back pain and function: a prospective study. Ann Intern Med. 1998;128(10):793–800.
15. Hurxthal LM. Measurement of anterior vertebral compressions and biconcave vertebrae.

Am J Roentgenol Radium Therapy, Nucl Med. 1968;103(3):635–44.
16. Lunt M, Ismail AA, Felsenberg D, Cooper C, Kanis JA, Reeve J, et al. Defining incident vertebral deformities in population studies: a comparison of morphometric criteria. Osteoporos Int. 2002;13(10):809–15.
17. Gaitanis IN, Hadjipavlou AG, Katonis PG, Tzermiadianos MN, Pasku DS, Patwardhan AG. Balloon kyphoplasty for the treatment of pathological vertebral compressive fractures. Eur Spine J. 2005;14(3):250–60.
18. Maynard AS, Jensen ME, Schweickert PA, Marx WF, Short JG, Kallmes DF. Value of bone scan imaging in predicting pain relief from percutaneous vertebroplasty in osteoporotic vertebral fractures. AJNR Am J Neuroradiol. 2000;21(10):1807–12.
19. Park SY, Lee SH, Suh SW, Park JH, Kim TG. Usefulness of MRI in determining the appropriate level of cement augmentation for acute osteoporotic vertebral compression fractures. J Spinal Disord Tech. 2013;26(3):E80–5.
20. Lin HH, Chou PH, Wang ST, Yu JK, Chang MC, Liu CL. Determination of the painful level in osteoporotic vertebral fractures – retrospective comparison between plain film, bone scan, and magnetic resonance imaging. J Chin Med Assoc. 2015;78(12):714–8.
21. Lenchik L, Rogers LF, Delmas PD, Genant HK. Diagnosis of osteoporotic vertebral fractures: importance of recognition and description by radiologists. AJR Am J Roentgenol. 2004;183(4):949–58.
22. Laredo JD, Lakhdari K, Bellaiche L, Hamze B, Janklewicz P, Tubiana JM. Acute vertebral collapse: CT findings in benign and malignant nontraumatic cases. Radiology. 1995;194(1):41–8.
23. Cuenod CA, Laredo JD, Chevret S, Hamze B, Naouri JF, Chapaux X, et al. Acute vertebral collapse due to osteoporosis or malignancy: appearance on unenhanced and gadolinium-enhanced MR images. Radiology. 1996;199(2):541–9.
24. Lakadamyali H, Tarhan NC, Ergun T, Cakir B, Agildere AM. STIR sequence for depiction of degenerative changes in posterior stabilizing elements in patients with lower back pain. AJR Am J Roentgenol. 2008;191(4):973–9.
25. Jung HS, Jee WH, McCauley TR, Ha KY, Choi KH. Discrimination of metastatic from acute osteoporotic compression spinal fractures with MR imaging. Radiographics. 2003;23(1):179–87.
26. Tsujio T, Nakamura H, Terai H, Hoshino M, Namikawa T, Matsumura A, et al. Characteristic radiographic or magnetic resonance images of fresh osteoporotic vertebral fractures predicting potential risk for nonunion: a prospective multicenter study. Spine (Phila Pa 1976). 2011;36(15):1229–35.
27. Kanchiku T, Imajo Y, Suzuki H, Yoshida Y, Taguchi T. Usefulness of an early MRI-based classification system for predicting vertebral collapse and pseudoarthrosis after osteoporotic vertebral fractures. J Spinal Disord Tech. 2014;27(2):E61–5.
28. Yuh WT, Zachar CK, Barloon TJ, Sato Y, Sickels WJ, Hawes DR. Vertebral compression fractures: distinction between benign and malignant causes with MR imaging. Radiology. 1989;172(1):215–8.
29. Collier BD Jr, Fogelman I, Brown ML. Bone scintigraphy: part 2. Orthopedic bone scanning. J Nucl Med. 1993;34(12):2241–6.
30. Matin P. The appearance of bone scans following fractures, including immediate and long-term studies. J Nucl Med. 1979;20(12):1227–31.
31. Masala S, Schillaci O, Massari F, Danieli R, Ursone A, Fiori R, et al. MRI and bone scan imaging in the preoperative evaluation of painful vertebral fractures treated with vertebroplasty and kyphoplasty. In Vivo. 2005;19(6):1055–60.
32. Brown DB, Gilula LA, Sehgal M, Shimony JS. Treatment of chronic symptomatic vertebral compression fractures with percutaneous vertebroplasty. AJR Am J Roentgenol. 2004;182(2):319–22.
33. Jordan E, Choe D, Miller T, Chamarthy M, Brook A, Freeman LM. Utility of bone scintigraphy to determine the appropriate vertebral augmentation levels. Clin Nucl Med. 2010;35(9):687–91.
34. Benz BK, Gemery JM, McIntyre JJ, Eskey CJ. Value of immediate preprocedure magnetic resonance imaging in patients scheduled to undergo vertebroplasty or kyphoplasty. Spine (Phila Pa 1976). 2009;34(6):609–12.
35. Kim JH, Kim JI, Jang BH, Seo JG. The comparison of bone scan and MRI in osteoporotic compression fractures. Asian Spine J. 2010;4(2):89–95.
36. Bierry G, Venkatasamy A, Kremer S, Dosch JC, Dietemann JL. Dual-energy CT in vertebral compression fractures: performance of visual and quantitative analysis for bone marrow edema demonstration with comparison to MRI. Skelet Radiol. 2014;43(4):485–92.
37. Wang CK, Tsai JM, Chuang MT, Wang MT, Huang KY, Lin RM. Bone marrow edema in vertebral compression fractures: detection with dual-energy CT. Radiology. 2013;269(2):525–33.
38. Petritsch B, Kosmala A, Weng AM, Krauss B, Heidemeier A, Wagner R, et al. Vertebral compression fractures: third-generation dual-energy CT for detection of bone marrow edema at visual and quantitative analyses. Radiology. 2017;284(1):161–8.
39. Fogelman I, Boyle IT. The bone scan in clinical practice. Scott Med J. 1980;25(1):45–9.
40. Aggarwal A, Salunke P, Shekhar BR, Chhabra R, Singh P, Bhattacharya A, et al. The role of magnetic resonance imaging and positron emission tomography-computed tomography combined in differentiating benign from malignant lesions contributing to vertebral compression fractures. Surg Neurol Int. 2013;4(Suppl 5):S323–6.
41. Link TM, Guglielmi G, van Kuijk C, Adams JE. Radiologic assessment of osteoporotic vertebral fractures: diagnostic and prognostic implications. Eur Radiol. 2005;15(8):1521–32.

42. Kubota T, Yamada K, Ito H, Kizu O, Nishimura T. High-resolution imaging of the spine using multidetector-row computed tomography: differentiation between benign and malignant vertebral compression fractures. J Comput Assist Tomogr. 2005;29(5):712–9.
43. Uetani M, Hashmi R, Hayashi K. Malignant and benign compression fractures: differentiation and diagnostic pitfalls on MRI. Clin Radiol. 2004;59(2):124–31.
44. Linn J, Birkenmaier C, Hoffmann RT, Reiser M, Baur-Melnyk A. The intravertebral cleft in acute osteoporotic fractures: fluid in magnetic resonance imaging-vacuum in computed tomography? Spine (Phila Pa 1976). 2009;34(2):E88–93.
45. Baur A, Stabler A, Arbogast S, Duerr HR, Bartl R, Reiser M. Acute osteoporotic and neoplastic vertebral compression fractures: fluid sign at MR imaging. Radiology. 2002;225(3):730–5.
46. Malghem J, Maldague B, Labaisse MA, Dooms G, Duprez T, Devogelaer JP, et al. Intravertebral vacuum cleft: changes in content after supine positioning. Radiology. 1993;187(2):483–7.
47. Carroll KW, Feller JF, Tirman PF. Useful internal standards for distinguishing infiltrative marrow pathology from hematopoietic marrow at MRI. J Magn Reson Imaging. 1997;7(2):394–8.
48. Ishiyama M, Fuwa S, Numaguchi Y, Kobayashi N, Saida Y. Pedicle involvement on MR imaging is common in osteoporotic compression fractures. AJNR Am J Neuroradiol. 2010;31(4):668–73.
49. Shih TT, Huang KM, Li YW. Solitary vertebral collapse: distinction between benign and malignant causes using MR patterns. J Magn Reson Imaging. 1999;9(5):635–42.
50. Leeds NE, Kumar AJ, Zhou XJ, McKinnon GC. Magnetic resonance imaging of benign spinal lesions simulating metastasis: role of diffusion-weighted imaging. Top Magn Reson Imaging. 2000;11(4):224–34.
51. Yuzawa Y, Ebara S, Kamimura M, Tateiwa Y, Kinoshita T, Itoh H, et al. Magnetic resonance and computed tomography-based scoring system for the differential diagnosis of vertebral fractures caused by osteoporosis and malignant tumors. J Orthop Sci. 2005;10(4):345–52.
52. Takigawa T, Tanaka M, Sugimoto Y, Tetsunaga T, Nishida K, Ozaki T. Discrimination between malignant and benign vertebral fractures using magnetic resonance imaging. Asian Spine J. 2017;11(3):478–83.
53. Le Bihan DJ. Differentiation of benign versus pathologic compression fractures with diffusion-weighted MR imaging: a closer step toward the "holy grail" of tissue characterization? Radiology. 1998;207(2):305–7.
54. Baur A, Stabler A, Bruning R, Bartl R, Krodel A, Reiser M, et al. Diffusion-weighted MR imaging of bone marrow: differentiation of benign versus pathologic compression fractures. Radiology. 1998;207(2):349–56.
55. Baur A, Huber A, Durr HR, Nikolaou K, Stabler A, Deimling M, et al. [Differentiation of benign osteoporotic and neoplastic vertebral compression fractures with a diffusion-weighted, steady-state free precession sequence]. Rofo. 2002;174(1):70–5.
56. Byun WM, Shin SO, Chang Y, Lee SJ, Finsterbusch J, Frahm J. Diffusion-weighted MR imaging of metastatic disease of the spine: assessment of response to therapy. AJNR Am J Neuroradiol. 2002;23(6):906–12.
57. Maeda M, Sakuma H, Maier SE, Takeda K. Quantitative assessment of diffusion abnormalities in benign and malignant vertebral compression fractures by line scan diffusion-weighted imaging. AJR Am J Roentgenol. 2003;181(5):1203–9.
58. Balliu E, Vilanova JC, Pelaez I, Puig J, Remollo S, Barcelo C, et al. Diagnostic value of apparent diffusion coefficients to differentiate benign from malignant vertebral bone marrow lesions. Eur J Radiol. 2009;69(3):560–6.
59. Geith T, Schmidt G, Biffar A, Dietrich O, Durr HR, Reiser M, et al. Comparison of qualitative and quantitative evaluation of diffusion-weighted MRI and chemical-shift imaging in the differentiation of benign and malignant vertebral body fractures. AJR Am J Roentgenol. 2012;199(5):1083–92.
60. Tang G, Liu Y, Li W, Yao J, Li B, Li P. Optimization of b value in diffusion-weighted MRI for the differential diagnosis of benign and malignant vertebral fractures. Skelet Radiol. 2007;36(11):1035–41.
61. Chan JH, Peh WC, Tsui EY, Chau LF, Cheung KK, Chan KB, et al. Acute vertebral body compression fractures: discrimination between benign and malignant causes using apparent diffusion coefficients. Br J Radiol. 2002;75(891):207–14.
62. Zhou XJ, Leeds NE, McKinnon GC, Kumar AJ. Characterization of benign and metastatic vertebral compression fractures with quantitative diffusion MR imaging. AJNR Am J Neuroradiol. 2002;23(1):165–70.
63. Sung JK, Jee WH, Jung JY, Choi M, Lee SY, Kim YH, et al. Differentiation of acute osteoporotic and malignant compression fractures of the spine: use of additive qualitative and quantitative axial diffusion-weighted MR imaging to conventional MR imaging at 3.0 T. Radiology. 2014;271(2):488–98.
64. Dietrich O, Biffar A, Reiser MF, Baur-Melnyk A. Diffusion-weighted imaging of bone marrow. Semin Musculoskelet Radiol. 2009;13(2):134–44.
65. Ragab Y, Emad Y, Gheita T, Mansour M, Abou-Zeid A, Ferrari S, et al. Differentiation of osteoporotic and neoplastic vertebral fractures by chemical shift {in-phase and out of phase} MR imaging. Eur J Radiol. 2009;72(1):125–33.
66. Erly WK, Oh ES, Outwater EK. The utility of in-phase/opposed-phase imaging in differentiating malignancy from acute benign compression fractures of the spine. AJNR Am J Neuroradiol. 2006;27(6):1183–8.
67. Zajick DC Jr, Morrison WB, Schweitzer ME, Parellada JA, Carrino JA. Benign and malignant processes: normal values and differentiation with chemi-

cal shift MR imaging in vertebral marrow. Radiology. 2005;237(2):590–6.
68. Douis H, Davies AM, Jeys L, Sian P. Chemical shift MRI can aid in the diagnosis of indeterminate skeletal lesions of the spine. Eur Radiol. 2016;26(4):932–40.
69. Kim DH, Yoo HJ, Hong SH, Choi JY, Chae HD, Chung BM. Differentiation of Acute Osteoporotic and Malignant Vertebral Fractures by Quantification of Fat Fraction With a Dixon MRI Sequence. AJR Am J Roentgenol. 2017;209(6):1331–9.
70. Chen WT, Shih TT, Chen RC, Lo HY, Chou CT, Lee JM, et al. Blood perfusion of vertebral lesions evaluated with gadolinium-enhanced dynamic MRI: in comparison with compression fracture and metastasis. J Magn Reson Imaging. 2002;15(3):308–14.
71. Biffar A, Dietrich O, Sourbron S, Duerr HR, Reiser MF, Baur-Melnyk A. Diffusion and perfusion imaging of bone marrow. Eur J Radiol. 2010;76(3):323–8.
72. Geith T, Biffar A, Schmidt G, Sourbron S, Durr HR, Reiser M, et al. Quantitative analysis of acute benign and malignant vertebral body fractures using dynamic contrast-enhanced MRI. AJR Am J Roentgenol. 2013;200(6):W635–43.
73. Savvopoulou V, Maris TG, Koureas A, Gouliamos A, Moulopoulos LA. Degenerative endplate changes of the lumbosacral spine: dynamic contrast-enhanced MRI profiles related to age, sex, and spinal level. J Magn Reson Imaging. 2011;33(2):382–9.
74. Arevalo-Perez J, Peck KK, Lyo JK, Holodny AI, Lis E, Karimi S. Differentiating benign from malignant vertebral fractures using T1 -weighted dynamic contrast-enhanced MRI. J Magn Reson Imaging. 2015;42(4):1039–47.
75. Zhuang H, Sam JW, Chacko TK, Duarte PS, Hickeson M, Feng Q, et al. Rapid normalization of osseous FDG uptake following traumatic or surgical fractures. Eur J Nucl Med Mol Imaging. 2003;30(8):1096–103.
76. Shon IH, Fogelman I. F-18 FDG positron emission tomography and benign fractures. Clin Nucl Med. 2003;28(3):171–5.
77. Bredella MA, Essary B, Torriani M, Ouellette HA, Palmer WE. Use of FDG-PET in differentiating benign from malignant compression fractures. Skelet Radiol. 2008;37(5):405–13.
78. Cho WI, Chang UK. Comparison of MR imaging and FDG-PET/CT in the differential diagnosis of benign and malignant vertebral compression fractures. J Neurosurg Spine. 2011;14(2):177–83.
79. Bohdiewicz PJ, Wong CY, Kondas D, Gaskill M, Dworkin HJ. High predictive value of F-18 FDG PET patterns of the spine for metastases or benign lesions with good agreement between readers. Clin Nucl Med. 2003;28(12):966–70.
80. Kato K, Aoki J, Endo K. Utility of FDG-PET in differential diagnosis of benign and malignant fractures in acute to subacute phase. Ann Nucl Med. 2003;17(1):41–6.
81. Shin DS, Shon OJ, Byun SJ, Choi JH, Chun KA, Cho IH. Differentiation between malignant and benign pathologic fractures with F-18-fluoro-2-deoxy-D-glucose positron emission tomography/computed tomography. Skelet Radiol. 2008;37(5):415–21.
82. Tokuda O, Harada Y, Ueda T, Ohishi Y, Matsunaga N. Malignant versus benign vertebral compression fractures: can we use bone SPECT as a substitute for MR imaging? Nucl Med Commun. 2011;32(3):192–8.

10 Natural History and Long-Term Sequelae of Vertebral Compression Fractures

John A. Buza III and Emmanuel Menga

Introduction

Osteoporotic vertebral compression fractures (VCFs) are increasing in prevalence with the aging population [1]. The majority of these fractures are treated conservatively, and therefore, understanding the natural history and long-term sequelae of these fractures is important for the practitioner. The clinical consequences of VCF can include pain, poor physical functioning, kyphosis, loss of appetite, depression, and increased mortality. One of the primary concerns following VCF is the risk of subsequent VCF at a different vertebral level. In recognizing these clinical sequelae, the practitioner can optimize the care of the patient presenting with VCF. This chapter is aimed at presenting the natural history and long-term sequelae associated with these common fractures.

J. A. Buza III
Department of Orthopedic Surgery, NYU Langone Orthopedic Hospital, NYU Langone Medical Center, New York, NY, USA

E. Menga (✉)
Department of Orthopaedic Surgery, University of Rochester Medical Center, Rochester, NY, USA

Presentation of Vertebral Compression Fracture

The natural history and expected clinical course following VCF largely depend on the nature of the initial presentation. Not all patients with symptomatic VCF are clinically diagnosed. VCFs typically either present as an acute symptomatic clinical event or are detected incidentally on plain radiographs. In those patients with an acute onset of back pain and the finding of VCF, the episode of acute pain typically lasts for a minimum of 2 weeks. Patients with VCF detected incidentally on imaging may experience little or no symptoms. These patients may report a prior episode of back pain for which they did not seek medical care or report no history of prior back pain at all. With a usually short duration of pain and a typically good response to analgesics, it is likely many VCFs are not detected clinically. In a population-based study, Cooper et al. found that 16% of VCF diagnoses were made incidentally during radiographic investigations into unrelated disorders, while 84% of patients with clinically diagnosed VCFs were associated with pain [2]. Elderly patients with chronic back pain may present with multiple vertebral compression fractures, vertebral height loss, low bone mineral density, and worsening structural changes or deformity.

A. E. Razi, S. H. Hershman (eds.), *Vertebral Compression Fractures in Osteoporotic and Pathologic Bone*, https://doi.org/10.1007/978-3-030-33861-9_10

Pain Associated with Acute Vertebral Compression Fracture

The pain associated with acute VCF is often described as an intense, deep pain at the site of fracture [3]. The pain is intermittent or chronic and is worse with sitting, standing, or any movement, including walking and bending. Pain symptoms are often relieved with lying down and pain medication. On examination, the patient may report tenderness to deep palpation over the spine and may also report paraspinal muscle spasm. VCF may be associated with either unilateral or bilateral radiculopathy, with pain radiating along the dermatomal nerve root distribution.

Despite the high incidence and prevalence of VCF, surprisingly little is known about the long-term course of pain for these fractures. It is generally believed that the pain related to this fracture is self-limiting and resolves after an average period of 2 weeks to 3 months [3, 4]. It is also generally believed that VCF only results in chronic pain in select patients with multiple VCF, height loss, and low bone mineral density [4]. Several early studies evaluated the natural history of pain in the first month following VCF [5, 6] – these studies found that the pain associated with an acute fracture may not significantly decrease during the first 7–10 days. In a study of 56 hospitalized patients with an acute vertebral fracture, Lyritis et al. found that self-reported pain had decreased by only 22% at day 7 following a fracture [5]. By day 14 following a fracture, pain had decreased by only 33% [5]. In a study of 21 patients with acute VCF, Gennari et al. found that there was no significant decrease in pain (as measured by visual analogue scale [VAS]) until day 15 after a fracture [6]. By day 30, pain had decreased by approximately 40% [6].

More recent studies have examined the course of pain following VCF at longer follow-up. Venmans et al. analyzed the natural course of conservatively treated osteoporotic VCF from the VERTOS trial (A Trial of Vertebroplasty for Painful Chronic Osteoporotic Vertebral Fractures) with a follow-up period of 1 year [7]. Of 95 patients treated without surgery, 38 patients (40%) had severe pain (defined as VAS pain scores ≥4) at the last follow-up interval of 12 months, despite the use of increased pain medication [7]. The authors concluded that a substantial percentage of patients with acute VCF have continued severe pain at 1 year following fracture [7]. Suzuki et al. followed 107 patients for a total of 12 months following presentation to the emergency unit with a finding of an acute VCF [8]. The authors analyzed pain, disability (von Korff pain and disability scores), ADL (Hannover ADL score), and quality of life (QoL) (EQ-5D) at 3 weeks and 3, 6, and 12 months [8]. In this study, the largest improvement in pain and disability scores occurred between the 3-week and 3-month visit, representing an average improvement of only 10–15% [8]. The authors found that even at 1 year following a VCF, the majority of patients had a high degree of pain and disability. The average pain scores at 1 year following a VCF were similar to preoperative scores of patients with herniated lumbar disk and lumbar spinal stenosis and those on 100% disability [8, 9]. The authors concluded that for the majority of patients, an acute VCF was the beginning of a long-lasting and severe deterioration of health.

It has previously been estimated that up to one-third of the approximately 700,000 osteoporotic vertebral compression fractures develop chronic pain [10]. The study by Suzuki et al. demonstrates that this percentage may be an underestimation, as more than 75% of patients in their study had severe pain at a minimum of 1 year following the fracture [8]. A 2005 study by Hasserius et al. also demonstrated an increased incidence of chronic back pain after VCF. Two hundred fifty-seven patients with VCF were followed as part of the European Vertebral Osteoporosis Study (EVOS) [11]. Of the 76 patients that were alive at 12-year follow-up, 56 were available to participate in an examination and questionnaire. Of these patients, more than 70% of the women had severe chronic back pain, which was significantly higher than age-matched controls [11]. These studies suggest that an acute VCF does not lead to a short self-limited episode of pain but may represent the beginning of a painful condition that can potentially last for a decade or more.

Physical Consequences of Vertebral Compression Fracture

Several studies have examined the clinical consequences of both acute and chronic VCFs [3, 4, 11–13]. A VCF frequently leads to increased kyphosis, which accounts for the significant long-term consequences of these fractures. VCFs result in anterior compression of the vertebral body, which moves the center of gravity forward, thereby creating a large bending moment. This bending moment must be counterbalanced by the posterior ligaments and musculature, which may result in chronic back pain and fatigue. The anterior compression on the vertebral body also results in an uneven transmission of loads to the intervertebral disks and end plates, which, along with loss of disk height, results in increased loads on the vertebral body. These increased loads lead to an increased risk of additional VCFs and worsening kyphosis [13].

In patients with multiple VCFs, the kyphosis of the thoracic spine may exceed 50 degrees [13] which may result in a loss of overall height for the individual. As vertebral height is lost, there is a reduction in the size of both the abdominal and thoracic cavities [4], and the 12th rib may come to rest on the iliac crest. In addition, patients may develop a protuberant abdomen, which can result in early satiety after eating and secondary weight loss [4]. Reduction in the size of the thoracic cavity may lead to reduced exercise tolerance as a result of restricted lung volume. Studies have demonstrated that a single thoracic vertebral compression fracture causes an approximate 10% loss of forced vital capacity [12]. In patients with pre-existing pulmonary conditions or lung diseases, this loss of vital capacity may be clinically significant [12]. The Study of Osteoporotic Fractures Research Group found that women with one or more VCFs have an age-adjusted relative risk of mortality from pulmonary causes that is approximately 2–2.7 times higher than women without VCFs [14].

Due to the possible deformity and back pain associated with chronic VCFs, patients may have difficulty with sitting or standing for prolong periods of time and may be most comfortable in bed. A kyphotic posture may force a patient to bend their knees and tilt the pelvis to maintain sagittal balance. This may result in muscle fatigue, gait abnormalities and, as a result, an increased risk of falls and additional fractures [15]. In addition, exercise is poorly tolerated, and lifting and bending are avoided. The decreased physical activity likely contributes to the worsening of osteoporosis. Many patients experience a distorted body image and poor self-esteem, leading to depression [3, 4]. In addition, the chronic pain associated with VCFs may have significant psychological consequences, including social isolation, increased anxiety, poor self-esteem, insomnia, and depression [15–17].

Disability After Vertebral Compression Fracture

The true amount of disability following VCF is difficult to quantify and may depend on the patient and the severity of fractures. Holbrook et al. performed some of the early work on this subject and estimated that a recognized VCF results in approximately 2 weeks of bed rest and 1 month of restricted activity [18]. In a series of 204 women between the age of 55 and 75 with a VCF, Ettinger et al. reported 8.4% of patients with moderate to severe vertebral deformity required help at home [19].

Ettinger et al. performed a larger cross-sectional study of 2992 women aged 65–70 years and found that the degree of disability may be directly related to the severity of VCF [20]. The authors measured the radiographic vertebral dimensions of T5–L4 and determined the degree of deformity by measuring the number of standard deviations (SD) that the ratio differed from the mean ratio calculated for the same vertebral level in the age-matched general population. The severity of deformity was then correlated with back disability in six ADLs and back pain. The authors reported 39.4% of the cohort had no vertebral deformity, while 10.2% had a deformity ≥4 SD from the mean [20]. The authors also reported that vertebral deformities with <4 SD from the mean were not associated with an increase in either pain or disability. Women with deformity ≥4 SD had a 2.6 (95% CI, 1.7–3.9) times increased risk of disability involving the back and a 1.9 (95% CI, 1.5–2.4) times increased risk of moderate to severe back pain [20]. They concluded vertebral deformities with vertebral height ratios less than 4 SD below the mean were associated with substantial pain and disability [20]. This study demonstrates that the severity of VCFs should be considered when assessing patients for risk of disability.

While early studies focused on the disability in the first several months following a VCF, more recent studies have demonstrated the long-term disability associated with these fractures. Both prospective and retrospective studies have shown that the deterioration of both health and QoL after a VCF can last for many years [11, 21–23]. In the Rancho Bernardo Study, a total of 1010 patients with osteoporotic fractures were followed for an average of 6.7 years (range, 1–17 years) following an initial fracture [24]. The authors found that women with a history of VCF had up to a seven times increased odds of reporting difficulties with a variety of activities than those without VCFs [24]. In a similar study, Ensrud et al. found that the odds of impaired ADLs (defined as difficulty with ≥3 physical ADLs) was 2.3 times higher among those with a clinically diagnosed VCF compared to controls [25].

Compared to other fragility fractures, VCFs appear to have a more deleterious effect on a patient's quality of life. This effect on QoL was reported in two prospective studies from Sweden [22, 26]. Both studies suggested a VCF had a more negative impact on a patient's quality of life than any other type of osteoporotic fracture, including hip fractures [22, 26].

Risk of Subsequent Fracture Following Vertebral Compression Fracture

One of the most significant consequences of a VCF is the risk of a subsequent VCF at another vertebral level. The Vertebral Efficacy with Risedronate Therapy (VERT) trial demonstrated a 1 in 5 risk of a subsequent VCF within 12 months following an incidental finding of a VCF among postmenopausal women [27]. The authors reported a fivefold increased risk of a subsequent VCF at 12 months in patients found to have one or more VCFs at baseline compared to patients without VCFs at baseline (relative risk [RR], 5.1; 95% confidence interval [CI], 3.1–8.4; $P < 0.001$) [27]. This study highlights the importance of early intervention in any patient who sustains a VCF.

Previous fractures and low bone density are both known risk factors for a subsequent VCF [28]. In a series of 1098 women between the ages of 43 and 80 years (mean, 63.3 years), Ross et al. reported that women with low bone mass had a sevenfold increased risk of VCF [28]. Women with a low bone mass and a single previous VCF were at a 25-fold increased risk of a subsequent VCF [28]. Therefore, in addition to a history of a previous VCF, practitioners should be particularly wary when these patients also have a low BMD.

Conclusion

The natural history of VCFs depends largely on the initial presentation. VCFs are frequently defined as a radiographic finding; however, many VCFs are clinically asymptomatic and many are undiagnosed. VCFs characterized by both an episode of acute pain and vertebral height loss may result in chronic pain and disability. The notion that VCF is a self-limiting condition with a relatively positive prognosis has been challenged by multiple studies with long-term follow-up reporting significant pain, disability, and impact to patients' quality of life and physical health. Vertebral height loss is a significant predictor of associated disability. The long-term sequelae of VCFs are characterized by additional VCFs, loss of vertebral height, and worsening disability in many patients.

References

1. Johnell O, Kanis JA. An estimate of the worldwide prevalence and disability associated with osteoporotic fractures. Osteoporos Int. 2006;17(12):1726–33.

2. Cooper C, Atkinson EJ, O'Fallon WM, Melton LJ 3rd. Incidence of clinically diagnosed vertebral fractures: a population-based study in Rochester, Minnesota, 1985–1989. J Bone Miner Res. 1992;7(2):221–7.
3. Leidig G, Minne HW, Sauer P, et al. A study of complaints and their relation to vertebral destruction in patients with osteoporosis. Bone Miner. 1990;8(3):217–29.
4. Silverman SL. The clinical consequences of vertebral compression fracture. Bone. 1992;13(Suppl 2):S27–31.
5. Lyritis GP, Tsakalakos N, Magiasis B, Karachalios T, Yiatzides A, Tsekoura M. Analgesic effect of salmon calcitonin in osteoporotic vertebral fractures: a double-blind placebo-controlled clinical study. Calcif Tissue Int. 1991;49(6):369–72.
6. Gennari C, Agnusdei D, Camporeale A. Use of calcitonin in the treatment of bone pain associated with osteoporosis. Calcif Tissue Int. 1991;49(Suppl 2):S9–13.
7. Venmans A, Klazen CA, Lohle PN, Mali WP, van Rooij WJ. Natural history of pain in patients with conservatively treated osteoporotic vertebral compression fractures: results from VERTOS II. AJNR Am J Neuroradiol. 2012;33(3):519–21.
8. Suzuki N, Ogikubo O, Hansson T. The course of the acute vertebral body fragility fracture: its effect on pain, disability and quality of life during 12 months. Eur Spine J. 2008;17(10):1380–90.
9. Hansson TH, Hansson EK. The effects of common medical interventions on pain, back function, and work resumption in patients with chronic low back pain: a prospective 2-year cohort study in six countries. Spine. 2000;25(23):3055–64.
10. Phillips FM. Minimally invasive treatments of osteoporotic vertebral compression fractures. Spine. 2003;28(15 Suppl):S45–53.
11. Hasserius R, Karlsson MK, Jonsson B, Redlund-Johnell I, Johnell O. Long-term morbidity and mortality after a clinically diagnosed vertebral fracture in the elderly – a 12- and 22-year follow-up of 257 patients. Calcif Tissue Int. 2005;76(4):235–42.
12. Leech JA, Dulberg C, Kellie S, Pattee L, Gay J. Relationship of lung function to severity of osteoporosis in women. Am Rev Respir Dis. 1990;141(1):68–71.
13. Cortet B, Roches E, Logier R, et al. Evaluation of spinal curvatures after a recent osteoporotic vertebral fracture. Joint Bone Spine. 2002;69(2):201–8.
14. Kado DM, Browner WS, Palermo L, Nevitt MC, Genant HK, Cummings SR. Vertebral fractures and mortality in older women: a prospective study. Study of Osteoporotic Fractures Research Group. Arch Intern Med. 1999;159(11):1215–20.
15. Gold DT. The clinical impact of vertebral fractures: quality of life in women with osteoporosis. Bone. 1996;18(3 Suppl):185S–9S.
16. Roberto KA. Women with osteoporosis: the role of the family and service community. Gerontologist. 1988;28(2):224–8.
17. Ross PD, Ettinger B, Davis JW, Melton LJ 3rd, Wasnich RD. Evaluation of adverse health outcomes associated with vertebral fractures. Osteoporos Int. 1991;1(3):134–40.
18. Holbrook TLGK, Kelsey JL, Stauffer RN. The frequency of occurrence, impact, and cost of musculoskeletal conditions in the United States. Chicago: American Academy of Orthopaedic Surgeons; 1985.
19. Ettinger B, Block JE, Smith R, Cummings SR, Harris ST, Genant HK. An examination of the association between vertebral deformities, physical disabilities and psychosocial problems. Maturitas. 1988;10(4):283–96.
20. Ettinger B, Black DM, Nevitt MC, et al. Contribution of vertebral deformities to chronic back pain and disability. The Study of Osteoporotic Fractures Research Group. J Bone Miner Res. 1992;7(4):449–56.
21. Hall SE, Criddle RA, Comito TL, Prince RL. A case-control study of quality of life and functional impairment in women with long-standing vertebral osteoporotic fracture. Osteoporos Int. 1999;9(6):508–15.
22. Hallberg I, Rosenqvist AM, Kartous L, Lofman O, Wahlstrom O, Toss G. Health-related quality of life after osteoporotic fractures. Osteoporos Int. 2004;15(10):834–41.
23. Cockerill W, Lunt M, Silman AJ, et al. Health-related quality of life and radiographic vertebral fracture. Osteoporos Int. 2004;15(2):113–9.
24. Greendale GA, Barrett-Connor E, Ingles S, Haile R. Late physical and functional effects of osteoporotic fracture in women: the Rancho Bernardo Study. J Am Geriatr Soc. 1995;43(9):955–61.
25. Ensrud KE, Nevitt MC, Yunis C, et al. Correlates of impaired function in older women. J Am Geriatr Soc. 1994;42(5):481–9.
26. Borgstrom F, Zethraeus N, Johnell O, et al. Costs and quality of life associated with osteoporosis-related fractures in Sweden. Osteoporos Int. 2006;17(5):637–50.
27. Lindsay R, Silverman SL, Cooper C, et al. Risk of new vertebral fracture in the year following a fracture. JAMA. 2001;285(3):320–3.
28. Ross PD, Davis JW, Epstein RS, Wasnich RD. Pre-existing fractures and bone mass predict vertebral fracture incidence in women. Ann Intern Med. 1991;114(11):919–23.

Medical, Interventional, and Orthotic Management of Osteoporotic Vertebral Compression Fractures

11

Kartik Shenoy and Yong H. Kim

Introduction

Osteoporotic vertebral compression fractures (OCVFs) are the most common type of osteoporotic fractures seen in the elderly. Although many of these individuals may sustain a fracture, only around one third seek medical care [1]. Patients report back pain, and the true diagnosis can be easily missed or misdiagnosed as a back strain. These fractures can be a significant source of pain and dysfunction and can lead to a variety of complications. Acutely, ileus, urinary retention, and even spinal cord compression can occur. Conservatively treated OVCFs can result in kyphosis, depression, and chronic pain [2].

Initial management of these fractures is focused on pain control, but the long-term management should be focused on prevention and treatment of the underlying osteoporosis. Some patients may require surgical intervention, ranging from simple procedures such as vertebroplasty or kyphoplasty to major reconstructive surgery. Each patient deserves a tailored treatment plan with a focus on multimodal pain control and the involvement of both surgical and medical teams to develop an appropriate approach specific to each patient. In some cases, psychological treatment may be needed for depression with regard to function, appearance, and pain. The majority of patients can be treated with conservative management; however in some cases, surgical intervention may be warranted.

Pharmacologic Treatment

Pain control is critical to the early management of OVCFs. Proper pain control allows for early mobilization and rehabilitation which facilitates an earlier return to function and a higher quality of life. Prolonged bed rest and inactivity can lead to worsening osteoporosis in these already compromised patients. Treatment requires a multimodal approach, and as such, there are a number of pharmacologic pain relievers which can be used; however, the side effect profiles must be carefully considered, particularly in the elderly population. Acute pain from OVCFs typically lasts between 6 and 12 weeks [3, 4]. Initial analgesia should attempt to avoid using narcotics unless absolutely necessary. First-line medications include acetaminophen and nonsteroidal anti-inflammatory drugs (NSAIDs). The acute phase of pain is partially due to the inflammatory response associated with the injury, and therefore NSAIDs can be very effective. In the elderly,

K. Shenoy (✉)
Department of Orthopaedic Surgery, Rothman Orthopaedic Institute, Philadelphia, PA, USA

Y. H. Kim
Department of Orthopedic Surgery, NYU Langone Orthopedic Hospital, NYU Langone Medical Center, New York, NY, USA
e-mail: YONG.KIM@NYUMC.ORG

A. E. Razi, S. H. Hershman (eds.), *Vertebral Compression Fractures in Osteoporotic and Pathologic Bone*, https://doi.org/10.1007/978-3-030-33861-9_11

NSAIDs pose the risk of gastrointestinal bleeding and acute kidney injury. Selective cyclooxygenase-2 inhibitors can be used in place of NSAIDs to mitigate the aforementioned side effects [5].

When the pain is severe, narcotic pain medications can be administered in addition to nonnarcotic medication. Patients, family members, and healthcare staff must be aware of the side effects of narcotics including mental status changes, respiratory depression, nausea, and constipation [6]. As an adjunct, muscle relaxants can be beneficial since paraspinal muscle spasms can be very painful. Muscle relaxants are particularly useful in the first 1–2 weeks following a fracture. Similar to narcotic medications, patients must be monitored for side effects including drowsiness, dizziness, dependence, and abuse.

Radicular pain can also result from OVCFs due to general inflammation or retropulsion of fragments with resultant nerve root irritation. Furthermore, collapse of the vertebral body puts the exiting bilateral nerve roots at risk for compression in the setting of a narrowed foramen. NSAIDs can be helpful for initial inflammatory-type radicular pain, but other medications such as antidepressants and anticonvulsants can be helpful for neuropathic pain control. There are many types of neuropathic pain, and the majority of studies have focused on diabetic neuropathy and fibromyalgia; nevertheless, these medications have been utilized for patients with neuropathic pain following OVCFs. Within the antidepressant class of medications, tricyclic antidepressants (TCAs) and selective serotonin-norepinephrine reuptake inhibitors (SSNRIs) have been effective [7, 8]. TCAs block norepinephrine and serotonin reuptake inhibition for the treatment of depression; however, the mechanism of action through which tricyclics provide analgesia is unclear. It is thought that they are part of neuromodulatory serotonergic and noradrenergic pathways resulting in the recruitment of the endogenous opioids [9, 10]. However, TCAs are not without side effects as anticholinergic symptoms such as drowsiness, dizziness, dry mouth, and blurry vision can occur which can be dangerous in the elderly. These effects can be mitigated by initiating therapy with low doses and slowly titrating until effective. In an effort to avoid the adverse effects of TCAs, selective serotonin reuptake inhibitors were studied; however, given that they only worked on the serotonin pathway, they had limited utility in pain control. Therefore, the newer SSNRIs such as duloxetine and venlafaxine have been evaluated and were reported to be effective for neuropathic pain control [11]. Additionally, they have proven efficacy in the treatment of chronic low back pain and can serve a dual purpose in the treatment of OVCFs [12].

Anticonvulsants, specifically gabapentin and pregabalin, are also used in the treatment of neuropathic pain. They are calcium channel alpha-2-delta ligands and can provide analgesia while simultaneously treating comorbid depression, anxiety, and sleep disturbance, thereby allowing an increased quality of life [13]. There is evidence to support the treatment of neuropathic pain with these agents; however there is weak evidence for the use of gabapentinoids for low back pain. These drugs are generally well tolerated, but a common side effect is sedation. Both drugs must be titrated to the patient's needs, and they should always be discontinued in a tapered fashion to avoid seizures.

When the above measures do not provide sufficient pain control, calcitonin can be used as an adjunct to provide analgesia [14]. Calcitonin is an antiresorptive agent which can be given for acute pain when first-line agents fail, but it should be discontinued after 6–12 weeks [15, 16] for concern that there may be increased rates of cancer associated with its use [17].

In summary, when considering medications for pain control, the treatment must be individualized according to the patient's symptoms, comorbidities, and preferences. Although many guidelines provide recommendations for many of the aforementioned pharmacologic pain control modalities, the recommendations are weak at best; nevertheless, they are currently the best options currently available for the treatment of pain associated with OVCFs.

Injections

In difficult cases where acute pain is not relieved by the aforementioned techniques or when a patient develops chronic back pain, injections can be helpful for pain control. Conservative care is considered to have failed when there is continued severe pain at 2 weeks despite treatment or when pain does not improve despite treatment for 4 weeks [18]. There are a number of different injections that can be performed to assist in pain management and improve overall function. As back pain is the most common complaint, facet injections and medial branch nerve blocks can help to alleviate pain. Many authors have theorized that the pain from OVCFs is multifactorial and may not be just from the fracture itself [19–23]. It is thought that facet joints are subjected to abnormal loads due to the increased flexion moment from compression of the anterior column [21, 24]. In a study by Wilson et al., they report that the pain generators following OVCFs are multifactorial and that facet joint injections were able to control pain in about one third of patients. In this same study, they reported that patients who failed facet joint injection were more likely to experience relief from vertebroplasty as the anterior column was more likely to be the pain generator [21]. Wang et al. have published the only prospective, randomized controlled study comparing facet block and vertebroplasty for pain relief and found that in the first week, vertebroplasty had better pain relief but after 1 month and at the final follow-up at 12 months, there was no difference in pain relief between the two groups [25].

As an alternative to facet joint injections, medial branch nerve blocks have also been explored as a treatment option following OVCFs [26]. The nerve block prevents ascending pain signals from the facet joint from reaching the brain. Park et al. reported their 1-year retrospective experience on medial branch blocks for patients who failed conservative treatment or had chronic pain following vertebroplasty and found patients experienced significant pain relief and functional recovery.

In the acute setting, patients may occasionally have radicular pain following an OVCF for which epidural or nerve root injections can help with intractable pain and speed recovery [19]. Kim et al. reported on up to four selective nerve root injections at a time in patients with bilateral, multilevel disease at 2-week intervals with a maximum of three sessions – they reported that 78% of patients had good to excellent results [18]. There is also literature to support that in patients with OVCFs at L3 or L4, a selective L2 nerve root block can be performed for temporary pain relief. The sensory fibers from these vertebrae enter the paravertebral sympathetic trunks and then enter the L2 dorsal root ganglion. The effects of these injections were clinically significant at 2 weeks but not significant at 1 month [27, 28].

For pain suspected of originating from the anterior column of the vertebral body, gray ramus communicans nerve blocks have been done since these nerves provide the greatest innervation to the intervertebral disc and adjacent structures. Given that this injection is more anterior, there is a risk of pneumothorax in the thoracic spine and bowel perforation, intravascular injection, and kidney puncture in the lumbar spine [29, 30]. The potential risk frequently outweighs the potential benefit from this procedure; more studies need to be done to better assess the safety and efficacy of this procedure.

As there are many options for spinal injections, it is important to thoroughly evaluate the patient to accurately determine the sources of pain. When considering injection, the surgeon must weigh the risks and benefits. Steroids, which are often used in these injections, can also further exacerbate the osteoporosis. Some authors have found that spinal injections can put patients at an increased risk for future vertebral compression fractures. A study by Mandel et al. found that each successive epidural steroid injection increased the risk of fragility fracture by 20%; therefore the risks and benefits must be weighed when performing these injections [31]. Additionally, each injection carries its own inherent risks which should be discussed with the patient during the decision-making process.

Bracing

Spinal orthoses can be used in the acute, subacute, or chronic phases of treatment following an OVCF for pain control. The goal is to provide support, limit motion at the injury site, and improve posture, all in an effort to reduce pain and prevent deformity. Braces must be tailored to the patient's needs, and most importantly, patients must be compliant for the brace to be effective. Furthermore, the brace should be affordable and easy to put on and take off. As the pain subsides, the brace can be slowly weaned off with a total brace time of 2–3 months following the fracture [32].

Although bracing is commonly used in the treatment of OVCFs, the evidence regarding their utility is uncertain [27, 33, 34]. There is evidence for bracing following traumatic fractures but not for OVCF [32]. The options for bracing include flexible, semirigid, and rigid braces, and each comes in a variety of custom and prefabricated models. Thoracolumbar orthoses including the Jewett (Fig. 11.1), cruciform anterior spinal hyperextension (Fig. 11.2), and Knight-Taylor braces have been advocated by some authors [2, 35–37]. The more commonly available standard thoracolumbar and thoracolumbosacral orthoses (Fig. 11.3) can also be used; however

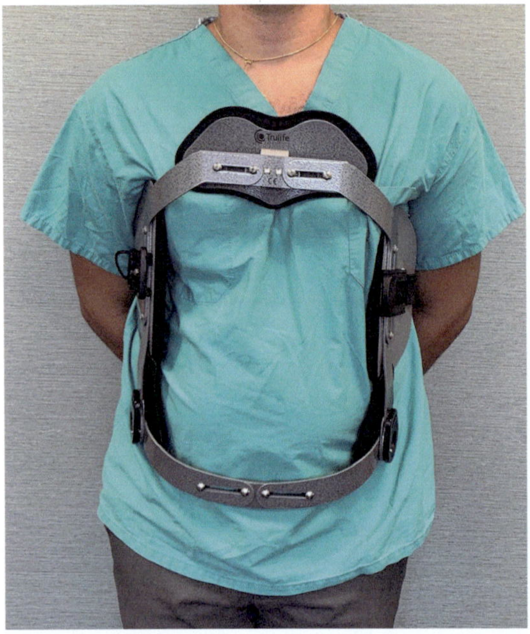

Fig. 11.1 Jewett brace

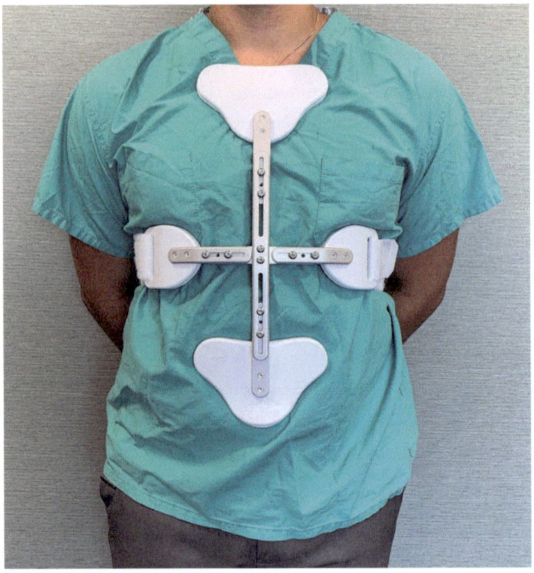

Fig. 11.2 Cruciform anterior spinal hyperextension (CASH) brace

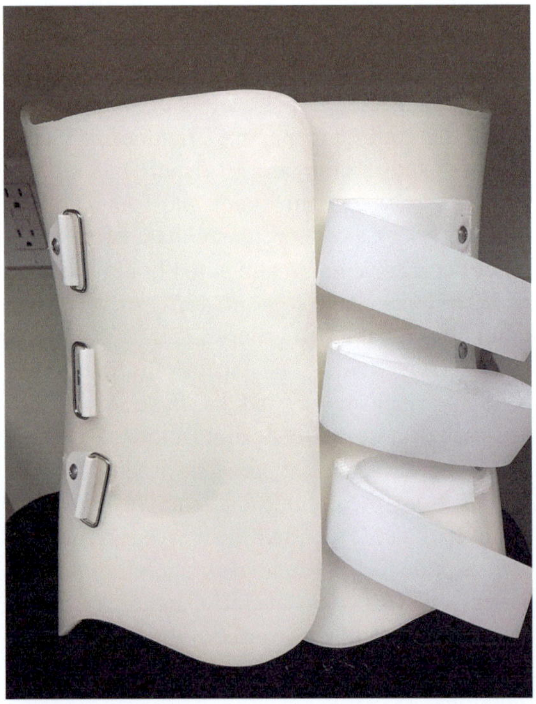

Fig. 11.3 Thoracolumbosacral orthosis (TLSO)

they are frequently cumbersome and can be difficult to put on and off. When to apply the brace, what type of brace to use, and how long to wear the brace are still questions that need to be answered formally.

In the initial 3 months following an OVCF, there is a paucity of literature looking at the direct effects of bracing; however, the majority of literature that discusses treatment options for OVCFs include bracing in the algorithm. Studies looking at three-point orthoses (3-POs) and corsets have shown varying results as to which is the preferred method of bracing in the acute treatment phase. Murata et al. found that rigid external supports are more likely to prevent deformity and nonunion compared to flexible corsets, whereas Meccariello et al. found that flexible corsets in comparison to 3-POs showed greater improvements in quality of life and function with less complications while providing equivalent stabilization effects [38, 39]. Prospective studies looking at conservative treatment with and without bracing are needed to better elucidate the effects of specific orthoses.

The strongest evidence exists for the use of bracing after the acute period. In patients who develop kyphosis, the utility of a semirigid backpack thoracolumbar orthosis has been described. Two studies by Pfeifer et al. demonstrated using a thoracolumbar orthosis in the 6-month period following an OVCF resulted in increased core strength, decreased kyphosis, decreased pain, and improved function and quality of life [40, 41].

Like other treatments, bracing also has its risks. Rigid braces can result in decubitus ulcers and infections. Although the studies above reported increased strength following bracing, some braces have been reported to result in weakening of the axial musculature and decreased pulmonary function. There is also the theoretical potential for fracture at the proximal and distal ends of the brace as there is an abrupt change in stiffness. Therefore, when bracing is used, patients and caregivers must be counseled on monitoring for side effects, and the duration of use should be limited.

As there are many brace options available, the decision to prescribe a particular brace should be based on patient comfort, compliance, and cost until there is clear evidence that one brace is superior.

Psychological Treatment

Quality of life following an OVCF has been well studied and was shown to be negatively impacted [42–45]. In particular, following the resolution of pain, patients often have psychological impairment. Patients have reported anxiety and depression and, as a result of kyphosis, abdominal protrusion, and activity limitation, can also have diminished self-esteem [44]. Additionally, a fear of falling, embarrassment, and frustration have been reported [43, 46].

Orthopedic surgeons play a role in the treatment of the above conditions primarily through recognition of the condition in follow-up, but also in making referrals to person-centered and other supportive interventions for continued treatment following an OVCF. During follow-up, the surgeon must make it a point to inquire about patients' quality of life and psychological issues as many patients may not openly offer this information [43]. When abnormal moods and fear of functional impairments are identified, consultation with a physical therapist, psychologist, or psychiatrist may be warranted. In a study by Olsen et al., an exercise and education program led by a physical therapist showed a significant decrease in the fear of falling [47]. Gold et al. showed that a physical therapist-led class was able to not only teach exercises but also stress reduction techniques, relaxation techniques, and lifestyle modifications to address psychological symptoms [48].

References

1. Cooper C, Atkinson EJ, O'Fallon WM, Melton LJ 3rd. Incidence of clinically diagnosed vertebral fractures: a population-based study in Rochester, Minnesota, 1985-1989. J Bone Miner Res. 1992;7:221–7.

2. Prather H, Watson JO, Gilula LA. Nonoperative management of osteoporotic vertebral compression fractures. Injury. 2007;38(Suppl 3):S40–8.
3. Kim DH, Silber JS, Albert TJ. Osteoporotic vertebral compression fractures. Instr Course Lect. 2003;52:541–50.
4. Silverman SL. The clinical consequences of vertebral compression fracture. Bone. 1992;13(Suppl 2):S27–31.
5. Chou R, Huffman LH, American Pain S, American College of P. Medications for acute and chronic low back pain: a review of the evidence for an American Pain Society/American College of Physicians clinical practice guideline. Ann Intern Med. 2007;147:505–14.
6. Longo UG, Loppini M, Denaro L, Maffulli N, Denaro V. Conservative management of patients with an osteoporotic vertebral fracture: a review of the literature. J Bone Joint Surg Br. 2012;94:152–7.
7. Dworkin RH, O'Connor AB, Audette J, Baron R, Gourlay GK, Haanpaa ML, et al. Recommendations for the pharmacological management of neuropathic pain: an overview and literature update. Mayo Clin Proc. 2010;85:S3–14.
8. McCleane G. Antidepressants as analgesics. CNS Drugs. 2008;22:139–56.
9. Benbouzid M, Gaveriaux-Ruff C, Yalcin I, Waltisperger E, Tessier LH, Muller A, et al. Delta-opioid receptors are critical for tricyclic antidepressant treatment of neuropathic allodynia. Biol Psychiatry. 2008;63:633–6.
10. Bohren Y, Tessier LH, Megat S, Petitjean H, Hugel S, Daniel D, et al. Antidepressants suppress neuropathic pain by a peripheral beta2-adrenoceptor mediated anti-TNFalpha mechanism. Neurobiol Dis. 2013;60:39–50.
11. Watson CP, Gilron I, Sawynok J, Lynch ME. Nontricyclic antidepressant analgesics and pain: are serotonin norepinephrine reuptake inhibitors (SNRIs) any better? Pain. 2011;152:2206–10.
12. Skljarevski V, Zhang S, Desaiah D, Alaka KJ, Palacios S, Miazgowski T, et al. Duloxetine versus placebo in patients with chronic low back pain: a 12-week, fixed-dose, randomized, double-blind trial. J Pain. 2010;11:1282–90.
13. Mehta S, McIntyre A, Dijkers M, Loh E, Teasell RW. Gabapentinoids are effective in decreasing neuropathic pain and other secondary outcomes after spinal cord injury: a meta-analysis. Arch Phys Med Rehabil. 2014;95:2180–6.
14. Ameis A, Randhawa K, Yu H, Cote P, Haldeman S, Chou R, et al. The Global Spine Care Initiative: a review of reviews and recommendations for the non-invasive management of acute osteoporotic vertebral compression fracture pain in low- and middle-income communities. Eur Spine J. 2018;27(Suppl 6):861–9.
15. Knopp JA, Diner BM, Blitz M, Lyritis GP, Rowe BH. Calcitonin for treating acute pain of osteoporotic vertebral compression fractures: a systematic review of randomized, controlled trials. Osteoporos Int. 2005;16:1281–90.
16. Knopp-Sihota JA, Newburn-Cook CV, Homik J, Cummings GG, Voaklander D. Calcitonin for treating acute and chronic pain of recent and remote osteoporotic vertebral compression fractures: a systematic review and meta-analysis. Osteoporos Int. 2012;23:17–38.
17. Overman RA, Borse M, Gourlay ML. Salmon calcitonin use and associated cancer risk. Ann Pharmacother. 2013;47:1675–84.
18. Kim DJ, Yun YH, Wang JM. Nerve-root injections for the relief of pain in patients with osteoporotic vertebral fractures. J Bone Joint Surg Br. 2003;85:250–3.
19. Georgy BA. Interventional techniques in managing persistent pain after vertebral augmentation procedures: a retrospective evaluation. Pain Physician. 2007;10:673–6.
20. Bogduk N, MacVicar J, Borowczyk J. The pain of vertebral compression fractures can arise in the posterior elements. Pain Med. 2010;11:1666–73.
21. Wilson DJ, Owen S, Corkill RA. Facet joint injections as a means of reducing the need for vertebroplasty in insufficiency fractures of the spine. Eur Radiol. 2011;21:1772–8.
22. Kim TK, Kim KH, Kim CH, Shin SW, Kwon JY, Kim HK, et al. Percutaneous vertebroplasty and facet joint block. J Korean Med Sci. 2005;20:1023–8.
23. Mitra R, Do H, Alamin T, Cheng I. Facet pain in thoracic compression fractures. Pain Med. 2010;11:1674–7.
24. Lehman VT, Wood CP, Hunt CH, Carter RE, Allred JB, Diehn FE, et al. Facet joint signal change on MRI at levels of acute/subacute lumbar compression fractures. AJNR Am J Neuroradiol. 2013;34:1468–73.
25. Wang B, Guo H, Yuan L, Huang D, Zhang H, Hao D. A prospective randomized controlled study comparing the pain relief in patients with osteoporotic vertebral compression fractures with the use of vertebroplasty or facet blocking. Eur Spine J. 2016;25:3486–94.
26. Solberg J, Copenhaver D, Fishman SM. Medial branch nerve block and ablation as a novel approach to pain related to vertebral compression fracture. Curr Opin Anaesthesiol. 2016;29:596–9.
27. Esses SI, McGuire R, Jenkins J, Finkelstein J, Woodard E, Watters WC 3rd, et al. The treatment of symptomatic osteoporotic spinal compression fractures. J Am Acad Orthop Surg. 2011;19:176–82.
28. Ohtori S, Yamashita M, Inoue G, Yamauchi K, Suzuki M, Orita S, et al. L2 spinal nerve-block effects on acute low back pain from osteoporotic vertebral fracture. J Pain. 2009;10:870–5.
29. Chandler G, Dalley G, Hemmer J, Seely T. Comparison of Thoracic versus Lumbar Gray Ramus Communicans Nerve Block in the treatment of painful osteoporotic vertebral compression fracture. Pain Physician. 2000;3:240.
30. Chandler G, Dalley G, Hemmer J Jr, Seely T. Gray ramus communicans nerve block: novel treatment approach for painful osteoporotic vertebral compression fracture. South Med J. 2001;94:387–93.

31. Mandel S, Schilling J, Peterson E, Rao DS, Sanders W. A retrospective analysis of vertebral body fractures following epidural steroid injections. J Bone Joint Surg Am. 2013;95:961–4.
32. Chang V, Holly LT. Bracing for thoracolumbar fractures. Neurosurg Focus. 2014;37:E3.
33. Kim HJ, Yi JM, Cho HG, Chang BS, Lee CK, Kim JH, et al. Comparative study of the treatment outcomes of osteoporotic compression fractures without neurologic injury using a rigid brace, a soft brace, and no brace: a prospective randomized controlled non-inferiority trial. J Bone Joint Surg Am. 2014;96:1959–66.
34. Parreira PCS, Maher CG, Megale RZ, March L, Ferreira ML. An overview of clinical guidelines for the management of vertebral compression fracture: a systematic review. Spine J. 2017;17:1932.
35. Garg B, Dixit V, Batra S, Malhotra R, Sharan A. Non-surgical management of acute osteoporotic vertebral compression fracture: a review. J Clin Orthop Trauma. 2017;8:131–8.
36. Wu SS, Lachmann E, Nagler W. Current medical, rehabilitation, and surgical management of vertebral compression fractures. J Womens Health (Larchmt). 2003;12:17–26.
37. Liaw MY, Chen CL, Chen JF, Tang FT, Wong AM, Ho HH. Effects of Knight-Taylor brace on balance performance in osteoporotic patients with vertebral compression fracture. J Back Musculoskelet Rehabil. 2009;22:75–81.
38. Meccariello L, Muzii VF, Falzarano G, Medici A, Carta S, Fortina M, et al. Dynamic corset versus three-point brace in the treatment of osteoporotic compression fractures of the thoracic and lumbar spine: a prospective, comparative study. Aging Clin Exp Res. 2017;29:443–9.
39. Murata K, Watanabe G, Kawaguchi S, Kanaya K, Horigome K, Yajima H, et al. Union rates and prognostic variables of osteoporotic vertebral fractures treated with a rigid external support. J Neurosurg Spine. 2012;17:469–75.
40. Pfeifer M, Kohlwey L, Begerow B, Minne HW. Effects of two newly developed spinal orthoses on trunk muscle strength, posture, and quality-of-life in women with postmenopausal osteoporosis: a randomized trial. Am J Phys Med Rehabil. 2011;90:805–15.
41. Pfeifer M, Begerow B, Minne HW. Effects of a new spinal orthosis on posture, trunk strength, and quality of life in women with postmenopausal osteoporosis: a randomized trial. Am J Phys Med Rehabil. 2004;83:177–86.
42. Suzuki N, Ogikubo O, Hansson T. Previous vertebral compression fractures add to the deterioration of the disability and quality of life after an acute compression fracture. Eur Spine J. 2010;19:567–74.
43. Cook DJ, Guyatt GH, Adachi JD, Clifton J, Griffith LE, Epstein RS, et al. Quality of life issues in women with vertebral fractures due to osteoporosis. Arthritis Rheum. 1993;36:750–6.
44. Gold DT. The clinical impact of vertebral fractures: quality of life in women with osteoporosis. Bone. 1996;18:185S–9S.
45. Lyles KW, Gold DT, Shipp KM, Pieper CF, Martinez S, Mulhausen PL. Association of osteoporotic vertebral compression fractures with impaired functional status. Am J Med. 1993;94:595–601.
46. Ettinger B, Block JE, Smith R, Cummings SR, Harris ST, Genant HK. An examination of the association between vertebral deformities, physical disabilities and psychosocial problems. Maturitas. 1988;10:283–96.
47. Olsen CF, Bergland A. The effect of exercise and education on fear of falling in elderly women with osteoporosis and a history of vertebral fracture: results of a randomized controlled trial. Osteoporos Int. 2014;25:2017–25.
48. Gold DT, Shipp KM, Pieper CF, Duncan PW, Martinez S, Lyles KW. Group treatment improves trunk strength and psychological status in older women with vertebral fractures: results of a randomized, clinical trial. J Am Geriatr Soc. 2004;52:1471–8.

12

Outcomes of Non-operative Management and Vertebral Augmentation of Vertebral Compression Fractures

Robert A. McGuire Jr and Joseph M. Zavatsky

The primary goals of treatment for VCFs are pain relief and restoration of vertebral body height. There are also secondary benefits of fracture treatment – preservation of the independence of the individual with the fracture, protection of pulmonary function, and avoidance of medical complications following the fracture. There are several treatment options available for these patients. Fortunately, the majority of these fractures heal uneventfully with conservative management which typically consists of rest, short-term activity modification, bracing for comfort, and short-term use of calcitonin [1–4].

For those patients who have unrelenting pain or progressive collapse of the vertebral body, cement augmentation is an option.

The concept of vertebroplasty was initiated in France in 1987 for the treatment of symptomatic vertebral hemangioma [5]. This consisted of injection of a PMMA cement through a large needle in the vertebral body performed either unilaterally or bilaterally (Fig. 12.1). Improvement of pain was not found to correlate with the amount of cement injected, so this procedure could be done under local anesthesia and at a very low cost. The concept of vertebroplasty does not address the spinal deformity and uses high pressure cement in a very liquid form and therefore has a greater potential for leakage outside the vertebral body into the spinal canal and surrounding soft tissues.

The concept of kyphoplasty, which uses a bone tamp or balloon introduced into the vertebral body to create a cavity for implantation of the cement [6], is more expensive to use but has the potential to improve the kyphotic angle through the cavity creation and placement of a large volume of cement into the re-expanded

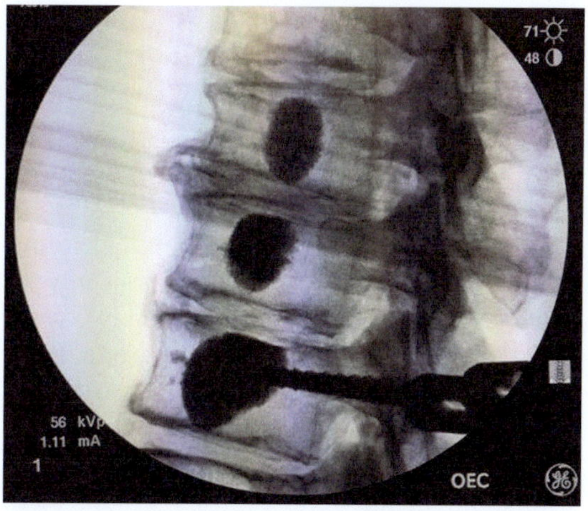

Fig. 12.1 This lateral radiograph reveals consistent flow through the cancellous interstices of the vertebral body. This is done by using cement in a very liquid consistency, whereas the consistency of the cement is doughy in kyphoplasty and is not likely to be extruded into the canal

R. A. McGuire Jr (✉)
Department of Orthopaedic Surgery, University of Mississippi Medical Center, Jackson, MS, USA
e-mail: rmcguire@umc.edu

J. M. Zavatsky
Spine and Scoliosis Specialists, Tampa, FL, USA

A. E. Razi, S. H. Hershman (eds.), *Vertebral Compression Fractures in Osteoporotic and Pathologic Bone*, https://doi.org/10.1007/978-3-030-33861-9_12

fractured vertebra. Additionally, the cement is thicker in viscosity which minimizes the risk of extrusion.

Three periods of time will be used to evaluate the evidence available for treating these fractures non-operatively and with cement augmentation using the two above techniques. We will use the available literature prior to the publication of the AAOS guidelines, the literature used for the production of the AAOS guidelines, and then the literature published after the AAOS guideline publication.

Pre-AAOS Guideline Evidence

Hulme et al. performed a systematic review of 69 clinical studies comparing the use of vertebroplasty and kyphoplasty [7]. Review of these clinical studies revealed no randomized or prospective articles at that time and very few prospective cohort studies. There were 22 kyphoplasty studies with 1288 patients, and the vertebroplasty group consists of 44 studies with 2958 patients. From the data analysis of this study, pain relief was achieved in 92% of patients who were treated with kyphoplasty, with the visual analog scale decreasing from 7.15 to 3.4. In the vertebroplasty group, 87% achieved some relief of their pain with the VAS decreasing from 8.2 to 3.0. There were a limited number of studies that involved the physical function, but it was felt that pain relief resulted in improvement of function in most patients.

When evaluating height restoration, measurement techniques vary greatly from study to study, so it is difficult to compare the two techniques directly. In the kyphoplasty group, there was an average of 6.6 degrees of kyphosis correction, and in 34% of the studies, there was no appreciable improvement in angular or height restoration. In the vertebroplasty group, there also was a 6.6 degree kyphosis correction with 39% exhibiting no appreciable improvement in the kyphosis.

Reported complications consisted predominantly of cement leakage, which was noted 9% of the time in the kyphoplasty group and 41% of the time in the vertebroplasty group. Most of these cement leakages, however, were clinically asymptomatic in both groups. The most notable complication in both groups was the occurrence of fractures occurring at levels next to the treated level. This occurred in 15% of patients in the kyphoplasty group and 12.9% of patients in the vertebroplasty group.

Taylor [8, 9] and Liu [10] also published studies which were consistent with the finding of the Hulme [7] study. Liu et al. [10] recommended vertebroplasty to be used in the treatment of VCF based on the higher cost of the kyphoplasty. Eck et al. [11] performed a meta-analysis of the literature comparing the two procedures; the findings of their study found an improvement of 4.6 points on the visual analog scale following kyphoplasty and 5.68 points following vertebroplasty. New fractures were also noted in 4.1% of those patients treated with kyphoplasty and 7.6% treated with vertebroplasty. They also noted cement leakage occurring in 7% of patients treated with kyphoplasty and 19.7% with vertebroplasty.

In conclusion, when evaluating the data from studies comparing vertebroplasty to kyphoplasty, pain relief was similar in both procedures, functional improvement was tied to pain relief, and cement leakage was higher following vertebroplasty but, in most cases, was clinically irrelevant. The ability to restore height was only seen within the first 3–6 months and was somewhat better with kyphoplasty.

When evaluating these techniques to conservative management, a study by Diamond et al. [12] using a nonrandomized trial found that after cement augmentation, there was an earlier improvement in pain scores as well as improved physical function in those patients treated with vertebroplasty as compared to the control group. The benefits were usually seen within 24 hours, and patients treated with vertebroplasty seemed to have a more rapid rehabilitation and lower complication rate. The benefits however were only short term – after 6 weeks, compared to the control group, patients treated with vertebroplasty were noted to be fairly similar in all outcome measures.

Rousing et al. [13] found that compared to non-operative treatment, vertebroplasty was successful in improving pain early, but no difference was found between the two groups at 3 months. Wardlaw et al. [14] published the results of a randomized trial comparing kyphoplasty to non-operative management and found that kyphoplasty was better than non-operative treatment with respect to pain improvement and functional outcomes at 1 month, but those improvements were less apparent at 12 months. McGirt et al. [15] published a systematic review using level 1 evidence and found that compared to non-operative treatment, vertebroplasty and kyphoplasty showed better results in the first 2 weeks after the procedure. The level 2 and level 3 evidence revealed that patients who underwent kyphoplasty or vertebroplasty had improved pain at 6 months, but none of the studies showed overwhelming differences between conservative and surgical management after that period of time. From the above studies, there appears to be some evidence that early treatment with cement augmentation results in improved pain control, but as time progresses, these differences become negligible.

AAOS Guidelines

The American Academy of Orthopaedic Surgeons convened a committee which met in 2009 and 2010 to evaluate the existing body of published evidence in order to develop guidelines for the treatment of osteoporotic vertebral compression fractures. The resulting guidelines were published in 2011 [16, 17]. What was noted at that time was the fact that there were very few level 1 studies which could be used to develop these guidelines. Buchbinder et al. [18] performed a multicenter, randomized, double-blind, placebo-controlled study looking at outcomes at 1 week and 1, 3, and 6 months. The primary outcome evaluated with this study was overall pain relief at 6 months. Seventy-eight participants were enrolled, 38 were treated with vertebroplasty, and 40 underwent a sham procedure; 91% completed the 6-month study. This level 1 study found no benefit of vertebroplasty over sham surgery at any time point. Kallmes et al. [19] also published a randomized, prospective, multicentered study on patients that had failed medical treatment with fractures less than 1 year old; the primary outcome measures were scored on the modified disability questionnaire, and patients rated their pain during the preceding 24 hours. Over 1800 patients were screened with 431 of the patients being eligible; 70% declined participation in the study. In the end, there were only 131 patients enrolled in the study, and it was found that 43% of the control group crossed over to surgery by 3 months due to unrelenting pain. The findings reported showed a trend toward clinically meaningful improvement in the vertebroplasty group compared to the control group (61% vs. 48%); however there was no statistical significance demonstrated at any point in time.

Based on the two studies in the *New England Journal of Medicine*, the AAOS guidelines that were developed recommended against vertebroplasty; this was based on the two level 1 and three level 2 studies with a strong consensus opinion. Strangely enough, kyphoplasty was noted to have weak support based on two level 1 studies. When comparing kyphoplasty to vertebroplasty, three studies showed inconsistent results, and therefore, no recommendation could be made.

Post-AAOS Guidelines

Since the publication of the AAOS guidelines, there have been multiple studies comparing vertebroplasty to conservative treatment. Klazen et al. [20] published the Vertos II study which enrolled 431 patients; 229 patients improved with non-operative management, and 202 were randomized to receive cement augmentation. Cement augmentation resulted in significant pain relief at 1 month, and similar results were maintained at 1 year. Farrokhi et al. [21] also published a randomized controlled study of vertebroplasty compared to medical management and found that after vertebroplasty there was a significant decrease in pain and a significant improvement in the quality of life at 1 week;

this effect was sustained over 36 months. Berenson et al. [22, 23] published a randomized, controlled trial of cancer patients who sustained a fracture and randomized them to either kyphoplasty or nonsurgical treatment. Patients who underwent kyphoplasty showed a substantial and statistically significant improvement as compared to the nonsurgical control group. Eddin et al. [24] published a study evaluating the mortality risk following VCF in Medicare patients following operative versus non-operative treatment. They found that after 4 years, the survival rate for patients treated non-operatively was 50% compared to the operatively treated group which was 60.8%. When comparing vertebroplasty and kyphoplasty, there was a 57.3% survival rate in patients treated with vertebroplasty and 62.8% in patients treated with kyphoplasty.

Anderson et al. [25] published a meta-analysis of eight prospective randomized trials comparing vertebral augmentation to conservative treatment. The meta-analysis revealed greater pain relief, functional recovery, and quality of life with cement augmentation as compared to conservative treatment. Similar results were noted by Yang et al. [26], after they followed 107 patients for 1 year. Wang et al. [27] looked at studies comparing vertebroplasty to kyphoplasty for single-level compression fractures. They evaluated 8 studies involving 845 patients and found that there were no differences in long-term VAS scores, ODI scores, and short- or long-term SF 36 scores, or differences in adjacent segment fracture rates with either of these procedures. The study did however show kyphoplasty to be superior in correcting the kyphotic angle and vertebral body height as compared to vertebroplasty.

In summary, recent studies have shown that vertebroplasty and kyphoplasty can be used for the treatment of patients with osteoporotic compression fractures in patients who fail to improve with medical management. Determining who will benefit from cement augmentation versus conservative treatment is an ongoing issue and warrants further research.

Conclusion

Some patients with VCFs can benefit from cement augmentation. Studies show that the greatest benefit following cement augmentation is usually within the first 3 months following a fracture. Controversies exist in the literature with no study providing definitive evidence as to which patients will benefit most from cement augmentation. Patients who are immobilized due to chronic pain from their fracture should be offered the option of cement augmentation. Patients with pain from myeloma and lymphoma are also good candidates for treatment with cement augmentation. The use of kyphoplasty within 3 months of a VCF has the possibility of reducing kyphosis that resulted from the fracture. After 3 months, both vertebroplasty and kyphoplasty have a low likelihood of kyphosis correction.

References

1. Lyritis GP, Ioannidis GV, Karachalios T, Roidis N, Kataxaki E, Papaioannou N, Kaloudis J, Galanos A. Analgesic effect of salmon calcitonin suppositories in patients with acute pain due to recent osteoporotic vertebral crush fractures: a prospective double-blind, randomized, placebo-controlled clinical study. Clin J Pain. 1999;15(4):284–9.
2. Peichl P, Rintelen B, Kumpan W, Bröll H. Increase of axial and appendicular trabecular and cortical bone density in established osteoporosis with intermittent nasal salmon calcitonin therapy. Gynecol Endocrinol. 1999;13(1):7–14.
3. Pfeifer M, Begerow B, Minne HW. Effects of a new spinal orthosis on posture, trunk strength, and quality of life in women with postmenopausal osteoporosis: a randomized trial. Am J Phys Med Rehabil. 2004;83(3):177–86.
4. Papaioannou A, Adachi JD, Winegard K, Ferko N, Parkinson W, Cook RJ, Webber C, McCartney N. Efficacy of home-based exercise for improving quality of life among elderly women with symptomatic osteoporosis-related vertebral fractures. Osteoporos Int. 2003;14(8):677–82. Epub 2003 Jul 22.
5. Galibert P, Deramond H, Rosat P, Le Gars D. Preliminary note on the treatment of vertebral angioma by percutaneous acrylic vertebroplasty. Neurochirurgie. 1987;33(2):166–8. French.
6. Sietsma MS, Hosman AJ, Verdonschot NJ, Aalsma AM, Veldhuizen AG. Biomechanical evaluation of

the vertebral jack tool and the inflatable bone tamp for reduction of osteoporotic spine fractures. Spine (Phila Pa 1976). 2009;34(18):E640–4. https://doi.org/10.1097/BRS.0b013e3181b1fed8.
7. Hulme PA, Krebs J, Ferguson SJ, Berlemann U. Vertebroplasty and kyphoplasty: a systematic review of 69 clinical studies. Spine (Phila Pa 1976). 2006;31(17):1983–2001. Review.
8. Taylor RS, Taylor RJ, Fritzell P. Balloon kyphoplasty and vertebroplasty for vertebral compression fractures: a comparative systematic review of efficacy and safety. Spine (Phila Pa 1976). 2006;31(23):2747–55. Review.
9. Taylor RS, Fritzell P, Taylor RJ. Balloon kyphoplasty in the management of vertebral compression fractures: an updated systematic review and meta-analysis. Eur Spine J. 2007;16(8):1085–100. Epub 2007 Feb 3. Review. PubMed PMID: 17277923; PubMed Central PMCID: PMC2200787.
10. Liu JT, Liao WJ, Tan WC, Lee JK, Liu CH, Chen YH, Lin TB. Balloon kyphoplasty versus vertebroplasty for treatment of osteoporotic vertebral compression fracture: a prospective, comparative, and randomized clinical study. Osteoporos Int. 2010;21(2):359–64. https://doi.org/10.1007/s00198-009-0952-8. Epub 2009 Jun 10.
11. Eck JC, Nachtigall D, Humphreys SC, Hodges SD. Comparison of vertebroplasty and balloon kyphoplasty for treatment of vertebral compression fractures: a meta-analysis of the literature. Spine J. 2008;8(3):488–97. Epub 2007 May 29.
12. Diamond TH, Bryant C, Browne L, Clark WA. Clinical outcomes after acute osteoporotic vertebral fractures: a 2-year non-randomised trial comparing percutaneous vertebroplasty with conservative therapy. Med J Aust. 2006;184(3):113–7.
13. Rousing R, Andersen MO, Jespersen SM, Thomsen K, Lauritsen J. Percutaneous vertebroplasty compared to conservative treatment in patients with painful acute or subacute osteoporotic vertebral fractures: three-months follow-up in a clinical randomized study. Spine (Phila Pa 1976). 2009;34(13):1349–54. https://doi.org/10.1097/BRS.0b013e3181a4e628.
14. Wardlaw D, Cummings SR, Van Meirhaeghe J, Bastian L, Tillman JB, Ranstam J, Eastell R, Shabe P, Talmadge K, Boonen S. Efficacy and safety of balloon kyphoplasty compared with non-surgical care for vertebral compression fracture (FREE): a randomised controlled trial. Lancet. 2009;373(9668):1016–24. https://doi.org/10.1016/S0140-6736(09)60010-6.. Epub 2009 Feb 24.
15. McGirt MJ, Parker SL, Wolinsky JP, Witham TF, Bydon A, Gokaslan ZL. Vertebroplasty and kyphoplasty for the treatment of vertebral compression fractures: an evidenced-based review of the literature. Spine J. 2009;9(6):501–8. https://doi.org/10.1016/j.spinee.2009.01.003. Epub 2009 Feb 28. Review.
16. Esses SI, McGuire R, Jenkins J, Finkelstein J, Woodard E, Watters WC 3rd, Goldberg MJ, Keith M, Turkelson CM, Wies JL, Sluka P, Boyer KM, Hitchcock K. The treatment of symptomatic osteoporotic spinal compression fractures. J Am Acad Orthop Surg. 2011;19(3):176–82.
17. McGuire R. AAOS clinical practice guideline: the treatment of symptomatic osteoporotic spinal compression fractures. J Am Acad Orthop Surg. 2011;19(3):183–4.
18. Buchbinder R, Osborne RH, Ebeling PR, Wark JD, Mitchell P, Wriedt C, Graves S, Staples MP, Murphy B. A randomized trial of vertebroplasty for painful osteoporotic vertebral fractures. N Engl J Med. 2009;361(6):557–68. https://doi.org/10.1056/NEJMoa0900429.
19. Kallmes DF, Comstock BA, Heagerty PJ, Turner JA, Wilson DJ, Diamond TH, Edwards R, Gray LA, Stout L, Owen S, Hollingworth W, Ghdoke B, Annesley-Williams DJ, Ralston SH, Jarvik JG. A randomized trial of vertebroplasty for osteoporotic spinal fractures. N Engl J Med. 2009;361(6):569–79. https://doi.org/10.1056/NEJMoa0900563. Erratum in: N Engl J Med. 2012 Mar 8;366(10):970. PubMed PMID: 19657122; PubMed Central PMCID: PMC2930487.
20. Klazen CA, Lohle PN, de Vries J, Jansen FH, Tielbeek AV, Blonk MC, Venmans A, van Rooij WJ, Schoemaker MC, Juttmann JR, Lo TH, Verhaar HJ, van der Graaf Y, van Everdingen KJ, Muller AF, Elgersma OE, Halkema DR, Fransen H, Janssens X, Buskens E, Mali WP. Vertebroplasty versus conservative treatment in acute osteoporotic vertebral compression fractures (Vertos II): an open-label randomised trial. Lancet. 2010;376(9746):1085–92. https://doi.org/10.1016/S0140-6736(10)60954-3. Epub 2010 Aug 9.
21. Farrokhi MR, Alibai E, Maghami Z. Randomized controlled trial of percutaneous vertebroplasty versus optimal medical management for the relief of pain and disability in acute osteoporotic vertebral compression fractures. J Neurosurg Spine. 2011;14(5):561–9. https://doi.org/10.3171/2010.12.SPINE10286. Epub 2011 Mar 4.
22. Berenson J, Pflugmacher R, Jarzem P, Zonder J, Schechtman K, Tillman JB, Bastian L, Ashraf T, Vrionis F, Cancer Patient Fracture Evaluation (CAFE) Investigators. Balloon kyphoplasty versus non-surgical fracture management for treatment of painful vertebral body compression fractures in patients with cancer: a multicentre, randomised controlled trial. Lancet Oncol. 2011;12(3):225–35. https://doi.org/10.1016/S1470-2045(11)70008-0. Epub 2011 Feb 16.
23. Papanastassiou ID, Phillips FM, Van Meirhaeghe J, Berenson JR, Andersson GB, Chung G, Small BJ, Aghayev K, Vrionis FD. Comparing effects of kyphoplasty, vertebroplasty, and non-surgical management in a systematic review of randomized and non-randomized controlled studies. Eur Spine J. 2012;21(9):1826–43. Epub 2012 Apr 29. Review. PubMed PMID: 22543412.
24. Edidin AA, Ong KL, Lau E, Kurtz SM. Mortality risk for operated and nonoperated vertebral fracture

patients in the medicare population. J Bone Miner Res. 2011;26(7):1617–26. https://doi.org/10.1002/jbmr.353.
25. Anderson PA, Froyshteter AB, Tontz WL Jr. Meta-analysis of vertebral augmentation compared with conservative treatment for osteoporotic spinal fractures. J Bone Miner Res. 2013;28(2):372–82. https://doi.org/10.1002/jbmr.1762. Review.
26. Yang EZ, Xu JG, Huang GZ, Xiao WZ, Liu XK, Zeng BF, Lian XF. Percutaneous vertebroplasty versus conservative treatment in aged patients with acute osteoporotic vertebral compression fractures: a prospective randomized controlled clinical study. Spine (Phila Pa 1976). 2016;41(8):653–60. https://doi.org/10.1097/BRS.0000000000001298.
27. Wang H, Sribastav SS, Ye F, Yang C, Wang J, Liu H, Zheng Z. Comparison of percutaneous vertebroplasty and balloon kyphoplasty for the treatment of single level vertebral compression fractures: a meta-analysis of the literature. Pain Physician. 2015;18(3):209–22. Review.

13 Vertebroplasty Cement Augmentation Technique

A. Orlando Ortiz

Key Points

1. Careful patient selection is a prerequisite to performing a safe and effective vertebroplasty procedure.
2. Accurate needle placement whether unilateral or bilateral can be achieved with oblique "down-the-barrel" fluoroscopic imaging or with traditional frontal pedicle-targeting techniques.
3. Cement injection should be performed with meticulous imaging surveillance in order to avoid cement extravasation into the spinal canal, paraspinal veins, or intervertebral disk.
4. Complications in vertebroplasty, though uncommon, can be further reduced by attention to specific procedure details including use of proper fluoroscopic techniques, consistent needle insertion maneuvers with an active appreciation of all osseous landmarks during the procedure, and exquisite attention to the cement injection process.

A. O. Ortiz (✉)
Department of Radiology, Jacobi Medical Center, Bronx, NY, USA
e-mail: ortizo@nychhc.org

Introduction

It is now four decades since the first image-guided vertebroplasty procedure was performed in 1984 by Galibert and Deramond [1]. As compared to the standard vertebroplasty procedure which is most often performed percutaneously in the thoracic or lumbar spine to treat an osteoporotic vertebral compression fracture, this first image-guided vertebroplasty procedure was performed transorally in the upper cervical spine for a painful C2 hemangioma. Indeed, vertebroplasty is a percutaneous procedure in which a bone needle is advanced using image guidance into a vertebral body that has been fractured as a result of osteoporosis or, less commonly, neoplastic infiltration [2]. Acrylic bone cement, usually polymethyl methacrylate that is impregnated with barium for radiopacity, is injected through the bone needle into the vertebral body under direct imaging guidance [3]. The term vertebral augmentation is now used as the acrylic bone cement is considered an implant that augments the strength of the damaged vertebra.

The first image-guided vertebroplasty procedures that were performed in the United States commencing in 1993 were reported in 1997 [2]. Due to its early and dramatic success with respect to patient outcomes, this procedure was quickly adopted by those operators who perform percutaneous image-guided procedures. A review of the Medicare database from 2005 to 2008 showed

A. E. Razi, S. H. Hershman (eds.), *Vertebral Compression Fractures in Osteoporotic and Pathologic Bone*, https://doi.org/10.1007/978-3-030-33861-9_13

that 63,983 vertebroplasty procedures were performed over this 3-year period; in comparison 119,253 kyphoplasty procedures were performed over the same time period [4]. A review of the US National Inpatient Sample from 2005 to 2010 showed 81,790 vertebroplasty and 307,050 kyphoplasty procedures were performed [5]. Now, given that approximately 700,000 osteoporotic vertebral compression fractures occur each year within the United States, it is clear that cement augmentation is only performed on select patients. In other words, not every patient with an osteoporotic vertebral compression fracture is either a candidate for or requires a vertebral augmentation procedure.

Multiple osteoporotic vertebral compression fracture treatments are available. These are generally categorized into noninvasive and invasive treatment interventions. Noninvasive treatments for painful osteoporotic vertebral compression fractures include medical management and physical therapy. Medical management typically includes a trial of bedrest and analgesics. The use of a back brace or orthosis is another possible treatment intervention that might provide the patient some increased stability when they attempt to stand and ambulate. Physical therapy with spine rehabilitation is another treatment alternative that is sometimes employed to assist patients with basic ambulation and to reduce the loss of bone and muscle mass that is associated with prolonged inactivity. It must be emphasized that just because these treatment interventions are considered noninvasive does not mean that they do not have potential adverse implications for patient outcomes [6, 7]. Prolonged bedrest is associated with muscle wasting and further bone demineralization as well as the possibility of thromboembolic disease, pneumonia, or skin breakdown with decubitus formation. Further deterioration of the injured vertebra with progression of height loss and possible osseous retropulsion into the spinal canal may occur. The latter may be associated with spinal cord compression and neurologic compromise (Fig. 13.1). Progression of a kyphotic deformity may predispose the patient to poor balance and falls. The presence of one osteoporotic vertebral compression fracture increases the odds ratio of developing a second, often adjacent level, fracture in the same patient [8]. Analgesics often have significant side effects that are not well tolerated by elderly patients. Furthermore, because of analgesic dosing limitations, the patients often find that they have significant pain on a daily basis. The frequent and improper use of heating pads can be associated with skin irritation and mild burns. The challenge with physical therapy is that it can potentially increase axial loading in a

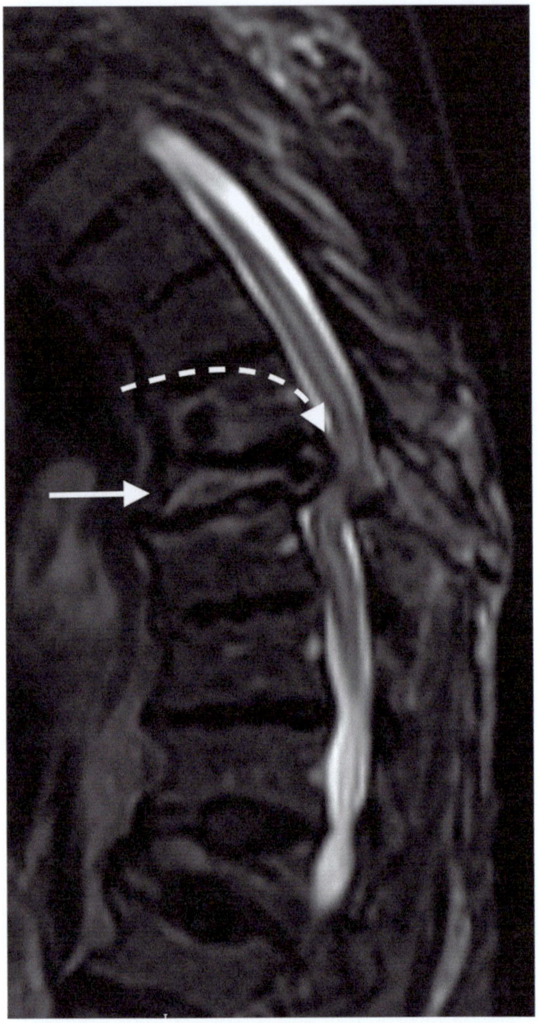

Fig. 13.1 A 97-year-old female with known T9 osteoporotic vertebral compression fracture being managed with bedrest and analgesics for 4 weeks is no longer able to stand or walk. T2-weighted sagittal MR image shows a marked compression deformity of the T9 vertebral body (arrow) with osseous retropulsion (curved arrow) and acute spinal cord compression

patient that is already compromised with a demineralized axial skeleton and possibly accelerate height loss in the compressed vertebral body. Noninvasive treatment strategies, therefore, are not necessarily benign.

The invasive treatment strategies for managing painful osteoporotic vertebral compression fractures include open spine surgery and percutaneous vertebral augmentation. Spine surgery with fixation and possible decompression and/or fusion is at the most invasive end of the treatment spectrum [9]. In general, many patients are not candidates for these open surgical procedures due to their pre-existing comorbidities. Furthermore, osteoporotic bone can pose a challenge to adequate spinal fixation with instrumentation. Nevertheless, in properly selected patients, this may be a necessary and viable treatment strategy, especially in patients with signs and symptoms related to spinal cord compression from retropulsed bone. Image-guided percutaneous vertebroplasty is an invasive procedure in which properly selected patients can achieve effective outcomes with respect to significant pain relief with low risk to the patient. Image-guided percutaneous vertebral augmentation has evolved into an important component of care for patients suffering from painful osteoporotic vertebral compression fractures [10].

Indication

Vertebroplasty is indicated to treat painful osteoporotic vertebral compression fractures of the thoracic and lumbar spine (Table 13.1). This indication requires that both a clinical and an

Table 13.1 Vertebroplasty: indications and contraindications

Indication	Contraindication
Painful osteoporotic vertebral compression fracture	Spinal cord compression
Painful pathologic vertebral compression fracture	Uncorrected coagulopathy
	Systemic infection
	Local infection: spine or skin
	Uncooperative patient

imaging component be addressed prior to considering a patient for this procedure. Patients with symptomatic osteoporotic vertebral fractures have significant mid or low back pain that is exacerbated by standing or any other type of activity; the pain is often relieved by lying down. On physical examination the patient may demonstrate exquisite point spinal tenderness at the level of the fracture and paraspinal tenderness in the area of the fracture; this clinical finding is even more apparent using fluoroscopic evaluation. The patient's pain diagram will indicate focal pain at the spinal level of the fracture, thoracic or lumbar, with anterior radiation along the ribs and/or anterior abdominal wall, respectively. The patient's pain should be significant, generally at least 7/10 on a numeric pain scale. There may be a transient or no response to narcotic analgesics. The onset of pain may be acute (measured in days) or be of subacute duration (approximately 3–12 weeks) and may be associated with an inciting event such as a fall or picking up a heavy object or a bumpy transportation ride. It is important to evaluate patients promptly after their fracture event because the opportunity for good outcomes in terms of pain relief and height maintenance of the injured vertebral body occur earlier in the patient's clinical course. Early intervention avoids the treatment challenges of further vertebral collapse and helps to prevent the formation of focal kyphosis. As the primary goal of vertebroplasty is pain relief, prudent patient selection requires that the patient have significant pain referable to their osteoporotic vertebral compression fracture. A secondary, nevertheless important clinical feature is that the patient should show evidence of having osteoporosis. If a history of osteoporosis is not already known, then the patient should undergo a bone density test in order to have a baseline value to monitor treatment; by definition, a compression fracture with a low energy mechanism by itself may be considered the confirmatory event. Obtaining the bone density test is the first step in initiating the medical management of the patient's osteoporosis.

The role of imaging in the evaluation of a suspected vertebral compression fracture is extremely important to patient selection. The patient's pain

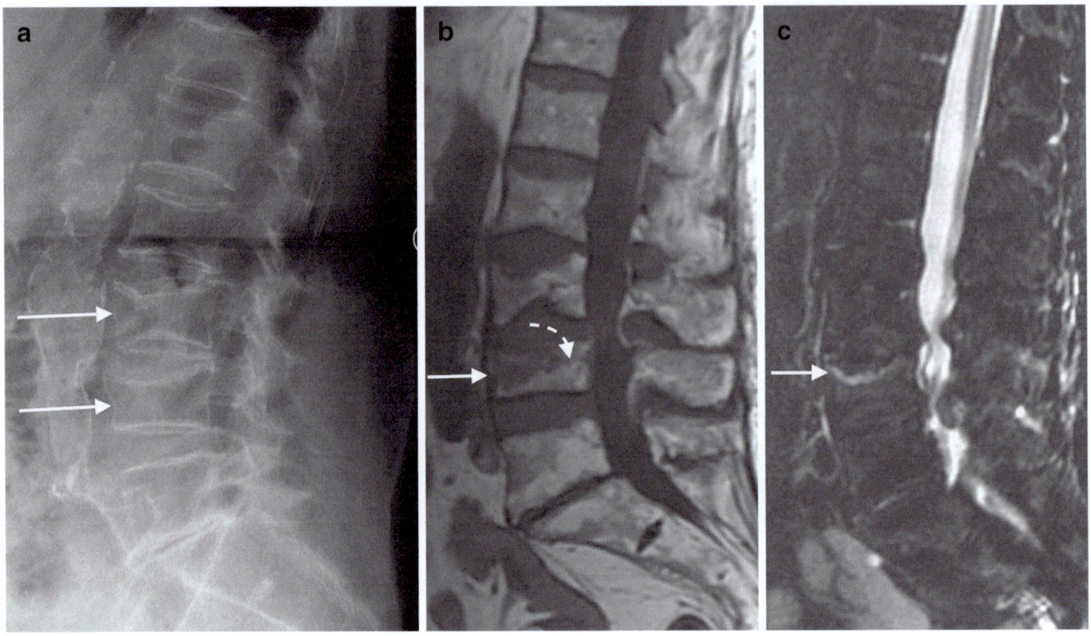

Fig. 13.2 A 93-year-old female with 1-month history of severe low back pain. (**a**) Lateral radiograph of the lumbar spine shows partial impaction vertebral compression deformities at L3 and L4 (arrows). (**b**) T1-weighted sagittal MR image obtained a few days later shows low signal intensity within the anterior aspect of the L4 vertebral body (arrow) as well as a fracture line (curved arrow); small Schmorl's nodes involve the superior and inferior endplates of L3. (**c**) Fat-suppressed T2-weighted sagittal MR image shows a horizontal hyperintense band of edema (arrow) adjacent to the superior endplate of L4 and consistent with a subacute L4 vertebral compression fracture

profile and clinical evaluation should correlate with the level of the fracture as seen on the imaging examination. Many patients initially undergo plain radiographic evaluation (Fig. 13.2). These radiographs can be helpful as they may quickly identify an isolated vertebral compression fracture in a patient with acute severe back pain. When multiple vertebral compression deformities are present, it may not be possible to identify recent fractures unless prior radiographic studies are available. More importantly, plain radiographs are notoriously insensitive and can miss acute fractures that have not yet demonstrated height loss. Magnetic resonance imaging (MRI) is the study of choice to evaluate patients with suspected vertebral compression fractures [11, 12]. Acute and subacute fractures can be readily identified due to the presence of marrow edema which manifests as hypointense signal on T1-weighted images and hyperintense signal on T2-weighted and inversion recovery sequences (Fig. 13.2). Vertebral body clefts, when present, are the result of avascular necrosis and are seen as fluid and/or gas containing collections located subjacent to a compressed vertebral endplate. MRI is used to evaluate whether there is spinal canal compromise by displaced fracture fragments and is also capable of identifying other potential pain generators such as disk herniations or facet joint pathology. MRI can also be used to help differentiate between osteoporotic and pathologic vertebral compression fractures. When the patient cannot undergo MR imaging, or when there is concern regarding the cortical integrity of the vertebral body, especially the posterior wall, computed tomography (CT) of the affected spine segment can be performed. CT is also helpful in identifying fracture lines, which may be a potential route for cement extravasation through the vertebral endplate or elsewhere. Vertebral endplate fractures are a very common component of osteoporotic vertebral compression fractures and, if not accounted for at the time of cement augmentation, can be associated with intra-diskal cement extravasation [13, 14]. As with plain radiographs, acute fractures may be missed on CT (Fig. 13.3). Recent advancements with dual energy CT

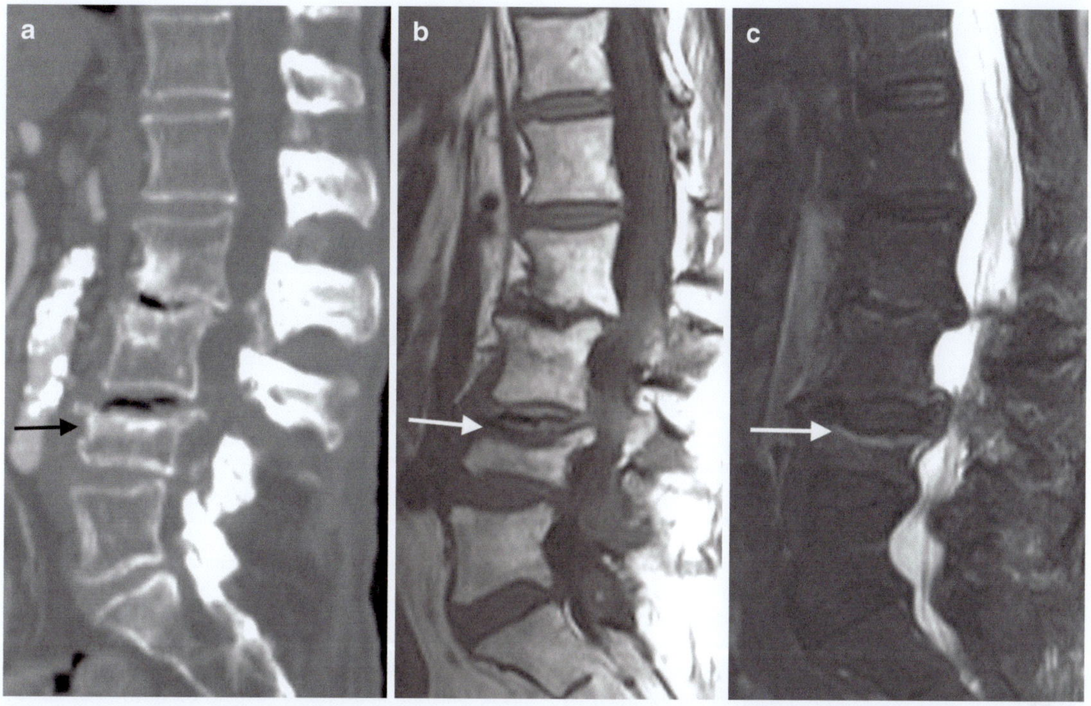

Fig. 13.3 An 86-year-old female with low back pain after lifting a box. (**a**) Midline sagittal CT reformation in bone window algorithm shows a partial impaction vertebral compression fracture that involves the superior endplate of L4 (arrow); on this isolated study, the L4 fracture is age-indeterminate. (**b**) T1-weighted sagittal MR image shows focal hypointensity within the superior endplate of L4 (arrow). (**c**) Fat-suppressed T2-weighted sagittal MR image shows a band of hyperintensity (arrow) within the superior endplate of L4. The findings are consistent with a subacute L4 vertebral compression fracture

technology may indeed show marrow edema; however, clinical investigations are still ongoing [15]. Skeletal scintigraphy can be used to identify acute or subacute osteoporotic vertebral compression fractures or pathologic fractures related to an underlying neoplasm. An acute or subacute osteoporotic vertebral compression fracture will present as a focal area of increased radiotracer uptake on the static images.

Fluoroscopy provides a quick clinical and imaging overview of a patient with a suspected osteoporotic vertebral compression fracture. Palpation of the spinous process of the fractured vertebra may result in reproduction of the patient's pain profile. In general, if there is pain provocation at the level of the patient's vertebral compression fracture, then that patient may be a candidate for vertebral augmentation. Fluoroscopic evaluation enables additional evaluation of a vertebral compression fracture for the purposes of treatment planning in terms of morphology, height loss, presence or absence of a cleft, location in the vertebral column, and size of the pedicles. The visibility of the bony landmarks can also be quickly assessed in patients with poor bone mineralization and/or a large body habitus. Fluoroscopy is able to dynamically evaluate patients with fracture instability associated with endplate motion, a phenomenon which is sometimes seen in the thoracic spine and related to respiratory motion (Fig. 13.4). At the time of the fluoroscopic evaluation, it is immediately determined if the patient is able to lie prone, if they are cooperative, and how much pain the patient is experiencing especially with transfer onto and off the fluoroscopy table. Regardless of the imaging pathway that is used, the imaging study or studies should demonstrate a recent vertebral compression fracture that correlates with the patient's clinical presentation.

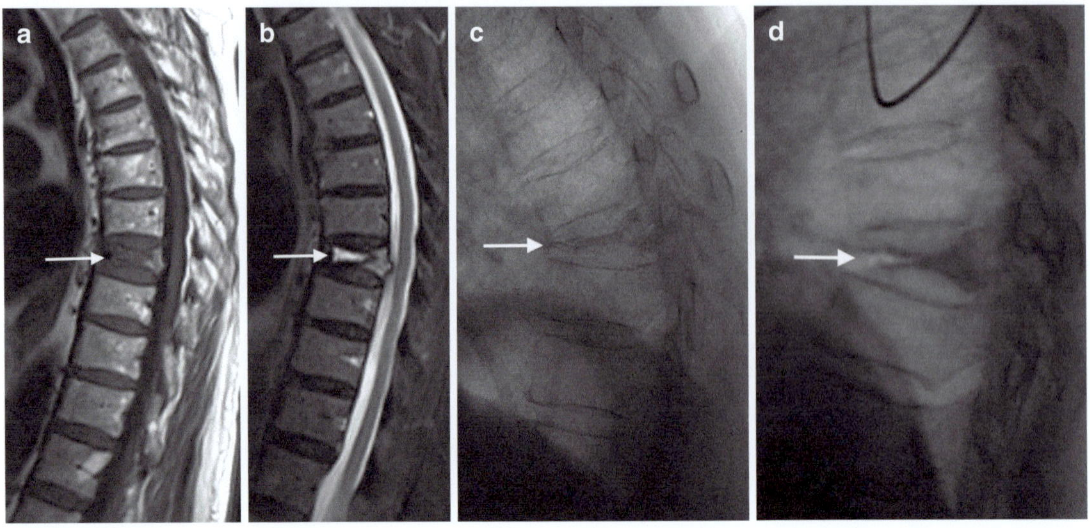

Fig. 13.4 An 83-year-old female with osteoporosis, who self-discontinued bisphosphonates, experienced sudden severe mid back pain 5 weeks earlier while attempting to bend over and put on her shoes. T1-weighted sagittal MR image (**a**) shows a partial impaction-type vertebral compression deformity at T9 (arrow) with low signal intensity consistent with edema. T2-weighted sagittal MR image (**b**) shows a hyperintense fluid cleft (arrow) within the vertebral body. The patient underwent conservative management, including physical therapy, but her pain persisted. Lateral radiograph of the thoracic spine (**c**) now shows a *vertebra plana* deformity (arrow) at T9 and osteopenia. Lateral fluoroscopic image (**d**) with the patient in the prone position shows focal expansion (arrow) of the T9 vertebral endplates which moved with the patients respirations

In addition to pain relief, another goal of vertebroplasty is to prevent further height loss in an already compromised and weakened vertebral body. This may retard the progression of kyphosis that is sometimes associated with wedging of the untreated fractured vertebral body. By avoiding further kyphosis, there may be fewer patient falls and fall-associated injuries.

The other treatment alternative to vertebroplasty is kyphoplasty or balloon-assisted vertebroplasty [3]. The latter procedure includes temporary inflation of a balloon tamp within the fractured vertebra in order to attempt to restore height and to create a space or cavity within the damaged vertebral. The cavity that is created by temporary balloon tamp inflation is the initial reservoir for injected cement and is thought to reduce the likelihood of cement extravasation beyond the vertebral body and may reduce the incidence of cement embolization due to high pressures. There are over 100 studies in the literature which compare vertebroplasty with kyphoplasty, and overall, both procedures are considered safe and effective. There are some advantages that vertebroplasty has over kyphoplasty . Since vertebroplasty entails one less step than kyphoplasty and tends to use smaller-gauge (e.g., 11- or 13-gauge) bone needles, it can be performed quite efficiently. Therefore, in patients who cannot tolerate a long procedure due to comorbidities, a vertebroplasty may be the better procedure. Also, smaller gauge needles might be useful in patients with a propensity to hemorrhage or in whom anticoagulation will be resumed shortly after the procedure.

Understanding the contraindications to cement augmentation is critical (Table 13.1). Cement augmentation is not indicated in patients with acute spinal cord compression (Fig. 13.1). Those patients require the immediate attention of a spine surgeon for possible decompression surgery. In the neurologically intact patient, the presence of bony retropulsion into the spinal canal is not a contraindication to cement augmentation [16] (Fig. 13.5). Cement augmentation is contraindicated in patients with uncorrected coagulopathy – the appropriate clinical steps must be taken in order to apply hold or bridging strategies in patients on anticoagulant and/or antiplatelet therapy so that this elective procedure can be performed safely [17]. Cement augmentation should not be performed in patients with concurrent sys-

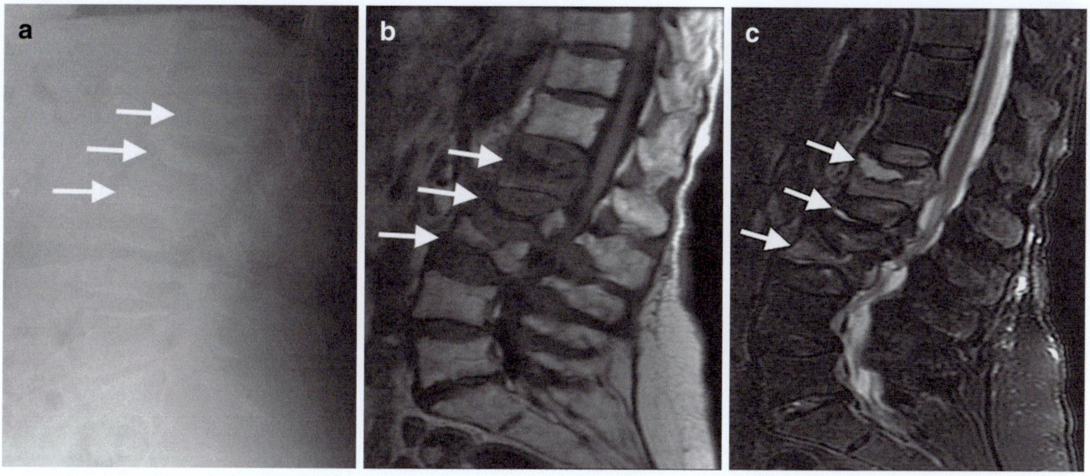

Fig. 13.5 An 89-year-old female with crippling low back pain that necessitated hospitalization. Lateral radiograph of the lumbar spine (**a**) shows diffuse osteopenia and multiple vertebral compression deformities (arrows) at L1, L2, and L3. T1-weighted sagittal MR image (**b**) shows hypointense signal (arrows) within portions of the affected vertebral bodies; a *vertebra plana* deformity is present at L2. T2-weighted sagittal MR image (**c**) shows hyperintense clefts (arrows) within L1 and L2 and edema within L3 (arrow)

temic infection – infections must first be treated, and the patient must be medically cleared prior to performing the procedure. Similarly, patients with spine infections are not candidates for cement augmentation. Because many patients with osteoporotic fractures are elderly and are often at prolonged bedrest, they may develop decubitus ulcers, especially at the apex of a kyphotic deformity. The procedure should be postponed in these patients until after these skin lesions undergo appropriate wound care therapy. The procedure cannot be performed in an uncooperative patient.

Careful patient selection is a prerequisite to performing a safe and effective cement augmentation procedure. The ideal candidate has a recent (acute or subacute) single-level osteoporotic vertebral compression fracture with focal severe pain that corresponds to the level of the fracture as seen on the imaging examination. Patients that were very active prior to sustaining their vertebral compression fracture tend to improve quicker and may have better outcomes than patients who are sedentary or chronically bedridden.

Vertebroplasty Technique

Prior to a vertebroplasty procedure, it is important that the patient refrain from oral intake for at least 8 hours. Laboratory parameters that are analyzed prior to the procedure include hematologic, coagulation, and renal profiles. Informed consent is obtained prior to the procedure. Vertebroplasty can be performed using either general intravenous anesthesia or intravenous sedation and local analgesia. Intravenous access is ideally obtained within the forearm or hand; the antecubital fossa should be avoided as the patient's arms are often bent when they are placed on the procedure table and this arm position may impede the function of the intravenous line. When patient comorbidities prevent the use of sedatives and analgesics, the procedure can be performed using local anesthetic agents alone. Vertebroplasty can be performed on an outpatient or an inpatient basis, depending upon the clinical situation. An intravenous antibiotic, for prophylaxis, is routinely given in our practice, within an hour of the start of the procedure. The physician should review the patient's imaging studies before the procedure and, whenever possible, have immediate access to the patient's key imaging studies at the time of the procedure. The use of a "time-out" with the procedural staff before the patient is prepped and sedated will assist in confirming the specific vertebral level(s) that will require treatment.

It is important that all vertebral augmentation procedures be performed using strict aseptic technique. This procedure is performed with imaging guidance, usually a multidirectional single or biplane fluoroscope, but some physicians prefer to perform the procedure using computed tomography or computed tomography with fluoroscopy. It is critical to have access to high-quality imaging so that key bony landmarks, including the spinous process, pedicles, and vertebral body margins, are readily visualized. The patients are carefully positioned in the prone position, and every attempt is made to bolster the patient to facilitate hyperextension at the level of the vertebral compression fracture. This maneuver has been reported to predispose to height restoration even with vertebroplasty [18]. The skin is then prepped and draped using strict sterile technique. For thoracic procedures it is important to make sure that all monitoring leads are placed outside of the fluoroscopic field of view. Once the patient is positioned and prepared, the vertebroplasty procedure can then be initiated; this consists of a two-step process: (1) needle placement and (2) cement injection (Table 13.2) [19, 20].

Table 13.2 Tips for improving patient outcomes with vertebroplasty

Patient selection
Severe axial back pain corresponding to the level of the vertebral compression fracture
Significant disability as seen on validated disability scales such as the Oswestry Disability Index or SF-36
Strict adherence to indications and contraindications
Optimized imaging
Operator is able to visualize all osseous landmarks on frontal and lateral fluoroscopic projections: pedicle outline, spinous process, vertebral body margins (anterior, posterior, lateral, superior, and inferior endplates)
Equipment for vertebroplasty
Bone needles: straight, curved
Needle approaches: transpedicular, parapedicular
Cement: opacified, high-viscosity
Cement injection: meticulous
Patient follow-up and evaluation
Monitor and document patient's pain profile and disability scores
Osteoporosis management
Current bone density test
Patients with osteoporosis will need to be on treatment
Physical therapy
Gait and balance training

Fig. 13.6 Step-by-step vertebroplasty. Oblique fluoroscopic image (**a**) shows needle placement (arrow) for anesthetic infiltration over the posterior surface of the pedicle (medial pedicle cortex indicated by small arrows). Oblique fluoroscopic image (**b**) during initial bone needle insertion (arrow) along lateral margin of the upper outer quadrant of the pedicle (p). Note the position of the pedicle relative to the superior endplate (dashed line) with the degree of obliquity indicated by the position of the spinous process (asterisk). Lateral fluoroscopic image (**c**) shows the position of the needle tip (arrow) on the posterior pedicle cortex. Lateral (**d**) and frontal (**e**) fluoroscopic images show the needle tip (arrow) entering the junction between the pedicle and posterior vertebral body. As shown on the frontal image, (**e**) the needle tip has not yet crossed the medial pedicle cortex (dashed line). Overhead photograph (**f**) of a vertebral body model to show the position of the needle tip (arrow) as it just enters the posterior vertebral body from the pedicle. The needle tip, as in (**d**) and (**e**), has not yet crossed the boundary (dashed line) of the medial pedicle cortex. Lateral (**g**) and frontal (**h**) fluoroscopic images show advancement of the needle tip (arrows) into the anterior one-third of the vertebral body just beyond the midline (dashed line). Lateral (**i**) and frontal (**j**) fluoroscopic images show coaxial replacement of the bone needle stylet with a cement introducer (large arrow); the bone needle cannula (small arrow) has been partially retracted into the posterior vertebral body. Lateral (**k**) and frontal (**l**) fluoroscopic images show obtained during the initial phase of cement injection the focal accumulation of opacified cement (dashed circle) just anterior to the cement introducer. Lateral (**m**) and frontal (**n**) fluoroscopic images show filling of the anterior vertebral body with cement (arrows) as the cement introducer is gradually retracted. Lateral fluoroscopic image (**o**) at the completion of injection shows removal of the cement introducer and replacement of the bone needle stylet. An endplate-to-endplate cement fill pattern (arrow) is seen within the anterior column. Frontal fluoroscopic image (**p**) shows midline and intravertebral location of the cement (arrow)

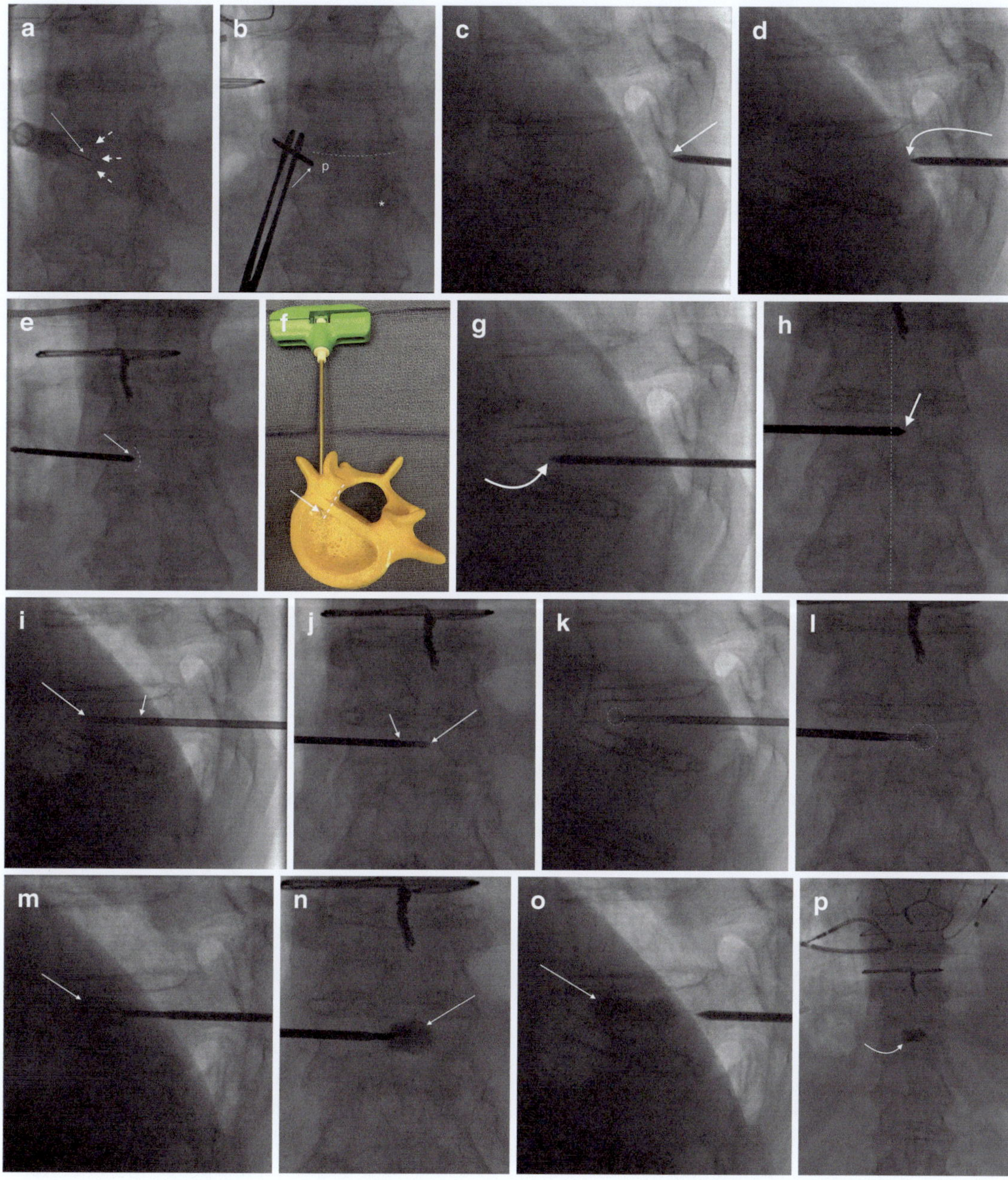
a
b
p
c
d
e
f
g
h
i
j
k
l
m
n
o
p

Equipment: Bone Needles

Bone needles for vertebroplasty range in size from 13 to 10 gauge and in length from 10 to 15 cm. The bone needle stylets consist of either beveled or diamond tips. The beveled tip does allow for slight steering of the bone needle as it is advanced into the vertebral body. Smaller gauge bone needles are often used to perform vertebroplasty within the upper thoracic spine where the pedicles are smaller. Larger gauge bone needles can accommodate biopsy cannulas or coaxial bone cannulas that can be used for cement injection. These large needles can also accommodate a curved bone needle that can be used to cross the midline of the anterior column using a unilateral approach [21]. Alternatively, the midline can be approached with a straight bone needle by using a lateral start point with a medial trajectory.

Needle Placement

Vertebroplasty is performed using either a unilateral or bilateral approach with the goal being to reach the anterior and paramedian aspect of the vertebral body (Fig. 13.6). A transpedicular route is often used as this "down-the-barrel" approach allows a relatively safe passage of the bone needle into the vertebral body. This is often performed with a 10-, 11-, or 13-gauge bone needle. A bone biopsy, when indicated, can be performed as the needle system is amenable to the coaxial insertion of a biopsy cannula. Appropriate alignment of the spine at the treatment level using patient positioning and positioning of the fluoroscope(s) is important in order to determine the optimal skin entry site(s) for the bone needle(s). A bone needle can be inserted into the vertebral body either by going directly through the pedicle (transpedicular) or by entering along the lateral margin of the pedicle (parapedicular). True extra-pedicular approaches, which completely avoid the pedicle, and involve insertion directly into the lateral aspect of the vertebral body, are infrequently used; when they are utilized, extra-pedicular approaches are most often used in the lumbar spine.

The author's preferred technique will be described here using a transpedicular approach. The fluoroscope is rotated such that the pedicle overlies vertebral body. In general, the craniocaudal angulation of the fluoroscope should place the pedicle within the upper one-third of the vertebral body (Fig. 13.6). Mediolateral rotation of the fluoroscope should place the pedicle in a slight "scottie-dog" configuration or within the lateral one-third of the vertebral body. The steeper the angulation of the fluoroscope, the more medial (relative to the midline) the needle will travel within the vertebral body. Some physicians will use this steeper angle in order to perform the procedure from a unilateral approach. A bilateral approach is preferred by some as it enables consistent access to both sides of the anterior aspect of the vertebral body. Regardless of the approach, sound fluoroscopic and radiation protection techniques should be utilized in order to minimize radiation exposure to the patient and to all personnel within the operative suite [22].

The skin is marked with a sterile marker at the site of intended skin entry. The skin is anesthetized with local anesthetic as are the subcutaneous tissues. A 22-gauge spinal needle is advanced to the periosteal surface of the posterior pedicle in order to anesthetize the periosteal entry site with local anesthetic. This serves as an opportunity to modify the subsequent bone needle insertion and trajectory if necessary and is also an important step for patient comfort. A small incision is made at the skin entry site using a #11 scalpel blade. The bone needle is advanced to the pedicle surface under imaging guidance (Fig. 13.6). A long clamp is used to hold the bone needle as it is advanced to the target entry site. The use of a sterile clamp keeps the operator's hands out of the fluoroscopy field. For transpedicular access, the upper outer quadrant is the initial entry site into the pedicle. The needle is advanced through the pedicle with a forward twisting motion; this enables the needle tip to cut through and penetrate the pedicle cortex. Another option is to use a surgical hammer to tap the bone needle handle in order to advance the bone needle. The bone needle is slowly advanced under fluoroscopic guidance into the posterior vertebral body (Fig. 13.6). The relationship of the bone needle tip with respect to the medial pedicle cortex and the posterior vertebral body should be continuously monitored with fluoroscopy in at least the frontal and lateral projections. On a frontal projection of the vertebral body, the bone needle should never cross the medial pedicle cortex until it has entered the posterior vertebral body as seen on a lateral projection (Fig. 13.6). If the bone needle tip crosses the medial pedicle cortex before it enters the vertebral body, then the bone needle is entering the spinal canal. Once the bone needle safely enters the posterior vertebral body, it can be advanced to the desired position within the vertebral body using both frontal and lateral fluoroscopic guidance. The target position for the needle tip is within the anterior one-third of the vertebral body as seen on the lateral projection and at last midway into the ipsilateral half of the vertebral body as seen on the frontal projection if using a bi-pedicular technique or at least just across the midline if using a unilateral approach (Fig. 13.7). Once the physician has optimized the needle position, cement injection may proceed.

If a satisfactory needle purchase on the posterior surface of the pedicle cannot be obtained or if the pedicle is of insufficient size to safely accommodate the bone needle, then a parapedicular approach can be used. Again, as soon as the needle tip reaches the medial border of the pedicle as seen on the frontal projection, its depth should be anterior to the posterior wall of the vertebral body as seen on the lateral projection. Some physicians prefer to use measurement techniques on the frontal projection in order to plan their trajectory through the pedicle into the vertebral body. This is an adaptation of percutaneous pedicle screw placement for establishing a bilateral transpedicular approach into the vertebral body using a well-aligned (parallel vertebral endplates) and centered frontal fluoroscopic projection with the spinous process equidistant between the pedicles [23]. The endplates of the affected

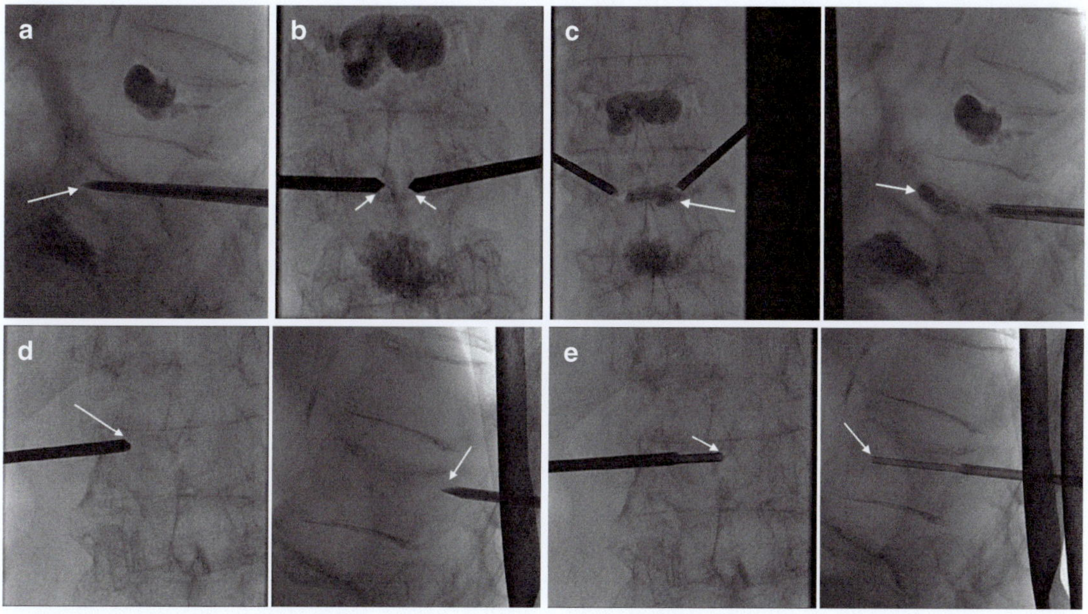

Fig. 13.7 Same patient as in Fig. 13.5. Lateral (**a**) and frontal (**b**) fluoroscopic images show bilateral transpedicular insertion of 11 gauge bone needles (arrows) into an L2 *vertebral plana* deformity. Frontal and lateral fluoroscopic images (**c**) show acrylic bone cement (arrows) that was injected through coaxial bone filler cannulas into the anterior column of the vertebral body. Frontal and lateral fluoroscopic images (**d**) show unilateral transpedicular 11 gauge bone needle insertion (arrow) into the L1 vertebral body. Frontal and lateral fluoroscopic images (**e**) show the coaxial exchange for a bone biopsy cannula (arrows) which was used to obtain three bone cores from this vertebral body

vertebral body should be aligned in a parallel orientation in both the frontal and lateral projections. The pedicles should be located within the upper half of the vertebral body on the frontal projection and should be aligned or overlapping on the lateral projection. The initial identification of the bone needle trajectory is performed using the frontal projection. The clamp or spinal needle can be used to identify the pedicle, and a skin mark is made using a sterile marker 1–2 cm lateral to the pedicle and slightly superior to the pedicle. The use of fluoroscopy, with frontal and lateral projections, during the application of local anesthetic with the spinal needle, will confirm that the appropriate skin entry site has been determined. The target point for bone needle insertion is at the intersection of the base of the transverse process and facet; this is the 10 or 11 o'clock position for the left pedicle and the 2 or 3 o'clock position for the right pedicle, as seen on the frontal projection with the patient prone. As the bone needle is advanced through the pedicle, it is directed toward the wall of the medial pedicle, just inside the medial wall of the pedicle. When the bone needle tip reaches approximately 3 mm beyond the junction of the pedicle and vertebral body as seen on the lateral projection, it should lie within the center of the pedicle, lateral to the medial pedicle wall, as seen on the frontal projection. With this technique, a bone needle can be safely placed within the paramedian aspect of each half of the vertebral body as seen on the frontal projection.

At the physician's discretion, a bone biopsy can be performed during the process of needle insertion; some prefer to perform a biopsy during all of their vertebral augmentation procedures [24]. It is reasonable to consider a biopsy procedure in patients with a prior history of cancer or imaging findings that are suspicious for pathologic fracture (Fig. 13.7). The biopsy can be performed using coaxial technique with a bone biopsy needle that is advanced through the cannula. The bone biopsy needle can be inserted once the initial bone cannula is situated within the substance of the pedicle in order to maximize the number of biopsy samples. When possible three bone cores should be obtained for pathologic analysis and submitted in a formalin specimen container [25]. If a bone aspirate is obtained, this should also be submitted for pathologic analysis as the sample may contain a diagnostic specimen.

Equipment: Bone Cements

The bone cements that are used for vertebroplasty are injected in a flowable state and become fully cured within the vertebral body within a short period of time (approximately 4–20 minutes, depending upon the manufacturer). The most common acrylic bone cement that is used for vertebroplasty is polymethyl methacrylate (PMMA). These cements have undergone significant improvements that have optimized their use in vertebral augmentation procedures. The polymethyl methacrylate is impregnated with sterile barium sulfate, approximately 30% weight/volume barium sulfate added to polymethyl methacrylate powder, for radio-opacification. A liquid monomer is added to the polymer powder and the two agents are mixed in a mixing chamber. The "working time" of the cement preparation is defined as the time when mixing is completed (anywhere from 30 seconds to a few minutes, depending on the manufacturer of the cement preparation) until the time that the cement hardens and can no longer be injected. These PMMA cement preparations offer reasonable working times, approximately 10–20 minutes depending on the ambient room temperature. Commercially available preparations provide pre-measured amounts of the two reagents and the mixing vehicles, either manual or motorized. All of this equipment has been pre-sterilized and is available for one-time use. A key advance with these medical grade acrylic bone cements has been the development of high-viscosity bone cements. The use of high-viscosity bone cement has the potential to decrease the likelihood of cement extravasation beyond the vertebral body [26]. Nevertheless, all cement injections should be performed with meticulous imaging surveillance in order to avoid cement extravasation into the spinal canal, paraspinal veins, or intervertebral disk.

Extensive attempts have been made to develop more biocompatible bone cements for vertebral augmentation [27]. One type of bone cement that can be used for vertebroplasty is bioceramic bone cement, which is composite acrylic bone cement that consists of cross-linked resins and glass ceramic particles [28]. Unlike PMMA, this cement is hydrophilic, a property which facilitates cement spread within the vertebral body. Also unlike PMMA, it is osteoconductive and stimulates bone apposition along its margins. In addition to these latter two properties, this cement functions similarly to cortical bone in terms of restoring compressive strength to the damaged vertebral body. An important advantage of this clinically available cement is its mix on demand feature that allows for multiple uses during one procedure; the cement cures within 3–4 minutes; hence it should be injected using a coaxial system (Fig. 13.8). Calcium phosphate cements have also been used for vertebroplasty procedures due to their biocompatibility and osteoconductivity and osteo-integrative properties. Unfortunately, many of these calcium phosphate cements provide poor structural reinforcement of the vertebral body. Attempts at developing other injectable cements such as calcium sulfate and magnesium sulfate cements have shown very limited applications.

Cement Injection

The cement, once prepared, can be injected with the cement delivery system that is supplied by the manufacturer – this often consists of a hydraulic plunger system that is activated by rotating the handle of the plunger. Alternatively, 1 mL syringes can be filled with cement, and these can be used to inject the cement through the bone needle and into the vertebral body. Another option involves the use of coaxial bone filler cannulas or cement introducers (Fig. 13.7). These bone filler devices are filled with the cement and then inserted coaxially through the bone needle. A small stylet is used to extrude cement from the bone filler device into the vertebral body. The syringe and bone filler device

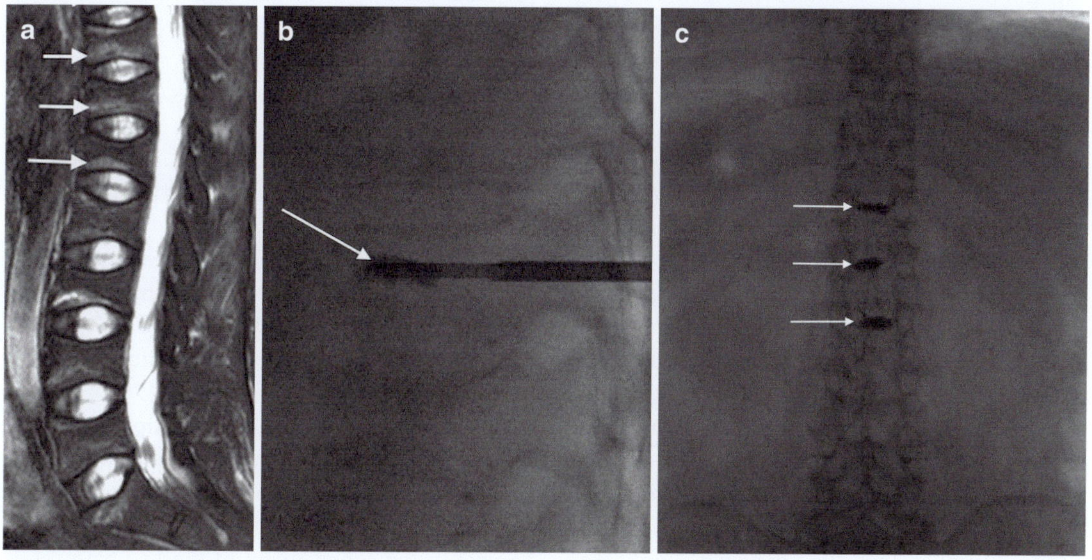

Fig. 13.8 A 28-year-old female with history of chronic steroid use for systemic lupus erythematosus and bedridden due to crippling back pain. T2-weighted sagittal MR image (**a**) shows multiple areas of T2 hyperintensity within the vertebral endplates (arrows) at the thoracolumbar junction. Lateral fluoroscopic image (**b**) during the injection of bioceramic cement (arrow) using coaxial technique. Frontal fluoroscopic image (**c**) shows bioceramic bone cement within the T11, T12, and L1 vertebral bodies (arrows). The patient experienced complete relief of her back pain symptoms

techniques offer tactile feedback during the cement injection process. The coaxial bone filler cannula technique offers the additional advantage of not obstructing the bone needle cannula with hardened cement and reduces the likelihood of a "cement tail" along the needle insertion tract. With this latter technique, the bone needle stylet is reinserted into the initially placed bone cannula (Fig. 13.6). This maneuver serves a dual purpose – to ascertain that no residual cement has entered the bone cannula forming a cement tail and to provide tamponade along the needle insertion tract facilitating hemostasis. With all of these injection vehicles, the goal is to deposit cement within the vertebral body to stabilize the anterior column. It is not necessary, and in fact, may be disadvantageous, to attempt to fill the entire vertebral body with bone cement. Another system utilizes the application of a radiofrequency pulse to immediately increase the cement viscosity at the time of injection; this system also requires a hydraulic injection device to deliver the very thick cement. A small volume of cement, in the range of 2.5–4.5 mL, is all that is required in order to restore vertebral body strength as shown in biomechanical studies [20]. The endpoints for stopping the cement injection include adequate, endplate-to-endplate filling of the anterior column of the vertebral body, cement entering the venous plexus within the posterior vertebral body, cement approaching or extending through a vertebral endplate defect, or cement extending beyond a vertebral body cortical margin in any direction.

Once cement injection is completed, the bone needle(s) can be removed. If there is a concern for cement extension along the bone needle insertion tract, then each bone needle is slowly retracted to the posterior pedicle. If there is no cement in the pedicle or bone needle cannula, then the bone needle can be safely removed. If there is cement within the pedicle and it extends into the cannula, then the physician should wait until the cement hardens (the specifications for cement hardening vary with the manufacturer of the cement). Once this occurs, safe retraction of the bone needle to the margin or edge of the posterior pedicle cortex is possible. A gentle rocking of the bone needle tip should sever the potential cement tail such that it is retained within the bone cannula and not in the patient's subcutaneous tissues. The latter is undesirable because the cement tail might irritate the soft tissues. After removal of the bone needle, hemostasis is achieved at the needle insertion site by firm hand compression for a few minutes.

After the procedure, the patient is transferred to a stretcher and allowed to recover in the supine position. The recovery time is approximately 3 hours and includes monitoring of the puncture site for swelling or active bleeding and monitoring of the patient's vital signs and pain profile. Patients are discharged home with discharge instructions and with a follow-up appointment. At our institution, we perform follow-up telephone calls 1 day and 1 week after the procedure and then see the patient in clinic for separate visits, at 3 weeks, 3 months, and 1 year. It is extremely important to see and examine the patient in follow-up. This helps to determine the success of the procedure, to evaluate for any adverse events, and to reinforce preventive measures such as osteoporosis management and physical therapy with gait and balance training (Table 13.2).

Special Situations

The occurrence of multiple synchronous or metachronous vertebral compression fractures in patients with osteoporosis is not uncommon. In one series in which multilevel vertebroplasty was performed, approximately one-third (27.2%) of 130 consecutive patients had 3 or more painful vertebral compression fractures [29]. In this series the patients had their multiple fractures treated in one session; up to six fractures were treated in one patient. There were no significant differences between the two patient groups with respect to the achievement of marked pain relief and no adverse outcomes. Another study showed that the pain relief and mobility improvement was equivalent in patients with multiple fractures treated in one session or in patients with fractures treated at different sessions as compared to

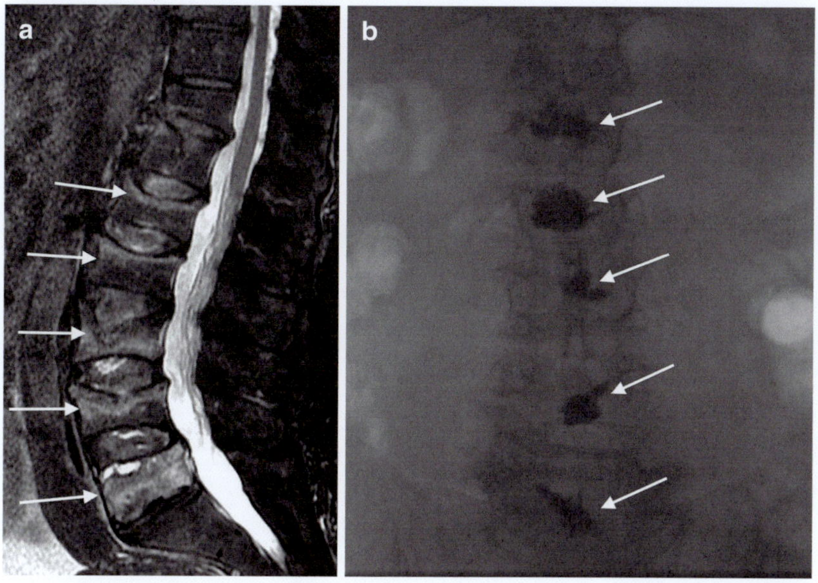

Fig. 13.9 A 79-year-old female with prior multiple falls with crippling low back pain. T2-weighted sagittal MR image (**a**) shows multiple partial vertebral compression deformities with T2 hyperintensity (edema) present in all five lumbar vertebra (arrows). The patient was treated as an outpatient with vertebroplasty in two sessions over a 2-week period, and all five lumbar vertebral bodies were stabilized (arrows) as shown on the frontal fluoroscopic image (**b**) with dramatic relief of her back pain symptoms

patients with a single treated fracture [30]. It is therefore possible to safely treat multiple osteoporotic vertebral compression fractures (Fig. 13.9). This treatment decision, however, will be influenced by the patient's comorbidities, their pre-procedure requirements for anticoagulation, and their ability to tolerate a longer and more extensive procedure. It is important to determine the causes of patients' osteoporosis and to treat accordingly. The use of a spine brace may be a reasonable temporary treatment intervention in those patients who are experiencing new vertebral compression fractures and in whom aggressive osteoporosis therapy is being initiated. At present, prophylactic vertebral augmentation, the protective treatment of non-fractured osteoporotic vertebra in patients highly susceptible to incident vertebral compression fractures, is not an indication for the performance of vertebral augmentation in the United States.

Another situation that can pose a challenge is the presence of rotatory scoliosis. This complex anatomy is best approached by utilizing the multiplanar capabilities of the fluoroscope to help position the patient such that satisfactory alignment of bony landmarks is achieved at the treatment level. Care must be taken during the initial bone needle placement and advancement in order to avoid the spinal canal. The position of the needle tip within the anterior column of the vertebral body should be confirmed with multiple projections prior to initiating cement injection. The presence of a *vertebra plana* deformity can pose a significant treatment challenge. In these patients, it is challenging to place even one bone needle within the limited volume of the residual vertebral body. Since the lateral portion of the vertebral body is usually more intact with respect to height preservation, it is recommended that a bilateral approach be used for patients with *vertebra plana* (Figs. 13.7 and 13.10). Smaller gauge needles may be helpful in traversing the narrow space between the collapsed vertebral endplates. Cement injection should occur slowly with small amounts (approximately 0.1 mL aliquots) injected at a time in order to minimize or avoid cement extravasation. This maneuver may also allow for gradual filling of any vertebral clefts

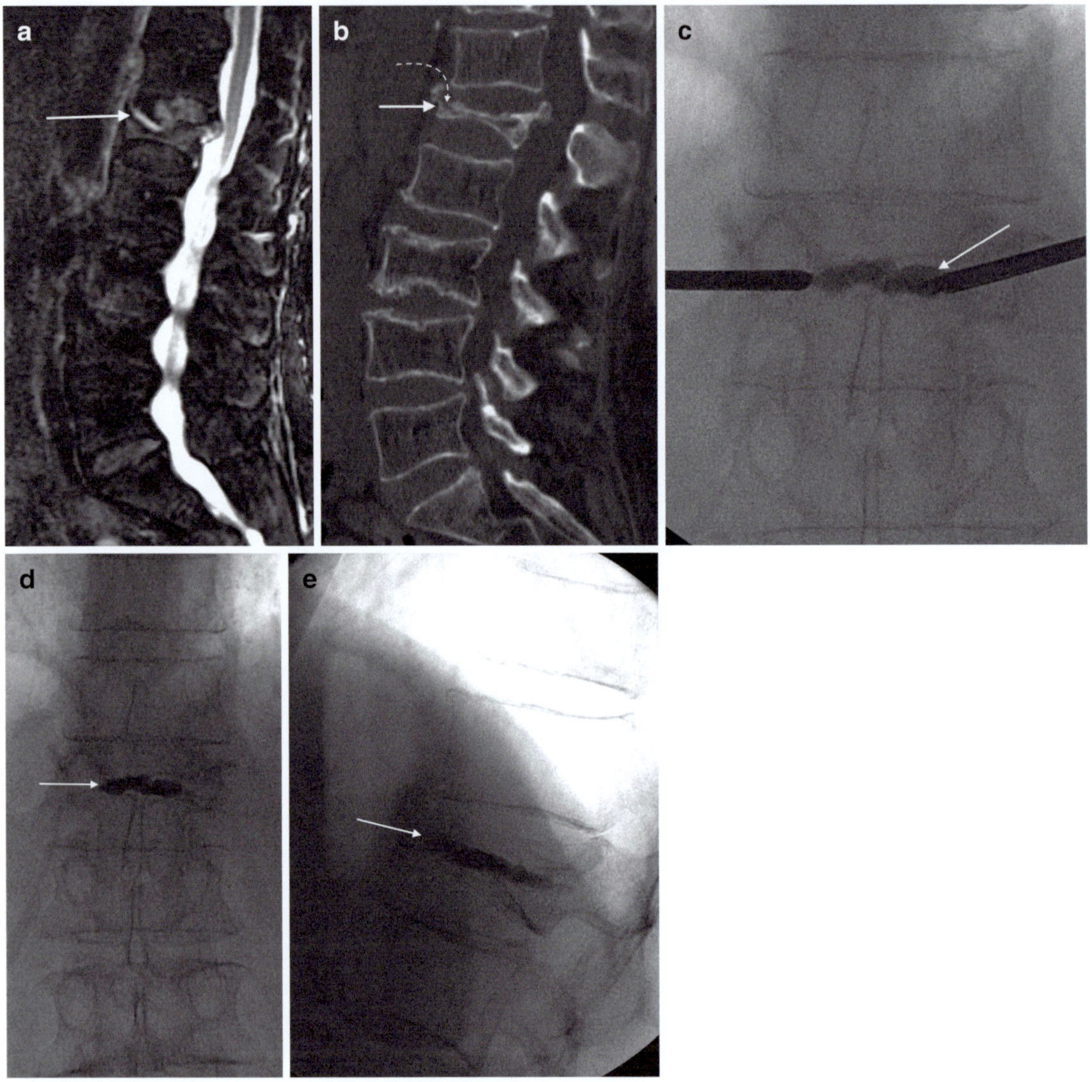

Fig. 13.10 An 80-year-old female with chronic low back pain of 5 months duration not responding to medical management and physical therapy. T2-weighted sagittal MR image (**a**) obtained 1 month after symptom onset shows a partial L1 vertebral compression deformity (arrow) which contains a small cleft and is associated with a superior endplate fracture and edema and morphologic alteration of the T12-L1 intervertebral disk. Midline sagittal CT reformation in bone window algorithm (**b**) obtained 4 months after symptom onset shows progression of the L1 vertebral compression deformity (arrow) with a fracture through the anterior aspect of the superior endplate (curved arrow). Frontal fluoroscopic image (**c**) obtained during a vertebroplasty procedure shows the sequential gradual injection of thick acrylic bone cement (arrow) using a bilateral transpedicular approach. Frontal (**d**) and lateral (**e**) fluoroscopic images show cement within the L1 vertebral body (arrows) and no evidence of cement extravasation. The patient responded favorably to this treatment

within the collapsed vertebral body. Sclerotic vertebral bodies can also be challenging to treat. These vertebrae may be sclerotic due to the presence of a chronic yet painful fracture or reflect the presence of a sclerotic bone lesion such as metastasis. It can be quite difficult to advance the bone needle into these painful sclerotic vertebral bodies. In these situations, the use of a mallet may prove useful to help advance the bone needle.

Vertebroplasty Complications and Their Treatment

Vertebroplasty complications can be categorized as either local or systemic (Table 13.3). The overall complication rate that is associated with vertebroplasty is <1% in those cases where osteoporotic fractures are being treated and <5% for the treatment of pathologic vertebral compression fractures [20, 31]. The most common event that occurs during vertebral augmentation procedures is cement leak, defined as extension of injected bone cement beyond the vertebral body margins [32]. Clinically significant cement leaks occur more frequently in patients with pathologic vertebral compression fractures. In patients with osteoporotic vertebral compression fractures, most leaks are local and asymptomatic [33]. It is only when the cement encroaches upon a neural structure that the cement leak becomes a complication of the procedure with the possibility of myelopathy or radiculopathy (Fig. 13.11). The extent of

Table 13.3 Vertebroplasty complications

Local complication	Management strategy
Vascular injury Direct: needle puncture Epidural hematoma Paraspinal hematoma Subcutaneous hematoma Indirect: coagulopathy	1. Review pre-op imaging 2. Use of fluoro-guided needle targeting 3. Check coagulation studies prior to the procedure 4. Use transient hold or bridging strategies for anticoagulants and antiplatelet medications 5. Monitor patients after their procedures and do examine their backs 6. Order emergent MRI for suspected epidural hemorrhage or CT for extra-spinal hemorrhage; check hematologic and coagulation profiles immediately
Neural injury Direct: needle puncture of nerve or spinal cord; dural puncture Indirect: mass effect from cement extravasation or hematoma	1. Review pre-op imaging to plan needle size and trajectory 2. Optimize patient position and fluoroscopy 3. Monitor needle insertion and advancement in multiple planes; respect the medial pedicle cortex 4. Monitor cement injection
Infection Cellulitis Infectious spondylitis	1. Strict aseptic technique 2. Pre-procedure antibiotic prophylaxis 3. Immediate patient follow-up for pain/fever 4. Order MRI with contrast and/or appropriate nuclear medicine study if patient cannot undergo MRI examination 5. Initiate antibiotic therapy if necessary
Intra-diskal cement	1.Review pre-op imaging and assess for endplate defects that may predispose to intra-diskal cement leak 2. Use high-viscosity cement
Others	
Pneumothorax Fragility fractures Ribs Sternum	Use proper targeting in the thoracic spine and at the thoracolumbar junction Careful patient transport and positioning
Systemic complication	**Management strategy**
Pulmonary embolism Cement Marrow fat	1.Use fluoroscopy when injecting cement 2. Use high-viscosity (thick) cement 3. Monitor patient's respiratory status just before, during, and after the procedure
Others	
Anesthesia complications Cardiovascular collapse Anaphylactic reaction to PMMA cement	1. Pre-operative anesthesia evaluation and use of American Society of Anesthesiology classification criteria 2. Use of local anesthetic only in very ill patients with multiple comorbidities

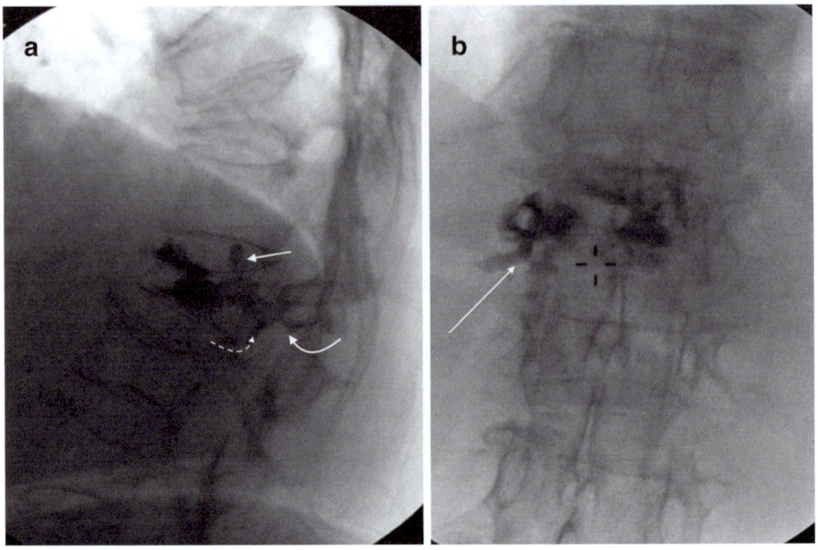

Fig. 13.11 Lateral (**a**) and frontal (**b**) fluoroscopic images show cement extravasation into the disk (small arrow), neural foramen (curved arrows), and paraspinal soft tissues (large arrow). The patient was symptomatic from the foraminal cement leak

neurologic compromise varies with the amount of extravasated cement; larger volumes of extravasation are associated with significant and possibly irreversible neurologic compromise unless immediate open surgical decompression is performed. Smaller amounts of cement leakage into the neural foramen, with cement extending through a fracture defect or through a foraminal vein, may be associated with transient irritation of the affected nerve root, and this may respond to a trial of oral steroids and/or a selective nerve root block (Fig. 13.11). If the radicular pain persists despite these interventions, the patient may require operative intervention to remove the extravasated cement fragment. Cement can also extend from the veins that communicate with the vertebral body and, particularly with low viscosity cement, may result in a pulmonary embolism. Cement embolism is rare and usually asymptomatic. Occasionally, especially in patients with compromised pulmonary function, cement emboli can produce symptoms. Again, it is important for the physician to actively monitor the cement injection, and injection should be stopped immediately if extravasation is seen. A combination of meticulous fluoroscopic monitoring, slow sequential injections of small aliquots of cement, and the use of high-viscosity cement all serve as valuable measures in reducing the likelihood of symptomatic cement extravasation. The other type of pulmonary embolism that may occur is fat embolism due to the displacement of marrow elements by injected cement. This is usually asymptomatic but could potentially cause respiratory compromise in patients who undergo multilevel vertebral augmentation.

Cement extension into the intervertebral disk should be avoided (Fig. 13.11). While this may initially appear to be an insignificant occurrence, there is an association with intra-diskal cement leak and a predisposition to an adjacent level vertebral compression fracture [34–36]. Percutaneous vertebroplasty itself is likely not a risk factor for new osteoporotic vertebral compression fractures [37]. High fracture severity grade, in other words those fractures with significant height loss, and the presence of vertebral clefts are risk factors that predispose to intra-diskal cement leaks [35]. Vertebral endplate defects are frequently seen in patients with osteoporotic vertebral compression fractures, and physicians should scrutinize the preoperative images to account for their presence and location [14]. The presence of abnormal T2 signal within a damaged disk adjacent to a damaged vertebral endplate may also predispose to intra-diskal cement leak [35, 38]. These pre-treatment imaging findings will enable closer monitoring of these areas during cement injection, thereby reducing the possibility of cement extravasation (Fig. 13.10).

Hemorrhage is also a potential complication of the vertebroplasty procedure. This may be due to direct vascular injury with a spinal or bone needle or, more frequently, may be associated with uncorrected coagulopathy. Vascular injury is more likely with an extra-pedicular or parapedicular approach as small vascular branches may travel near the lateral pedicle or vertebral body. A transpedicular approach is particularly desirable, when possible, especially in those patients who might be at a higher risk for a hemorrhagic complication such as those patients with transient correction of their anticoagulation status. Subcutaneous hematomas can occur and are often due to oozing of blood beneath the puncture site. This unpleasant complication is uncomfortable for the patient and can be minimized by firm hand compression at the puncture site for a few minutes immediately after removal of the bone needle. Following the procedure, the patient is instructed to lie on his/her back which helps to provide additional pressure on the puncture site. The puncture site should be monitored frequently for signs of swelling or active hemorrhage during the patient's recovery. Paraspinal hemorrhages are challenging to diagnose. Patients may complain of back pain and discomfort, and their vital signs can show hypotension and tachycardia. An emergent CT scan should be performed for suspected paraspinal hemorrhage. A patient with an expanding hematoma should be transferred to an intensive care unit with monitoring of their hematologic and coagulation status. If they are not responding to aggressive medical management, consideration ought to be given to an emergent angiogram with possible endovascular embolization. Acute epidural hemorrhage is a potential quality-of-life-threatening complication that usually requires a spinal MR for diagnosis; immediate spine surgical consultation for possible decompression of the epidural hematoma is warranted.

Infection is a potential complication of the cement augmentation procedure. In one series involving 1307 vertebral augmentation cases, 6 patients (0.46%) experienced postoperative infections [39]; several of the patients in this series had a pre-existing urinary tract infection. The most frequently encountered microorganism was *Staphylococcus*, but other organisms were also encountered. Nearly all of these patients required surgical debridement and stabilization at their prior augmentation site. At our institution, one post-augmentation infection was diagnosed 3 weeks post-procedure; this was successfully treated with a peripherally inserted central venous catheter and intravenous antibiotic therapy. A key to addressing potential post-vertebroplasty infections is patient optimization. Delaying this elective procedure in patients with suspected systemic or local infections (including urinary tract infections) until the infection has been successfully treated and the patient is medically cleared for their procedure is critical. Adherence to strict aseptic technique in the procedure suite is paramount. The use of pre-procedure intravenous antibiotic prophylaxis is highly recommended. Some physicians advocate the use of tobramycin powder in the cement mixture, especially for patients who are immunocompromised [32]. Post-procedure patient follow-up within the first month after the procedure is important as it may allow for earlier diagnosis and treatment of a spine infection. Since a spine infection is a clinical diagnosis, it may be necessary to obtain an infection laboratory panel (white blood cell count with differential, erythrocyte sedimentation rate, and C-reactive protein) and a contrast-enhanced MRI or nuclear medicine study (Gallium scan) in a patient in whom an infection is suspected.

The other types of complications that have been reported with the vertebroplasty procedure are exceedingly rare, but nonetheless significant. These include pneumothorax, cardiopulmonary collapse, anaphylactic reactions to the acrylic bone cement, and death.

Anesthesia-related complications may also occur and can be minimized by careful preoperative evaluation particularly in high-risk patients with multiple medical comorbidities. Other fragility fractures can occur in osteoporotic patients at the time of their transfer and positioning on the procedure table including rib fractures or sternal fractures. These are generally treated conservatively but can be a major source of patient discomfort.

Conclusions

Vertebroplasty has been shown to be effective in relieving pain associated with osteoporotic vertebral compression fractures [40] in patients who are inadequately treated with medication, bracing, and/or physical therapy. The pain relief is associated with a reduction in the use of analgesic medications and allows patients to return to their usual activities of daily living. These benefits are achieved in the setting of a low overall complication rate (less than 1%) [20]. Vertebroplasty is a palliative procedure and does not correct the underlying cause of the vertebral fracture; medical management of osteoporosis must therefore be initiated and continued.

References

1. Mathis JM, Belkoff SM, Deramond H. History and early development of percutaneous vertebroplasty. In: Mathis JM, Deramond H, Belkoff SM, editors. Percutaneous vertebroplasty and kyphoplasty. 2nd ed. New York: Springer; 2006. p. 3–7.
2. Jensen ME, Evans AE, Mathis JM, Kallmes DF, CLoft HJ, Dion JE. Percutaneous polymethylmethacrylate vertebroplasty in the treatment of osteoporotic vertebral compression fractures: technical aspects. AJNR Am J Neuroradiol. 1997;18:1897–904.
3. Mathis JM, Ortiz AO, Zoarski GH. Vertebroplasty versus kyphoplasty: a comparison and contrast. AJNR Am J Neuroradiol. 2004;25:840–5.
4. Edidin AA, Ong K, Lau E, Kurtz SM. Mortality risk for operated and nonoperated vertebral fracture patients in the Medicare population. J Bone Miner Res. 2011;26:1617–26.
5. Goz V, Errico TJ, Weinreb JH, Koehler SM, Hecht AC, Lafage V, et al. Vertebroplasty and kyphoplasty: national outcomes and trends in utilization from 2005 through 2010. Spine J. 2015;15:959–65.
6. Dittmer DK, Teasell R. Complications of immobilization and bed rest. Part 1: musculoskeletal and cardiovascular complications. Can Fam Physician. 1993;39:1428–32, 1435–7
7. Teasell R, Dittmer DK. Complications of immobilization and bed rest. Part 2: other complications. Can Fam Physician. 1993;39:1440–2, 1445–6
8. Lindsay R, Silverman SL, Cooper C, Hanley DA, Barton I, Broy SB, et al. Risk of new vertebral fracture in the year following a fracture. JAMA. 2001;285:320–3.
9. Ponnusamy KE, Iyer S, Gupta G, Khanna AJ. Instrumentation of the osteoporotic spine: biomechanical and clinical considerations. Spine J. 2011;11:54–63.
10. Jensen ME, McGraw JK, Cardella JF, Hirsch JA. Position statement on percutaneous vertebral augmentation: a consensus statement developed by the American Society of Interventional and Therapeutic Neuroradiology, Society of Interventional Radiology, American Association of Neurological Surgeons/ Congress of Neurological Surgeons, and American Society of Spine Radiology. J Vasc Interv Radiol. 2007;18:325–30.
11. Do HM. Magnetic resonance imaging in the evaluation of patients for percutaneous vertebroplasty. Top Magn Reson Imaging. 2000;11:235–44.
12. Tehranzadeh J, Tao C. Advances in MR imaging of vertebral collapse. Semin Ultrasound CT MR. 2004;25:440–60.
13. Jung JY, Lee MH, Ahn JM. Leakage of polymethylmethacrylate in percutaneous vertebroplasty: comparison of osteoporotic vertebral compression fractures with and without an intervertebral vacuum cleft. J Comput Assist Tomogr. 2006;30:501–6.
14. Ortiz AO, Bordia R. Injury to the vertebral endplate-disk complex associated with osteoporotic vertebral compression fractures. AJNR Am J Neuroradiol. 2011;32:115–20.
15. Karaca L, Yuceler Z, Kantarci M, Cakir M, Sade R, Calikoglu C, et al. The feasibility of dual-energy CT in differentiation of vertebral compression fractures. Br J Radiol. 2016;89:20150300.
16. Appel NB, Gilula LA. Percutaneous vertebroplasty in patients with spinal canal compromise. AJR Am J Roentgenol. 2004;182:947–51.
17. Hon M, Silbergleit R, Ortiz AO. Anticoagulation management. In: Ortiz AO, editor. Image-guided percutaneous spine biopsy. Cham: Springer; 2017. p. 13–30.
18. Teng MM, Wei CJ, Wei LC, Luo CB, Limg JF, Chang FC, et al. Kyphosis correction and height restoration effects of percutaneous vertebroplasty. AJNR Am J Neuroradiol. 2003;24:1893–900.
19. Kallmes D, Jensen ME. Percutaneous vertebroplasty. Radiology. 2003;229:27–36.
20. Mathis JM, Barr JD, Belkoff SM, Barr MS, Jensen ME, Deramond H. Percutaneous vertebroplasty: a developing standard of care for vertebral compression fractures. AJNR Am J Neuroradiol. 2001;22:373–81.
21. Brook AL, Miller TS, Fast A, Nolan T, Farinhas J, Shifteh K. Vertebral augmentation with a flexible curved needle: preliminary results in 17 consecutive patients. J Vasc Interv Radiol. 2008;19:1785–9.
22. Ortiz AO, Natarajan V, Gregorius D, Pollack S. Significantly reduced radiation exposure to operators during kyphoplasty and vertebroplasty procedures: methods and techniques. AJNR Am J Neuroradiol. 2006;27:989–94.
23. Magerl F. External skeletal fixation of the lower thoracic and the lumbar spine. In: Uhthoff HK, Stahl E, editors. Current concepts of external fixation of fractures. New York: Springer-Verlag; 1982. p. 353–66.
24. Muijs SP, Akkermans PA, van Erkel AR, Dijkstra SD. The value of routinely performing a bone biopsy during percutaneous vertebroplasty in treatment of

osteoporotic vertebral compression fractures. Spine. 2009;34:2395–9.
25. Ortiz AO, Marden J. Image-guided percutaneous spine and rib biopsy: tools and techniques. In: Ortiz AO, editor. Image-guided percutaneous spine biopsy. Cham: Springer; 2017. p. 35–70.
26. Georgy BA. Clinical experience with high-viscosity cements for percutaneous vertebral body augmentation: occurrence, degree, and location of cement leakage compared with kyphoplasty. AJNR Am J Neuroradiol. 2010;31:504–8.
27. He Z, Zhai Q, Hu M, Cao C, Wang J, Yang H, et al. Bone cements for percutaneous vertebroplasty and balloon kyphoplasty: current status and future developments. J Ortho Translat. 2015;3:1–11.
28. Middleton ET, Rajaraman CJ, O'Brien DP, Doherty SM, Taylor AD. The safety and efficacy of vertebroplasty using Cortoss cement in a newly established vertebroplasty service. Br J Neurosurg. 2008;22:252–6.
29. Mailli L, Filippiadis DK, Brountzos EN, Alexopoulou E, Kelekis N, Kelekis A. Clinical outcome and safety of multilevel vertebroplasty: clinical experience and results. Cardiovasc Intervent Radiol. 2013;36:183–91.
30. Gray LA, Ehteshami A, Gaughen JR, Kaufmann TJ, Kallmes DF. Efficacy of percutaneous vertebroplasty for multiple synchronous and metachronous vertebral compression fractures. AJNR Am J Neuroradiol. 2009;30:318–22.
31. Chandra RV, Meyers PM, Hirsch JA, Abruzzo T, Eskey CJ, Hussain MS, et al. Vertebral augmentation: report of the Standards and Guidelines Committee of the Society of NeuroInterventional Surgery. J Neurointerv Surg. 2014;6:7–15.
32. Mathis JM, Deramond H. Complications associated with vertebroplasty and kyphoplasty. In: Mathis JM, Deramond H, Belkoff SM, editors. Percutaneous vertebroplasty and kyphoplasty. 2nd ed. New York: Springer; 2006. p. 210–22.
33. Venmans A, Klazen CAH, Lohle PNM, van Rooij WJ, Verhaar HJJ, de Vries J, et al. Percutaneous vertebroplasty and pulmonary cement embolism: results from VERTOS II. AJNR Am J Neuroradiol. 2010;31:1451–3.
34. Lin EP, Ekholm S, Hiwatashi A, Westesson PL. Vertebroplasty: cement leakage into the disc increases the risk of new fracture of adjacent vertebral body. AJNR Am J Neuroradiol. 2004;25:175–80.
35. Nieuwenhuijse MJ, van Erkel AR, Dijkstra S. Cement leakage in percutaneous vertebroplasty for osteoporotic vertebral compression fractures: identification of risk factors. Spine J. 2011;11:839–48.
36. Syed MI, Patel NA, Jan S, Harron MS, Morar K, Shaikh A. Intradiskal extravasation with low-volume cement filling in percutaneous vertebroplasty. AJNR Am J Neuroradiol. 2005;26:2397–401.
37. Klazen CA, Venmans A, de Vries J, van Rooij WJ, Jansen FH, Blonk MC, et al. Percutaneous vertebroplasty is not a risk factor for new osteoporotic compression fractures: results from VERTOS II. AJNR Am J Neuroradiol. 2010;31:1447–50.
38. Hiwatashi A, Ohgiya Y, Kakimoto N, Westesson PL. Cement leakage during vertebroplasty can be predicted on preoperative MRI. AJR Am J Roentgenol. 2007;188:1089–93.
39. Abdelrahman H, Siam AE, Shawky A, Ezzati A, Boehm H. Infection after vertebroplasty or kyphoplasty. A series of nine cases and review of the literature. Spine J. 2013;13:1809–17.
40. Klazen CA, Lohle PN, de Vries J, Jansen FH, Tielbeek AV, Blonk MC, et al. Vertebroplasty versus conservative treatment in acute osteoporotic vertebral compression fractures (Vertos II): an open-label randomized trial. Lancet. 2010;276:1085–92.

14 Kyphoplasty Cement Augmentation Technique

Robert P. Norton

Indications

Kyphoplasty, a type of cement augmentation technique, is most commonly indicated for the treatment of painful osteoporotic compression fractures of the thoracic or lumbar spine which have failed nonsurgical management. Most authors recommend a minimum trial of conservative care for 1–3 weeks; however in situations of hospital admission with an inability to mobilize, kyphoplasty may be performed more urgently. Compression fractures left untreated may continue to be symptomatic for several months. In these situations, studies have shown excellent results in both early care (2–3 weeks) and later care (2–3 months) [1]. In addition, studies have indicated that kyphoplasty can lead to a reduced hospital length of stay and earlier mobilization [2], both of which may be cost-effective [3]. Other indications include painful pathologic fractures, aggressive hemangioma of the spine, and painful nonunion of vertebral fractures.

Relative contraindications to kyphoplasty include burst-type fracture patterns of the vertebral body with bony retropulsion into the spinal canal. These fractures are at risk of cement extravasation into the spinal canal and may result in neurologic compression. The presence of radiculopathy is another potential contraindication since kyphoplasty could exacerbate the radiculopathy if cement extravasation occurs. Collapse of greater than 70% of the vertebral body height can potentially make the procedure more difficult to be performed due to the difficult insertion angle required to get the trocar through the pedicle into the severely collapsed vertebral body. Additionally, collapsed vertebra has a limited area where cement may be injected. Lastly, a lack of a surgical backup plan to manage any potential complications is a relative contraindication to performing a kyphoplasty.

Absolute contraindications include asymptomatic fractures, an allergy to bone fillers or opacification agents, irreversible coagulopathy, or the presence of vertebral osteomyelitis.

Technique

A full work-up is required prior to performing a kyphoplasty. This includes radiographic imaging to identify the fracture level, as well as a recent MRI or bone scan to confirm that the fracture is acute or subacute. On MRI, acute fractures will show an increased signal intensity on the T2-weighted and STIR imaging sequences and a reduced signal on T1-weighted sequences. These findings are representative of edema within the vertebral body, confirming the acute process. Bone scan is recommended in those patients who have contradictions to an MRI. A bone scan will

R. P. Norton (✉)
Florida Spine Associates, Boca Raton, FL, USA

A. E. Razi, S. H. Hershman (eds.), *Vertebral Compression Fractures in Osteoporotic and Pathologic Bone*, https://doi.org/10.1007/978-3-030-33861-9_14

demonstrate increased uptake at the fracture site due to higher metabolic activity at that site. The nuances regarding radiographic findings of compression fractures are beyond the scope of this chapter but are found elsewhere in this book.

After a patient has met the criteria for kyphoplasty with a documented acute or subacute fracture on MRI or bone scan, the common risks, benefits, and expected outcome of the procedure are discussed with the patient. Traditionally, this procedure has been in done in the operating theater under anesthesia or with supervised sedation; however there has been a growing trend to do these procedures in the outpatient setting or in an office-based procedure room. It is the author's preference to perform kyphoplasty in an office-based procedure room using local anesthetic without sedation unless absolutely necessary.

The patient may be premedicated with Toradol injection along with IM antibiotic such as Ancef or clindamycin if penicillin allergy exists. Next, the patient is placed prone on a radiolucent operating table, and the back is cleansed with chlorhexidine or an appropriate alternative; he or she is then draped, and a time-out is performed. Supplies are set up ahead of time by the surgical technician (Fig. 14.1a, b).

Using fluoroscopy, the pedicles of the fractured vertebral body are marked out (Fig. 14.2). It is the author's preference to use a unilateral pedicle approach; however, a bipedicular approach may also be performed. The epidermis is then infiltrated with local anesthesia. Under image guidance, a spinal needle is inserted and docked over the lateral aspect of the facet joint and transverse process, which is the approximate entry point for the trocar when performing a transpe-

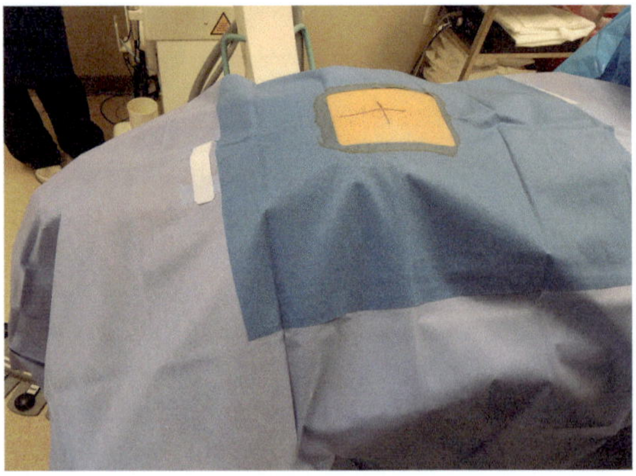

Fig. 14.2 Patient is prepped and draped with fluoroscopy in place. The vertical line represents the lateral boarder of the pedicle, and the horizontal line represents the midpoint of the pedicle

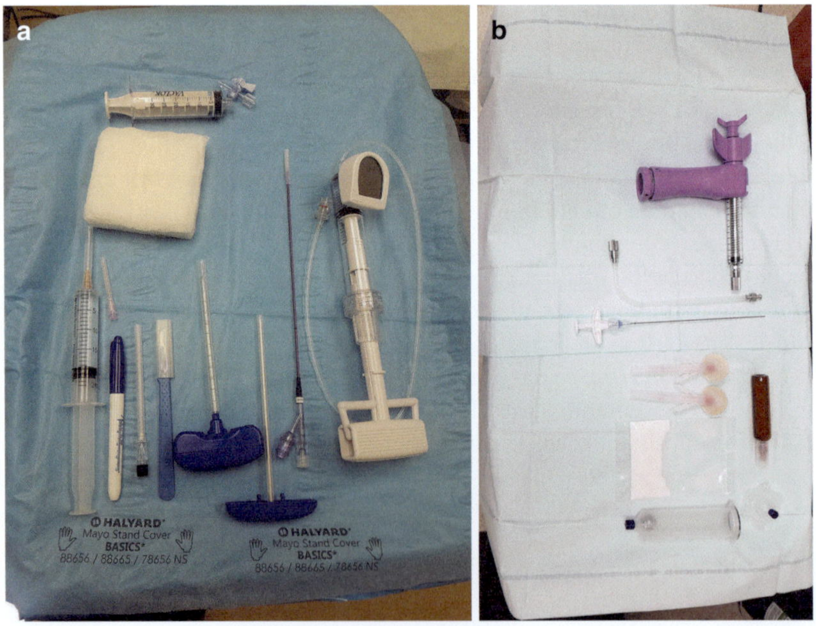

Fig. 14.1 (**a**) Operating room set up for equipment supplies needed, including syringe with anesthetic agents, spinal needle, marking pen, gauze pads, trocar (diamond and bevel tip), contrast, and balloon. (**b**) Remaining supplies including chlorhexidine swabs, bone cement supplies, injector gun with inner trocar, and extension tubing

dicular approach. This also serves to confirm the appropriate trajectory and the skin incision.

A transverse skin incision is then made – depending on the spinal level and body habitus – this may be anywhere from 1 to 5 cm lateral to the pedicle. The trocar is then inserted under fluoroscopy on the AP view and docked at the 9 o'clock position of the pedicle for a left-sided approach and the 3 o'clock position for a right-sided approach (Fig. 14.3a–c). This corresponds to the confluence of the superior articulating process of the facet joint, the midportion of the transverse process, and the pars interarticularis. The trocar should be advanced through the pedicle into the vertebral body and its position confirmed using both AP and lateral fluoroscopic imaging. There are two common types of trocar tip shapes – diamond and beveled. The beveled tip allows for more directional guidance and which one is used is a matter of preference. The trocars

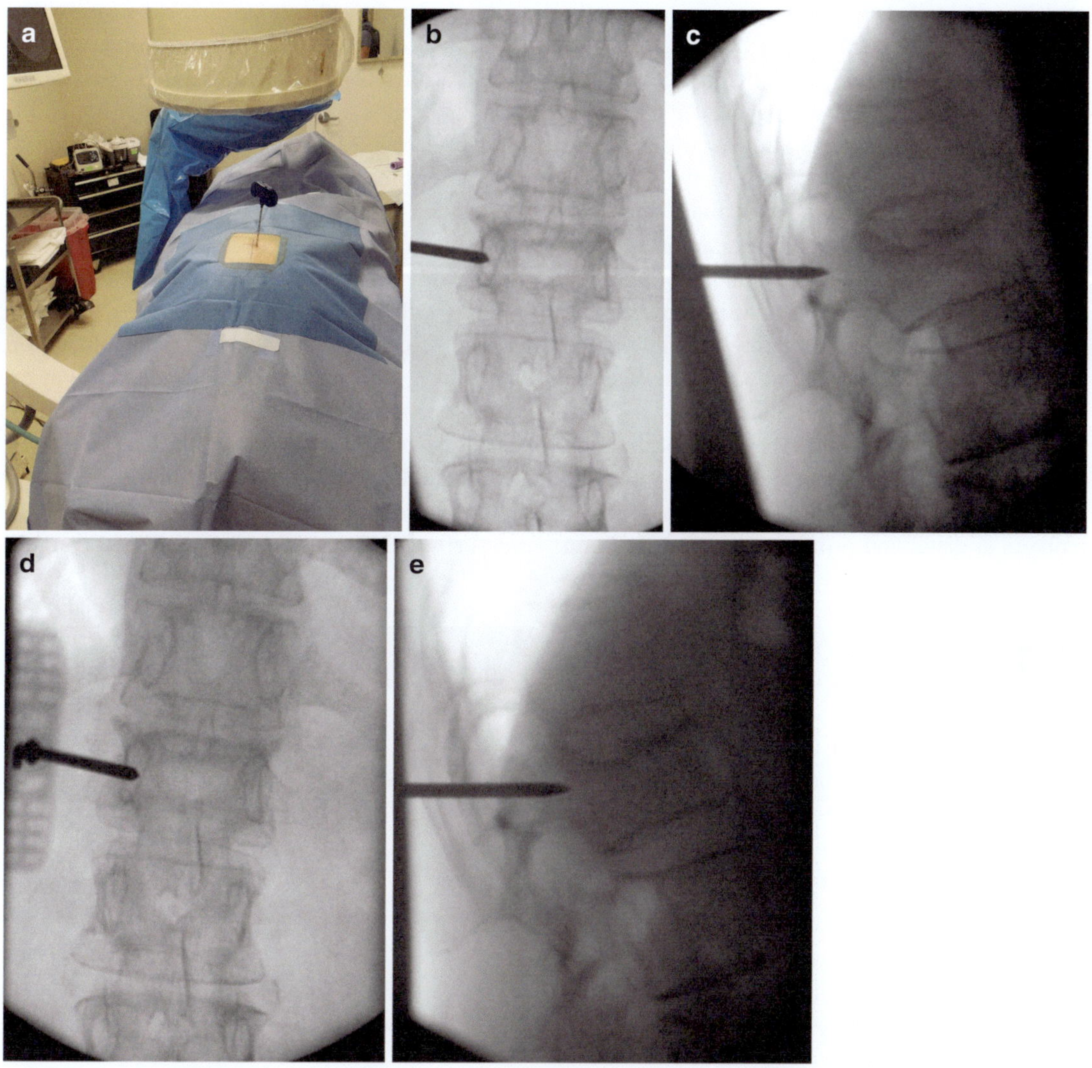

Fig. 14.3 (**a**) Trocar is inserted under fluoroscopic imaging guidance starting at the 9 o'clock position on the left pedicle of the fractured vertebral body. (**b**) AP fluoroscopy view of entry point of trocar. (**c**) Lateral fluoroscopy view of entry point of trocar. (**d**) AP fluoroscopy of trocar inserted through pedicle reaching vertebral body without breaching medial pedicle cortex. (**e**) Lateral fluoroscopy view of trocar advanced to vertebral body/pedicle junction

exist in various sizes – it is the author's preference to use 10-guage diamond tip trocar. Since osteoporotic bone is soft, the trocar can often be advanced with gentle rotation back and forth through the pedicle without the use of a mallet. It should be advanced through the pedicle to the medial border of the pedicle wall when viewed under AP imaging. The C-arm is then changed to the lateral position to confirm that the trocar is anterior to the pedicle-vertebral body junction. If not, it is essential to rotate the C-arm back to AP position to redirect the trocar appropriately (Fig. 14.3d, e). The trocar can be advanced into the vertebral body and medialized beyond the medial boarder of the pedicle once it is safely within the vertebral body. The trocar should be seated within the posterior third of the vertebral body, and the inner cannula is then removed. Either a hand drill or core biopsy cannula is then inserted and advanced anteromedially into the vertebral body, stopping prior to penetrating the anterior cortex on lateral imaging. At this point a biopsy may be taken if indicated or desired. Following this, a balloon catheter is inserted through the trocar into the vertebral body (Fig. 14.4a–c). The entire balloon must be inserted into the vertebral body; radiopaque markers at distal and proximal aspect of balloon serve to identify placement of balloon. Various balloon sizes exist; commonly a 10, 15, or 20 mm balloon is used. It is the author's preference to use a 10 mm balloon in the thoracic spine and a 15 mm balloon in the lumbar spine. The balloon is then slowly inflated with radiopaque contrast to the desired height or maximum pressure – this varies by manufacturer and system. Before removal, the balloon must be completely deflated to allow it to be pulled out of the trocar – this can be confirmed on lateral imaging.

At this point, the bone cement is prepared according to the specific manufacturer instructions. Various mixing and working times exist for different brands of the monomer and polymethylmethacrylate (PMMA). Care should be taken to have an optimal viscosity prior to cement injection, and it is the author's preference to have a viscosity similar to the consistency of toothpaste prior to injecting; there is a potential for extravasation with low-viscosity cement. Higher-viscosity cement can make the injection challenging and can reduce the chance that an adequate amount of cement is placed within the vertebral body. Various cement delivery systems are available – these include manual delivery plunger-based cannulas, as well as mechanically pressurized devices. The plunger-based cannula

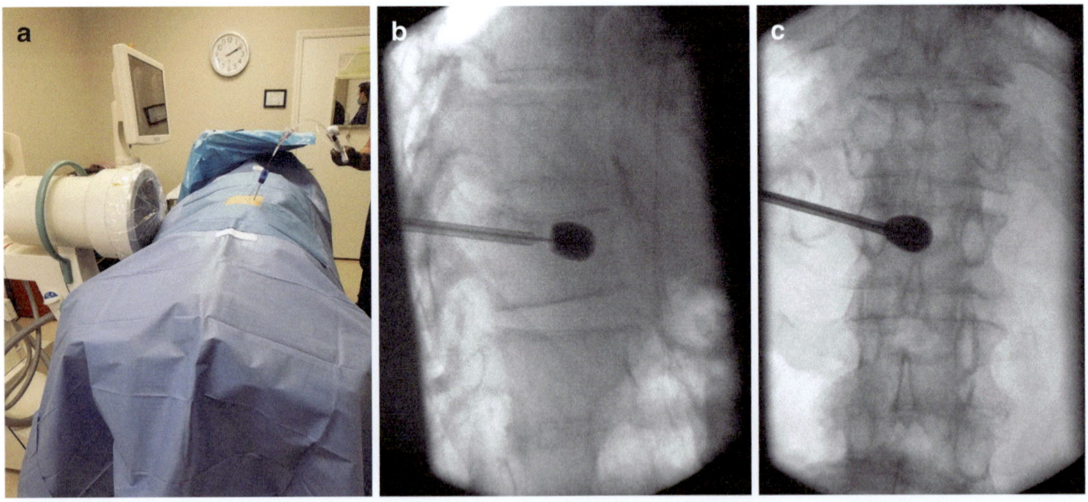

Fig. 14.4 (**a**) Balloon is inserted into vertebral body and inflated to create a cavity for the bone cement. (**b**) Lateral fluoroscopic view of balloon inserted and inflated with contrast to create cavity for bone cement placement. (**c**) AP fluoroscopy of balloon inserted and inflated with contrast to create cavity for bone cement placement

allows for direct injection of cement with less trailing of cement since cement delivery halts when the pressure is stopped. The disadvantage to this system is that it requires a longer duration of injection which can increase radiation exposure to the patient, surgeon, and staff. Multiple cannulas filled with cement are placed sequentially into the trocar, and a plunger is used to introduce cement into the void created by the balloon. With a mechanically pressurized system, a syringe connected to a handle is assembled with an extension line and nozzle which connects to a cannula that is inserted through the trocar. Pressure is created in the device, and cement is delivered into the void via a piston mechanism. These systems are generally easier and faster to use and involve less radiation exposure by decreasing the total time needed to deliver the cement and by increasing the working distance to the radiation source. The potential disadvantage with these devices is inadvertent excess cement injection due to the inability to stop cement flow instantaneously since pressure is built up in the system.

Regardless of the specific delivery system, it is important to inject the cement in an efficient and controlled manner. Multiple AP and lateral images are performed to ensure an appropriate vertebral body fill of cement without extravasation in the canal, adjacent disc space, or into nearby blood vessels (Fig. 14.5a, b). After cement injection is finalized, the introducer trocars are reinserted into the outer cannula and slowly removed together to ensure that the cement is not tracking back through the pedicle – the cement can follow the path of least resistance especially with low-viscosity cement.

Once the trocar is removed, final AP and lateral images are obtained. The incision is cleaned, and bandages are applied along with a dry, compressive bandage (Fig. 14.6). The patient is then appropriately observed post procedure.

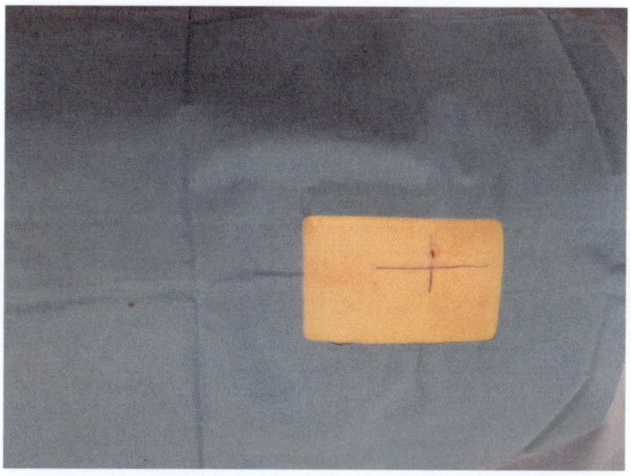

Fig. 14.6 When finished incision is approximately 4 mm in length and able to be closed with a bandage and dry compressive dressing

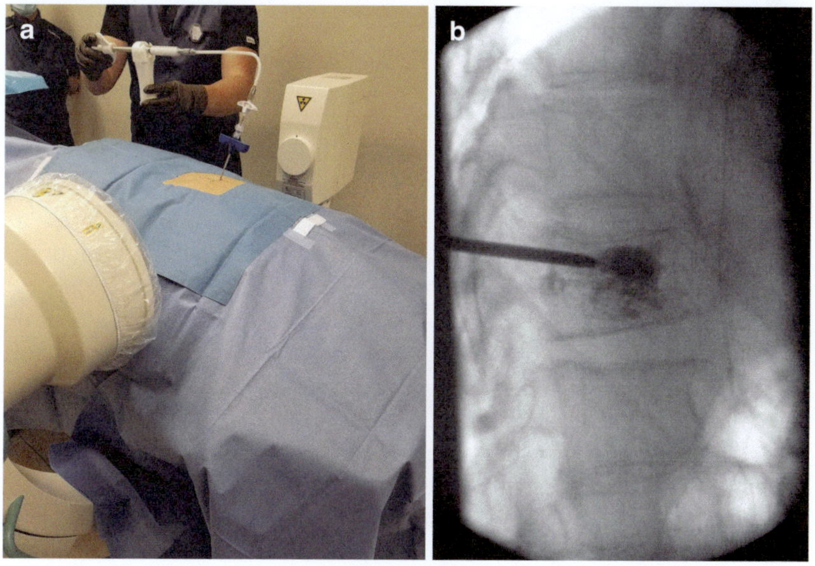

Fig. 14.5 (**a**) Bone cement is injected into the vertebral body using an injector gun and extension tubing to allow fluoroscopic imaging while standing further away from the radiation source. (**b**) Bone cement being injected through trocar

Tips

As with any procedure, there is a learning curve that must be overcome in order to reach maximal efficiency and safety with reproducible good surgical results. The following are some tips of the trade.

If performing a unipedicular kyphoplasty, the larger pedicle should be used for the approach. This will allow for easier access and an ability to medialize the trocar once in the vertebral body. If the pedicle is too small to allow safe placement of the trocar, an in-out-in technique can be utilized.

If there is a depressed fracture line of the superior end plate, care must be taken during the placement of cement to reduce the risk of intradiscal cement extravasation. In some situations, the balloon can be placed and expanded under the fractured superior end plate to partially reduce the collapse. This will help keep cement within the confines of the vertebral body.

Injection of cement at the appropriate viscosity is paramount. The bone cement will always follow the path of least resistance; therefore it is important to study the preoperative films closely to avoid placement of trocar tip in a location that may lead to extravasation of cement outside of the vertebral body. Prior to cement introduction, the consistency should be checked to ensure that is similar to that of toothpaste. The consistency of the cement is examined by pushing a small amount out of the tip of the delivery cannula. A good rule of thumb is that the surgeon should wait until the cement can stand on the end of the delivery cannula without falling over – at that point it is generally viscous enough for injection into the vertebral body.

To reduce the risk of extravasation when a clear fracture line is present, a small amount of cement may be injected at the start of the fracture line. Since the internal body temperature is higher than the room temperature, the cement will harden inside the body faster than the cement in the delivery system. This will create a "block" to cement extravasation through the fracture line.

Radiation exposure is known to be a major procedural hazard for patients, operating room staff, and physicians. Radiation precautions should be used and include a full lead apron and thyroid shield, as well as radiation-resistant eye protection and sterile gloves, if available. While localizing the entry point a sponge stick can be used to hold the trocar in place in order to distance the surgeon's hand from the radiation source.

Multilevel Compression Fractures

Patients with severe osteoporosis typically have multiple fractures in varying degrees of healing. Asymptomatic, healed fractures should not be treated with cement augmentation. However, there are patients who present with more than one acute fracture, often adjacent to each other or within the same region of the spine or at times in completely different locations. For those with both thoracic and lumbar acute compression fractures, the most symptomatic fractures should be addressed initially. It is reasonably safe to perform cement augmentation in up to three levels at the same time. Some recommend placing all the trocars prior to injecting cement to maximize efficiency. However, when multiple fractures are adjacent to each other, it might be difficult to insert multiple trocars without abutting each other. In these situations, alternating sides can be used while performing unipedicular kyphoplasty.

Complications

As with any surgical procedure, there are risks and complications associated with vertebral cement augmentation procedures. Most complications are secondary to cement extravasation. Using a low-viscosity cement and/or a higher injection volume will increase the risk of these complications. Post procedural CT scan studies have shown a surprisingly high rate of cement extravasation (18–88%) [4]. Fortunately, these incidental findings are often of minimal clinical significance. Cement extravasation can occur through the vertebral end plate into the disc space

(45%), into the paravertebral space (35%), into the epidural space (20%), and into the prevertebral region (18%). Despite these high rates of extravasation, less than 1% result in neurologic complications. Unfortunately, if a neurologic complication does occur, it can be permanent [5], and surgical intervention may be necessary to decompress the affected nerve root and/or spinal cord.

Embolization of cement may occur via inadvertent intravascular injection or through the introduction of a large cement load into the vertebral body. This may result in pulmonary embolism or passage through the heart into the arterial system. The incidence of cardiopulmonary embolism has been reported to range from 2% to 26% [6] – cardiopulmonary medical support may be necessary in these situations.

Hypotensive reaction to the monomer component of bone cement may occur as well. This typically occurs within the first few minutes of cement injection; therefore it is important to continuously monitor the heart rate, blood pressure, and oxygen saturation. The surgeon must be capable of providing immediate cardiopulmonary support if needed.

There has been much debate over the risk of adjacent vertebral fracture related to cement augmentation procedures. Biomechanically, there is an increased stiffness created by the cement augmentation which may translate to increased loads on adjacent segments and a theoretically increased risk of subsequent fracture. However, Anderson et al. [1] performed a meta-analysis of randomized controlled trials comparing kyphoplasty or vertebroplasty to nonsurgical care and found no increased risk of adjacent fracture following cement augmentation. Regardless of the treatment approach, both groups had about a 20% risk of developing a new fracture within 1 year. A systematic review by Zhang et al. [7] looking at risk factors for new osteoporotic compression fractures found low bone mineral density (BMD), low BMI, and intradiscal cement extravasation to be significant risk factors for the development of subsequent adjacent level compression fracture following a cement augmentation procedure.

Other potential complications include fracture of the rib, transverse process, or pedicle with trocar insertion, refracture of the vertebral body around the cement, and allergic reaction to bone cement.

References

1. Anderson PA, Froyshteter AB, Tontz WL Jr. Meta-analysis of vertebral augmentation compared with conservative treatment for osteoporotic spinal fractures. J Bone Miner Res. 2013;28(2):372–82.
2. Röllinghoff M, Zarghooni K, Schlüter-Brust K, et al. Indications and contraindications for vertebroplasty and kyphoplasty. Arch Orthop Trauma Surg. 2010;130(6):765–74.
3. Svedbom A, Alvares L, Cooper C, Marsh D, Ström O. Balloon kyphoplasty compared to vertebroplasty and nonsurgical management in patients hospitalised with acute osteoporotic vertebral compression fracture: a UK cost-effectiveness analysis. Osteoporos Int. 2013;24(1):355–67.
4. Martin DJ, Rad AE, Kallmes DF. Prevalence of extravertebral cement leakage after vertebroplasty: procedural documentation versus CT detection. Acta Radiol. 2012;53(5):569–72.
5. Patel AA, Vaccaro AR, Martyak GG, et al. Neurologic deficit following percutaneous vertebral stabilization. Spine (Phila Pa 1976). 2007;32(16):1728–34.
6. Wang LJ, Yang HL, Shi YX, Jiang WM, Chen L. Pulmonary cement embolism associated with percutaneous vertebroplasty or kyphoplasty: a systematic review. Orthop Surg. 2012;4(3):182–9.
7. Zhang Z, Fan J, Ding Q, Wu M, Yin G. Risk factors for new osteoporotic vertebral compression fractures after vertebroplasty: a systematic review and meta-analysis. J Spinal Disord Tech. 2013;26(4):E150–7.

15 Management of Spinal Deformity in the Setting of Osteoporotic Vertebral Compression Fractures

Michael P. Kelly

Introduction

Spinal deformity after osteoporotic fractures is an uncommon problem. It is most frequently observed in the setting of postfracture osteonecrosis (Kümmel disease), resulting in regional kyphosis. Thus, it is less frequently associated with a benign compression fracture and more frequently associated with osteoporotic burst fractures. Given the debilitated patient, this regional kyphosis often results in sagittal malalignment due to poor or inadequate compensatory mechanisms. In some cases, kyphosis with retropulsion of vertebral body fragments can result in neurological deficits requiring operative intervention. These cases are complex due to issues with comorbid conditions, difficulty of fixation points, the extent of fusion required, and achieving union of the instrumented levels. Given the rare overall occurrence of this condition, there is a paucity of high-quality data; thus decision-making often requires experience and conversation with other surgeons to achieve a good outcome.

M. P. Kelly (✉)
Department of Orthopedic Surgery, Washington University School of Medicine, Saint Louis, MO, USA
e-mail: kellymi@wustl.edu

Evaluation

Evaluation of a spinal deformity due to pathologic, osteoporotic insufficiency fractures is similar to the majority of other adult spinal deformity patients. One must question the progression of the deformity, as deformity that precedes the fracture may affect the choice of fusion levels. The history must include a review of prior spine surgeries and associated complications. In cases with severe sagittal plane malalignment, the surgeon should consider neurological disease such as Parkinson's disease and associated variants (Fig. 15.1). Camptocormia from neurological disease is a unique entity, often requiring extensive fusions (C2 to the sacrum), and surgical treatment can be wrought with complications. These patients often complain of being "pushed toward the ground." Prior to surgery, these diseases should be diagnosed and managed with the assistance of a neurologist. The history should also include any neurological complaints, including radiculopathy, signs of myelopathy, and queries regarding bowel and bladder habits. Appropriate patient counseling regarding expectations will improve satisfaction after treatment.

The physical examination begins with examination of the general patient condition. The body mass index is a simple guide to identify malnutrition. Malnutrition is characterized by a combination of weight loss, loss of muscle mass, loss of

A. E. Razi, S. H. Hershman (eds.), *Vertebral Compression Fractures in Osteoporotic and Pathologic Bone*, https://doi.org/10.1007/978-3-030-33861-9_15

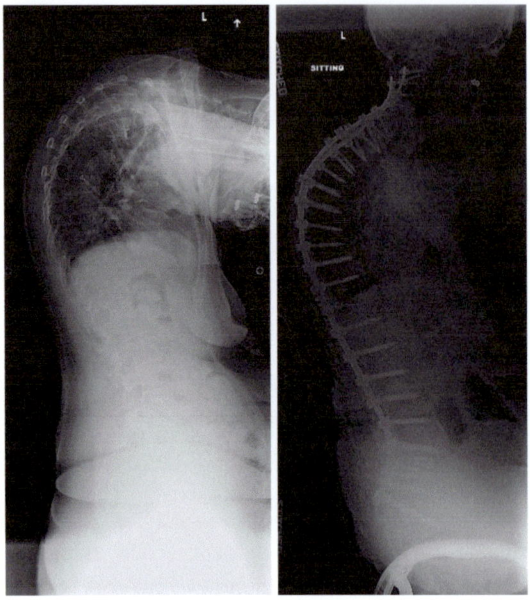

Fig. 15.1 Upright lateral and anteroposterior radiographs of a 67-year-old woman who presented with a chief complaint of kyphosis. Evaluation revealed osteoporotic compression deformities in the setting of Parkinson's disease. Treatment consisted of preoperative halo-gravity traction and C2-sacrum posterior spinal fusion

subcutaneous fat, worsened functional status, and poor caloric intake. In addition to judging the overall ability of the patient to tolerate an instrumented spinal fusion, adequate soft-tissue coverage for implants should be ensured. Frailty may be concomitant in patients presenting with osteoporotic spinal deformities. Identification of the malnourished and frail patient is necessary to assist with appropriate risk stratification and with the shared-decision-making process for these difficult patients. The five-time sit-to-stand (FTSTS) test and hand dynamometer strength testing are two measures easily obtained in the clinic. Appropriate FTSTS times are under 7 seconds for patients under the age of 70 and 10 seconds for those older. Grip strength threshold limits have been proposed, with 16 kg being appropriate for women and 27 kg for men.

Observation of the standing and supine alignment of the coronal and sagittal planes is critical. A supine examination helps reveal flexibility in the deformity, which will affect surgical planning. The extent of fusion will often be greater for those with sagittal plane malalignment and engaged compensatory mechanisms such as pelvic retroversion, hip flexion, and knee flexion. While standing, a Romberg test and examination of gait may help detect myelopathic symptoms and indicate the need for a decompression of the spinal cord, as it is not uncommon for subtle myelopathy to be ignored by patients. A routine neurological examination to document myotome and dermatome integrity is necessary, as always.

Radiographic Examination

Full-length standing and supine radiographs are required to appropriately treat spinal deformity. When available, standing "skull to foot" films allow for assessment of the engaged compensatory mechanisms in sagittal plane deformities (Fig. 15.2). Supine films allow for assessment of

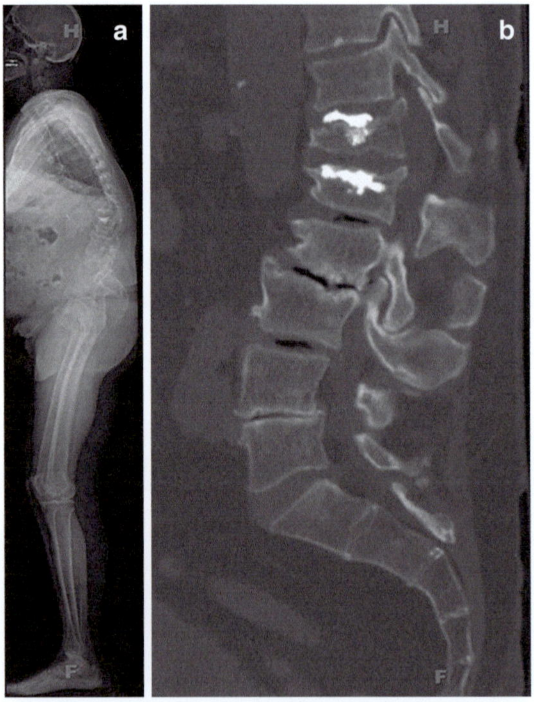

Fig. 15.2 (**a**) Standing, full-length lateral radiograph of a 64-year-old gentleman with thoracolumbar kyphosis secondary to osteoporotic fractures. Compensatory mechanisms engaged include knee flexion and upper cervical hyperextension. (**b**) Computed tomography scan of the lumbar spine showing compression deformities, status post cement augmentation, and multiple vacuum discs

rigidity of the deformity in both the coronal and sagittal planes. In the case of deformities driven by osteoporotic fractures, the supine film will assess the amount of regional correction that will be obtained simply by placing the patient prone on the operating table. It is not uncommon to plan for a three-column osteotomy (3CO) when upright, to find that the osteotomy is not needed. Radiographic measurements should include the pelvic incidence, supine lumbar lordosis (also available in a midsagittal computed tomography scan), and the T1 pelvic angle. Classification of patients according to the method of Roussouly may assist with the choice of fusion levels. Osteoporotic patients are at high-risk for proximal junctional failure through fracture, and inappropriate (too short) fusions will result in failure and early revision surgery.

Computed tomography scans offer detail regarding fixation points at the pedicle. In our experience, these patients tend to have larger pedicles, requiring larger than normal pedicle screw diameters. In general, we aim to fill 65–70% of the pedicle diameter. We avoid "fit and fill" as revision of a large, loose screw can be difficult should the patient go on to pseudarthrosis [1]. CT scans also offer the chance for opportunistic bone mineral density measurements, through the measurement of Hounsfield units (HU) within the vertebral body [2]. Measurements below 115HU may be consistent with the diagnosis of osteoporosis. Current technology does not allow for immediately actionable clinical information. However, immediate finite element modeling of the vertebral body architecture may offer surgeons data to assist with fusion level choices as well as suggest cement augmentation at weaker segments [3]. As previously mentioned, CT scans also offer data regarding the flexibility of the deformity, as they are obtained with the patient supine. One must be careful to check whether the head was placed on a pillow, or more, as this will underestimate flexibility, with a persistent forward head position and increased T1-pelvic angle. Both plain radiographs and CT scans should be evaluated for evidence of compression fractures away from the site of the spinal deformity. In some cases, these may help determine or dictate fusion levels (Fig. 15.3d).

Magnetic resonance imaging (MRI) is recommended for any cases where there will be manipulation of the spinal column. An MRI is required for any case with a preoperative neurological deficit. These images also allow for an opportunity to check the integrity of the paraspinal muscles. In cases of extreme atrophy and fat infiltration, we are inclined to choose longer fusions, as control of the sagittal plane by the patient may not be possible (Fig. 15.3e).

Medical Management

In an ideal situation, all patients with spinal deformities caused by insufficiency fractures would present already diagnosed with osteoporosis and with medical management. Unfortunately, this is not the case. Thus, ensuring that the patient understands that the presence of the insufficiency makes the diagnosis of osteoporosis, irrespective of any subsequent bone mineral density test, is essential so that they can engage in their own care for this disease. If a patient has not been evaluated for bone mineral density, we obtain a dual-energy x-ray absorptiometry (DEXA) exam of the hip, wrist, and lumbar spine. In cases of lumbar degeneration, osteophytes and sclerotic bone may overestimate the general quality of bone and disease state. As these patients have fractures, thus diagnosing the disease, we find the DEXA useful to see the true values of bone mineral density. In cases where the density is less than 0.60 gm/cm^2, concern for the ability to fix and hold the spine with pedicle screws exists. In these cases, one must consider cement augmentation or nonoperative care, as screw failures in a fragile patient could result in a worse overall condition. In addition to the DEXA, we check vitamin D levels, as hypovitaminosis D is frequently concomitant and is easily and affordably treated.

Our preferred method of pharmacologic treatment of osteoporosis in a spinal deformity patient is teriparatide, an anabolic agent. Teriparatide works through osteoclast stimulation, which

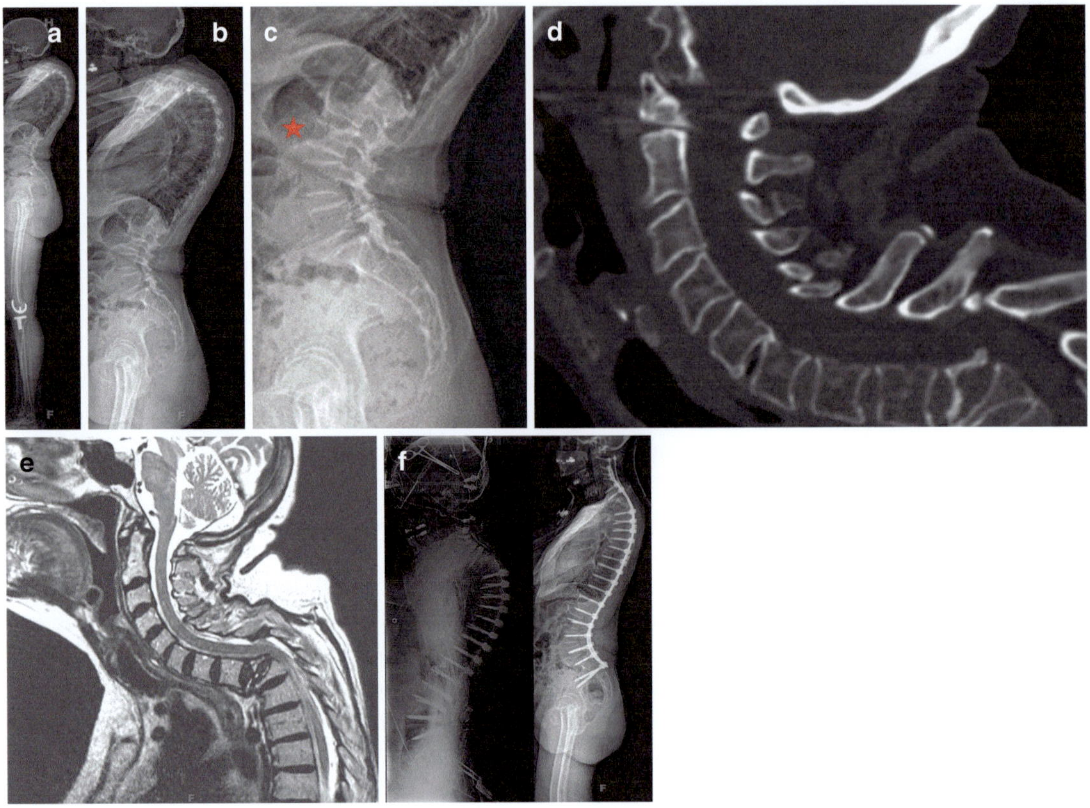

Fig. 15.3 (**a**) Standing, full-length lateral radiograph of a 78-year-old woman who presented with complaints of progressive kyphosis with progressive dysphonia and dysphagia. (**b**) Standing, 36″ cassette lateral radiograph revealing compression and vertebra plana of T2 and compression of C3 with 75° of kyphosis from T1 to T5. (**c**) Coned-down view of the lumbar spine in the previously described patient, showing a compression fracture of L3. This dictated fusion to the sacrum, with iliac instrumentation, to avoid distal failure through fracture. (**d**) Sagittal computed tomography (CT) scan of the cervicothoracic junction confirming vertebra plana with minimal retropulsion of the bone. For this reason, no anterior reconstruction was performed, and an "all-posterior" surgery with one single posterior column osteotomy with cantilever bending was the corrective maneuver. (**e**) Magnetic resonance imaging confirming draping of the spinal cord over the kyphosis. No cervical spinal stenosis was found. (**f**) Intraoperative radiographs showing correction using prone positioning with a four-pin halo holding the head. Postoperative radiographs show normal spinal alignment after C2-sacrum posterior spinal fusion

subsequently activate osteoblasts, encouraging bone turnover and formation. There are some data to suggest that teriparatide improves fusion rates, though more data, including appropriate dosing protocols, are needed [4]. Prolonged administration of teriparatide in animal models is associated with osteosarcoma formation. For this reason, teriparatide use is limited to 24 total months. In most cases, we require 3 months of therapy prior to surgery and request 3–6 months of teriparatide treatment after surgery. Patients are then switched to some other form of pharmacotherapy, preferably denosumab rather than a bisphosphonate. The pharmacologic treatments of osteoporosis are evolving rapidly, and research into the possible benefits, or detrimental effects, of these medications on bone mineral density and spinal fusion are needed.

Surgical Management

Surgical management of osteoporotic deformities is complicated by the multiple goals of surgery. Immobilization for pain relief is not adequate as a singular goal, as regional malalignment may lead to implant failure and revision surgery. Thus, goals of surgery are a stable and durable construct, with restoration of regional and global alignment and decompression of symptomatic neural compression. Given this, there are a number of surgical options, with both common and particular associated complications. Often, the surgical approach will be dictated by the deformity, patient factors such as frailty and bone density, and surgeon experience (Fig. 15.3f).

Historically, anterior procedures were advocated for cases with retropulsion of the vertebral body and neural compression. These surgeries involve both anterior column reconstruction with strut grafting or instrumentation, followed by anterior spinal instrumentation in the form of a plate and screws or a dual-rod construct. One benefit of anterior column reconstruction in non-osteoporotic burst fractures is that it will save fusion levels. Given the poor bone quality, anterior reconstructions are at risk for both subsidence of the interbody graft, be it allograft or metal, and for failure of the anterior vertebral body screws. If one feels that anterior reconstruction is required, a perfect endplate preparation is necessary, as any endplate defect will lead to subsidence with a high rate of failure. Bicortical purchase of anterior screws is necessary. Even with bicortical placement, anterior screws are at a higher risk for failure. The poor bone quality is manifest by thin cortices and low trabecular bone density, increasing the risk of screw loosening. The opportunity for direct decompression of the spinal canal is an advantage of the anterior approach. In the case of osteoporotic deformities, and as opposed to high-energy trauma, the neurological deficit is infrequently due to blunt impact and compression from the vertebral body fragments. Neurological deficits more frequently are insidious in onset with traction myelopathy developing over the deformity. Thus correction of the deformity, without attention to resection of the bony fragment, is likely to yield a satisfactory result.

Sudo et al. compared anterior and posterior thoracolumbar approaches for osteoporotic fractures with neurological deficits [5]. While both surgeries were able to decompress the neural elements and correct the spinal deformity, there were several benefits associated with posterior surgeries. Not surprisingly, anterior approaches had a pulmonary complication in one-third of the patients. In addition, estimated blood loss was lower in the posterior surgeries. Finally, patients with the lowest bone mineral density (<0.60 g/cm^2) or those with inadequate fusion levels were most likely to fail and undergo a second surgery. No patients in the posterior surgery group underwent a second surgery, and the authors report a low rate of complication (5%) in the posterior group. As a retrospective study, this likely underreports the risk of complication in these complicated patients and surgeries. Suk et al. described a more complicated cohort of patients and surgeries, with anterior-posterior surgery or posterior-based closing wedge osteotomies [6]. Complications related to surgery were more frequent, perhaps due to more severe deformity requiring a more complex surgery. The mean correction through a closing wedge osteotomy was 25°, four times greater than correction in the prior study. Finally, Krishnakumar and Lenke described a two-level vertebral column resection for a "sternum-into-abdomen" deformity [7]. This provided a 60° correction, though was complicated by high blood loss (3 L), pulmonary effusion requiring a chest tube, and a distal junctional fracture with kyphosis that was treated nonoperatively. As one can see, three-column osteotomies can provide excellent corrections and decompressions, though these surgeries are accompanied by an increased risk of perioperative complication.

Our preference for the management of spinal deformity in the setting of spinal stenosis (at the level of the spinal cord or cauda equina) is to use an "all-posterior technique." Frequently, the stenosis is due to retropulsion of the osteoporotic burst fracture and less frequently due to ligamentum flavum, as the segment may be in kyphosis. Thus, removal of the ventral bone and correction of the spinal deformity are the necessary components of the surgery. We will try to avoid a full laminectomy, as this will complicate achieving a fusion. Instead, we perform a hemilaminectomy and work through a transpedicular or posterolateral extra-cavitary approach to work ventral to the thecal sac. Removal of the pedicle gives access to the vertebral body, where we will create a void within the body into which the retropulsed fragments may be pushed using a downward curette or a Woodson elevator. Using the downward curette or Woodson elevator, one can work across the midline to the contralateral canal and fully decompress the spinal canal. This work should be done with a stabilizing rod engaged through the contralateral pedicle screws, with a minimum of two screws above and two below engaged to reduce the risk of screw failure. After decompressing the spinal canal, one is faced with the choice of how to treat the void created in the anterior and middle columns. We will frequently remove the majority of the disks above and below, so that there is an opportunity for anterior spinal fusion. In the thoracic spine, placing a mesh cage may be done after sacrificing a nerve root, though in cases of soft bone stock, we will often avoid anterior instrumentation as there is a high risk of subsidence through the end plates. In these cases, and in the majority of lumbar cases, we will pack the void with bone graft and cantilever around the decancellated vertebral body. This technique has been described in other spinal deformity pathologies, with good corrections and outcomes [8]. The contralateral lamina then serves as a bed for bone graft to increase the rate of a successful dorsal and posterolateral fusion.

In the absence of a kyphotic deformity, a dorsal decompression with fusion may be appropriate. A review of the preoperative imaging should lead the surgeon to the correct procedure to ensure adequate decompression of the neural elements and a stable result. In the case of a rigid segment, for example, anterior fusion occurred after healing of the burst, and then a decompression alone may suffice. In many instances, however, there are vacuum phenomena in the anterior and middle columns, similar to Kummel's disease, and decompression alone in the setting of this instability is unlikely to provide a durable, satisfactory result.

The choice of fusion levels in spinal deformities due to osteoporotic fracture should follow the tenets of adult spinal deformity surgery and not adult spinal trauma surgery [9]. That is, short segment fixation is unlikely to work in the setting of a longer-standing deformity. This is multifactorial, though changes in the posterior musculature affect the ability to stand upright and resist kyphosis. Short segment fixation may lead to early distal junctional failure in established sagittal plane deformities. The choice of the upper instrumented level (UIV) depends on the preexisting sagittal plane contour. The UIV should not be chosen within a kyphosis and should rather "cover" the kyphosis. Stopping within a kyphotic segment will leave a substantial risk for proximal junctional kyphosis requiring revision surgery. Thus, in cases of lumbar deformities, we will often stop at the lower thoracic spine (T10 or T11) if the proximal thoracic spine is not hyperkyphotic or if the patient does not have a high (>60 degrees) pelvic incidence. We avoid low thoracic UIV in the latter two cases because the reciprocal changes in thoracic kyphosis after fixing the lumbar deformity will increase the risk of a proximal junctional kyphosis. Thus, in these cases we will often extend the fusion to the upper thoracic spine, stopping at the first non-kyphotic segment.

The choice of the lower instrumented vertebra is more difficult. In older (>65 years of age) we will often fuse to the sacrum with iliac instrumentation. This is due to the likelihood of sagittal plane malalignment as the unfused segments degenerate, leading to poor patient-reported outcome scores and difficult revision surgeries. Iliac instrumentation is mandatory in these osteoporotic patients when fusing to the sacrum. The risk of sacral fracture is high, and management of these iatrogenic deformities is complicated, with substantial risk of associated morbidity. The choice of iliac screws versus S2-alar-iliac screws is left to the discretion and experience of the surgeon. If one uses S2-alar-iliac screws, then a minimum screw length of 80 millimeters (mm) and diameter of 8.0 mm is required. Shorter screws may not end ventral to the lumbosacral flexion point, rendering them useless and creating an opportunity for a sacral insufficiency fracture to propagate through the screw start site.

A lower instrumented vertebra (LIV) above the sacrum has potential risks and benefits to be discussed as a part of the informed-decision-making process. Fusions extended to the sacrum may have a higher rate of proximal junctional failure, perhaps increased in these patients with poor bone quality. Thus, avoiding the sacrum as the LIV may reduce proximal failures. However, there may be an increased risk of distal junctional failure, through a compression or burst fracture of the LIV. The force of the lever arm created by the long construct above may be too much for the weakened vertebral body to sustain. In general, we will choose a stable sagittal vertebra defined by a line drawn straight up from the posterior superior end plate of S1. In pediatric kyphosis surgery, the last "substantially" touched vertebra (line passes through the midpoint or dorsal to the midpoint) may have fewer distal junctional failures than a body touched in the anterior, inferior portion of the vertebral body.

Cement augmentation, in an addition to appropriately placed and sized pedicle screws, is a method that may improve fixation, thereby improving fusion rates, as well as minimizing the rate of proximal junctional failures. These are achieved by two distinct mechanisms. Augmentation of pedicle screw fixation is accomplished by placing a small amount of polymethyl methacrylate through the screw track prior to placement of the screw. In general, 1 to 3 cubic centimeters (cc) are used and the screw placed while the cement is still liquid. Biomechanical studies have suggested smaller (1 cc) volumes in the thoracic spine versus higher volume in the lumbar spine (3 cc) [10]. New pedicle screw designs include fenestrated and cannulated pedicle screws. Cement may be placed through the screws, extruding within the vertebral body. Both of these techniques have improved pullout strength versus non-augmented pedicle screws. Important to consider, given the cost of implants, is that there were no significant differences between an augmented solid screw and a fenestrated screw. Cement augmentation may be associated with embolic events, however [11]. While infrequently symptomatic (1–2%), pulmonary cement embolism is more likely when large numbers of screws are augmented; thus the use of cement augmentation should be judicious, with some preoperative planning.

Cement augmentation of the vertebral body (prophylactic vertebroplasty), distinct from screw augmentation, may reduce junctional failures, both proximal and distal to the UIV and LIV [12, 13]. Proximal junctional failure, with a vertebral compression fracture of the UIV or one above the UIV, is a vexing problem in osteoporotic spinal deformities. Several observational studies have found lower junctional fractures in the acute and subacute period, when the majority of adjacent segment failures occur. PMMA cement is applied using a syringe or commercially available cement delivery system, often with 2–3 cc of cement total, at the UIV, and the screws then placed. Cement is delivered to the level above the UIV as well, as junctional failures most frequently occur at one of these two levels. In some series, the rate of junctional failure is below 5%, though these findings are not universal. Raman et al. reported long-term (minimum 5 years) follow-up on one cohort of prophylactic vertebroplasty patients and noted that nearly 30% of patients developed proximal junctional kyphosis over time. Thus, cement augmentation may mitigate the risk of early failure, but it does not cure the disease of proximal failure, and long-term follow-up of these complicated patients is necessary.

Postoperative Care

Our postoperative care for these patients is not different from other adult spinal deformity patients. We do not use any sort of external orthosis as we believe this will lead to further deconditioning of the spinal extensors, critical to maintaining an erect posture. A front-wheeled walker is used for a minimum of 3 months after surgery. It is adjusted to the appropriate height, so that it encourages upright and lordotic standing and walking positions, to reduce the stresses across the cranial/caudal adjacent segments. One must ensure that the patient is not leaning forward onto the walker, with a kyphotic thoracic spine as this will lead to some form of junctional failure. The walker also helps minimize the risk of falls in the early postoperative period. Falls can be catastrophic, with implant failure, burst fractures, spondylolisthesis, and neurological injury. We do not use thoracolumbar orthoses in these patients. In select patients, a hard cervical orthosis may be used if fusion involves the cervicothoracic spine. We are cautious with our use of hard collars, though, given the generally debilitated state of these patients and the risks of pressure ulcers on the chin and/or occiput. Patients are seen at 6 weeks, 3 months, and 6 months after surgery. In some cases, where spinal alignment is appropriate, but a fracture occurs, we will have a vertebroplasty performed, as intraoperative vertebroplasty is not our standard of care.

As previously noted, long-term follow-up of these patients is needed to follow the unfused segments. Radiographic PJK is common and does not always need surgical intervention. However, some PJK may be a warning sign of a pending proximal failure with neurological compromise, and surgical treatment may be the conservative option in these cases.

Conclusion

The treatment of spinal deformities secondary to osteoporotic fractures requires experience with adult spinal deformity reconstructions. The tenets of adult deformity surgery are followed, with the increasing complexity of poor bone quality and neurological compromise from pathological burst fractures. Appropriate pharmacologic treatment of the osteoporosis is necessary in all cases, regardless of whether the patient moves forward with surgery. With modern techniques, "all-posterior" approaches allow for decompression and correction of deformity, particularly with three-column osteotomies. Cement augmentation of instrumented and non-instrumented levels may improve fixation and reduce failures after these large reconstructions. Given the aging population, surgeons should familiarize themselves with the concepts and techniques necessary to treat these complex patients and deformities.

Bibliography

1. Lai DM, et al. Effect of pedicle screw diameter on screw fixation efficacy in human osteoporotic thoracic vertebrae. J Biomech. 2018;70:196–203.
2. Kohan EM, et al. Lumbar computed tomography scans are not appropriate surrogates for bone mineral density scans in primary adult spinal deformity. Neurosurg Focus. 2017;43(6):E4.
3. Burch S, et al. Prevalence of poor bone quality in women undergoing spinal fusion using biomechanical-CT analysis. Spine (Phila Pa 1976). 2016;41(3):246–52.
4. Ebata S, et al. Role of weekly teriparatide administration in Osseous union enhancement within six months after posterior or transforaminal lumbar interbody fusion for osteoporosis-associated lumbar degenerative disorders: a multicenter, prospective randomized study. J Bone Joint Surg Am. 2017;99(5):365–72.
5. Sudo H, et al. Anterior decompression and strut graft versus posterior decompression and pedicle screw fixation with vertebroplasty for osteoporotic thoracolumbar vertebral collapse with neurologic deficits. Spine J. 2013;13(12):1726–32.
6. Suk SI, et al. Anterior-posterior surgery versus posterior closing wedge osteotomy in posttraumatic kyphosis with neurologic compromised osteoporotic fracture. Spine (Phila Pa 1976). 2003;28(18):2170–5.
7. Krishnakumar R, Lenke LG. "Sternum-into-abdomen" deformity with abdominal compression following osteoporotic vertebral compression fractures managed by 2-level vertebral column resection and reconstruction. Spine (Phila Pa 1976). 2015;40(18):E1035–9.
8. Zhang X, et al. Vertebral column decancellation: a new spinal osteotomy technique for correcting rigid thoracolumbar kyphosis in patients with ankylosing spondylitis. Bone Joint J. 2016;98-B(5):672–8.
9. Kuklo TR. Principles for selecting fusion levels in adult spinal deformity with particular attention to lumbar curves and double major curves. Spine (Phila Pa 1976). 2006;31(19 Suppl):S132–8.
10. Leichtle CI, et al. Pull-out strength of cemented solid versus fenestrated pedicle screws in osteoporotic vertebrae. Bone Joint Res. 2016;5(9):419–26.
11. Ulusoy OL, et al. Pulmonary cement embolism following cement-augmented fenestrated pedicle screw fixation in adult spinal deformity patients with severe osteoporosis (analysis of 2978 fenestrated screws). Eur Spine J. 2018;27(9):2348–56.
12. Raman T, et al. The effect of prophylactic vertebroplasty on the incidence of proximal junctional kyphosis and proximal junctional failure following posterior spinal fusion in adult spinal deformity: a 5-year follow-up study. Spine J. 2017;17(10):1489–98.
13. Theologis AA, Burch S. Prevention of acute proximal junctional fractures after long thoracolumbar posterior fusions for adult spinal deformity using 2-level cement augmentation at the upper instrumented vertebra and the vertebra 1 level proximal to the upper instrumented vertebra. Spine (Phila Pa 1976). 2015;40(19):1516–26.

16 Operative Treatment of Pathologic Compression Fractures of the Spine

Theodosios Stamatopoulos, Ganesh M. Shankar, and John H. Shin

Key Points

- Each patient requires a personalized evaluation of the mechanical, neurological, oncological, and functional impacts of the pathological fracture to help guide the decision for surgery.
- Multiple options for decompression and stabilization of pathological compression fractures are available including minimally invasive and open surgery.
- There is no gold standard stabilization technique. The safest approach is the one the surgeon is most familiar with.

Introduction

The management of tumors affecting the spinal column is complex and requires multidisciplinary and multimodal therapies. Historically, the treatment for fractures involving the spinal column due to cancer is associated with high morbidity [1]. The goal of intervention in these situations is to palliate the mechanical pain related to the fracture while minimizing the morbidity of the intervention. In patients suffering from cancer-related pain affecting the vertebrae and other bones, the restoration of stability in the spine can help improve pain and function. With advances in technology, spinal instrumentation, and fixation systems, there are now more ways to treat and address these fractures.

Regardless of whether the underlying tumor is a primary spinal column tumor such as chordoma or chondrosarcoma, or metastatic from another site, pathological fractures can occur in any vertebrae in the spinal column [2]. Because metastatic spinal column tumors are more common than primary spinal column tumors, the incidence of spinal metastases is certainly higher [3]. With the evolution of systemic cancer therapies including targeted therapies and immunotherapy, patients with metastatic cancer are living longer and with a greater burden of disease. As such, these patients may develop spinal and skeletal fractures which can produce significant pain and disability limiting ambulation and the ability to

T. Stamatopoulos
Department of Neurosurgery, Massachusetts General Hospital, Harvard Medical School, Boston, MA, USA

CORE-Center for Orthopedic Research at CIRI-AUTh, Aristotle University Medical School, Thessaloniki, Hellas, Greece

G. M. Shankar · J. H. Shin (✉)
Department of Neurosurgery, Massachusetts General Hospital, Harvard Medical School, Boston, MA, USA
e-mail: gshankar@mgh.harvard.edu; shin.john@mgh.harvard.edu

A. E. Razi, S. H. Hershman (eds.), *Vertebral Compression Fractures in Osteoporotic and Pathologic Bone*, https://doi.org/10.1007/978-3-030-33861-9_16

bear weight. With this in mind, the role of the spine surgeon is to thoughtfully consider methods and strategies to stabilize these fractures in order to restore function and palliate pain in these scenarios.

In principle, the management of metastatic spine tumors requires multidisciplinary input as to whether the patient can tolerate surgical intervention. Though imaging studies such as MRI, CT, and plain radiographs may demonstrate a fracture or fractures that correlate with the patient's symptoms, careful consideration of the morbidity of a planned intervention is necessary as complications associated with surgery can have a devastating effect on the patient's overall survival and outcome.

In this chapter, we will also discuss the role of radiation, specifically spine stereotactic radiosurgery (SRS), and its effects on the bone and associated risks for pathological fracture after treatment. Cement augmentation in the form of vertebroplasty or kyphoplasty can also be very effective for patients with vertebral fractures provided there is only minimal retropulsion and spinal cord, cauda equina, or nerve root compromise. Percutaneous techniques, like cement augmentation, are discussed elsewhere in this text book.

Evaluation

Incidence

According to the American Cancer Society, over 1.7 million new cancer cases are projected annually in the United States [1, 4]. Lung cancer and breast cancer are the most common cancers overall [5, 6]. With regards to sites of metastases, after the lungs and the liver, the skeletal system is the third most common site of metastasis, of which the spine is the most common (30–50%). Patients between 40 and 60 years old are most commonly affected, and from this group of patients, 10–30% will develop a clinical manifestation such as a pathological VCF and/or spinal cord compression. Additionally, surgery may be needed for SRS-induced VCF, which can occur in up to 39% of the patients treated [7]. The thoracic (60–70%) and lumbar (20–25%) spines are the most common sites of metastases, with the cervical spine (10%) and sacrum being affected less commonly.

Clinical Significance

VCF is a major problem that can occur at any time in the patient's cancer treatment. It is associated with functional impairment and/or deterioration with prolonged pain and inactivity [8]. VCFs are associated with spinal cord compression in 30–40% of cases and can lead to chronic pain, permanent weakness, and impairment of ambulation. Treatment goals have historically focused on preserving neurologic function, restoring mechanical stability, and providing pain relief [6, 9].

Continued developments in chemotherapy, immunotherapy, and radiotherapy have improved the treatment and survival of these patients. Despite these advances, systemic therapies are more effective for visceral than bone disease. This ultimately limits the effectiveness of these emerging therapies on painful spinal fractures. As such, for patients with panful VCF, surgical intervention is a consideration.

Pathologic Fracture After Spine Stereotactic Radiosurgery (SRS)

Radiation has a major role in the multimodal treatment of spinal tumors. Conventional fractionated radiation is associated with high-dose radiation delivery to adjacent anatomical structures including the skin, soft tissues, and solid body organs in the area of interest. Due to the fractionated nature of dose delivery and the volume of the radiation fields, each cancer type responds differently to conventional radiation, and accordingly, pain response and local tumor control are variables [10].

Stereotactic spine radiosurgery (SRS) has emerged as a powerful adjuvant not only postoperatively but also as a stand-alone treatment for spinal metastases [10–12]. With the advantages of minimizing radiation treatment-related complications and the accompanying high rates of tumor and pain control, SRS is now a therapy that complements other treatments in the spine [13]. With SRS, lesions are typically radiated in 1–5 fractions with highly conformal radiation beams. Tumors historically radioresistant to conventional fractionated radiation such as sarcoma, melanoma, and renal cell carcinoma (RCC) now demonstrate local tumor control rates up to 95% at 1 year following SRS [10]. Additionally, radiation-induced complications to surrounding tissue is minimized. The highly conformal treatment beams of SRS allow for limiting the dose exposure to surrounding vital organs (heart, lung, esophagus, kidney, skin, and spinal cord) [13–15]. This is particularly important in the postoperative setting where the radiation dose to the skin is minimized to prevent wound-healing issues. Because of the steep radiation dose falloff, the radiation dose to the vertebral column target and to the surrounding tissue, just millimeters away, is significant.

SRS is not complication-free, with VCF being a known posttreatment effect leading to potential instability [13, 16–18]. Compared to conventional radiotherapy where the incidence of postradiation VCF is lower than 5%, in SRS the incidence of VCF is up to 39% [7, 19]. Not all of these fractures are symptomatic, and it needs to be clarified that not all VCFs need to be treated. In fact, many pathological fractures that happen after SRS treatment can be followed with serial clinical follow-up and imaging. In cases where pain persists, further imaging is required to assess the extent of the fracture and whether cement augmentation or surgery is appropriate. If there is vertebral body height loss with minimal retropulsion of bone, cement augmentation through a percutaneous approach may be effective. If a spinal deformity or significant malalignment develops due to collapse and kyphosis, surgery may be needed.

According to the International Spine Research Consortium, the entire vertebra needs to be radiated in the event of a metastatic lesion [20, 21]. Although radiation of a specific spine level typically includes normal bone tissue and at least one vertebra above and below the lesion, VCFs occur almost only at the level of the metastasis. While spinal cord radiation dose tolerances have been reported, it is still unclear how much dose the spinal cord can actually tolerate. The data regarding dose tolerance is extrapolated from reported cases of spinal cord toxicity from SRS. There is variation in treatment protocols and dose constraints as published in the literature [10]. Depending on each institution's protocols, studies using different doses and fractions report conflicting tumor and pain response and total survival results. Radiation doses/fraction can vary between 30–40 Gy or 25–35 Gy/5 fractions, 30 Gy or 25–35 Gy/4 fractions, 24–30 Gy or 8–9 Gy/3 fractions, 24 Gy/2 fractions, and 18–24 Gy/1 fraction.

VCF following SRS tends to be dose-dependent (Table 16.1). Most post-SRS VCFs are reported in the thoracic and lumbar spines [6, 21–32]. VCFs can occur between 1.5 months and 2.5 years of follow-up but are mostly observed during the first year postradiation and specifically during the first 6–9 months, making VCF an acute or subacute complication [7, 13, 21, 26, 27, 31–33]. Specifically, the chances of a post-SRS VCF are less in single dosages of 16–18 Gy whereas >40% at multiple fractions over 20–24 Gy per dose [21]. From the first report of 39% VCF risk by Rose et al. in 2009, single- and multi-institutional studies have modified the radiation per fraction applied and narrowed VCF incidence down to 7.8% [7]. Using a single fraction protocol of 24 Gy, Virk S. et al. concluded that the cumulative 5-year incidence of VCF was 8.1% [31]. Sahgal et al. in multi-institutional study of Elekta Spine Radiosurgery Research Consortium including 410 lesions in 252 patients concluded that the risk of VCF is 14% [27]. In the largest series by Boyce-Fappiano et al. including 1070 lesions of 448 patients, it was found that SRS treatment of metastatic spine lesions led to an almost 12% (11.9%) VCF incidence [32].

Risk factors have been identified, although no commonly accepted factors exist. Associated risk factors include solitary, lytic lesions, and prescription doses higher than 24 Gy [10, 28, 30].

Table 16.1 Major studies describing the incidence of VCF after spine SRS as initial treatment

Author, year, ref.	Study type	Num. patients/ lesions	Mean imaging follow-up time in months	Mean/median time of VCF incidence after SRS in months (range)	Number of VCF (percentage of treated vertebra) De novo Progression of former	Number of cases and surgical interventions performed
Rose et al., 2009 [7]	Single-ICS prospective	62/71	13	25	27 (39%) 20 (74%) 7 (26%)	3 (4.8%) 1 VAT 2 surgery
Boheling et al., 2012, [26]	Single-ICS retrospective	93/123	14.9 (1–71)	14	25 (20%) 14 (11%) 11 (9%)	15 (16.1%) VAT
Sahgal et al., 2013, [27]	Multi-ICS	252/410	11.53 (0.03– 113.02)	2.46 (0.03–43.01)	57 (14%) 27 (6.5%) 30 (7.3%)	24 (9.5%) 17 VAT 1 percutaneous instrumentation 6 invasive instrumentation
Cunha et al., 2013, [28]	Single-ICS prospective	90/167	7.4 (NA)	2 (0.5–21.6)	19 (11%) 12 (7%) 7 (4%)	9 (10%) 6 VAT 3 spinal reconstructive surgery with instrumentation
Sung et al., 2014, [24]	Single-ICS prospective	72/72	11 (3–24)	2 (0.3–3.5)	26 (36%) NA NA	15 (20%) 10 VAT 5 fusion/instrumentation
Guckenberger et al., 2014, [25]	Multi-ICS retrospective	301/387	11.8	NA	30 (7.8%) 14 (3.6%) 16 (4.1%)	NA
Germano et al., 2017 [29]	Single-ICS prospective	79/143	16 (3–78)	NA	30 (21%) 9 (6.2%) 21 (14.7%)	14 (9.7%) 2 VAT 12 open surgery
Jawad et al., 2016, [21]	Multi-ICS retrospective	541/594	10.1 (0.03–57)	3 (1–36)	34 (5.7%) 18 (3%) 16 (2.7%)	36 (4%) 15 VAT 21 instrumentation

Virk S. et al., 2017, [31]	Single-ICS retrospective	323/551	12.6 (3.7–31.9)	13.2 months (6.3–28.7)	45 (8.1%) 28 (5%) 17 (3%)	26 cases (8%) 6 VAT 10 surgery 10 both
Boyce-Fappiano et al., 2017, [32]	Single-ICS retrospective	448/1070	11.53 (1.5–84)	2.7 (0.16–54.9)	127 (28.3%) 54 (12.1%) 73 (16.3%)	37 (8.2%) 21 VAT 16 instrumentation/fixation
Sun-Ho Lee et al., 2015, [33]	Single-ICS Prospective	79/79	24.05 (15.25)	5.7 (0.–34.1)	32 (40.5%) 20 (25.3%) 12 (15.2%)	15 cases (46.9%) 10 VAT 5 instrumentation
Thibault et al., 2014, [22]	Single-ICS retrospective on RCC	37/61	12.3 (1.2–55.4)	NA	10 (16.4%) 3 (4.9%) 7 (11.5%)	4 (6.6%) NA NA
Thibault et al., 2015, [35]	Multi-ICS retrospective on RCC	116/187	8.02 (0.03–75.9)	2.35 (0.03–43.1)	34 (18%) 31 (16.5%) 3 (1.6%)	NA

RCC renal cell carcinoma, *ICS* institutional cohort study, *VAT* vertebral augmentation techniques (kyphoplasty or vertebroplasty), *NA* not analyzed. The percentages refer to the total number of patients treated in each study

Additionally, the literature is consistent that SRS has no beneficial role in providing spinal stability [7, 26–30, 32]. Almost all studies confirm that a new post-SRS VCF is highly associated with the existence of fracture or spinal deformity before radiation [26–28, 34]. Lytic lesions and hypervascular lesions were found to significantly increase the chances of post-SRS VCF. Tumor growth against normal bone impairs the bone's mechanical properties; Thibault et al. observed that over 11.6% percentage of vertebral body involvement is predictive for imminent VCF post-SRS [24, 36]. Additionally, according to histopathological data, targeted radiation damages the collagen and causes necrosis and/or fibrosis, a phenomenon described as "osteoradionecrosis," which reduces spinal stability leading to insufficiency-VCF [18].

In the event of a post-SRS VCF, as described in Table 16.1, the most commonly used technique is percutaneous vertebral cement augmentation or conservative treatment. About half of patients will eventually need surgical intervention due to spinal instability, deformity, or pain. Patients who have a baseline fracture or spinal deformity are more likely to require surgery with instrumentation. Protective pre-SRS cement augmentation of metastatic lesions has been also proposed as a possible treatment algorithm [23, 26, 39] .

Medical Management and Optimization

Introduction

The presence of a spinal tumor, primary or metastatic, requires careful evaluation and treatment management [40]. Decision-making for surgical optimization is guided by algorithms evaluating the neurological, oncological, and spine-related aspects of the patient [38, 41, 42]. The NOMS algorithm guides the management of these patients. Specifically, these four initials assess the degree of epidural spinal cord compression, the radiosensitivity of the tumor, the mechanical stability of the level(s), and the extent of systemic disease [42].

Clinical Characteristics of Pathologic Spine Fractures

When symptomatic, pathologic spine fractures may present with constant, unremitting, or movement-related pain. Radiculopathy or myelopathy may occur as a result of the consequences of failure of the spinal column to withstand the loads associated with weight-bearing and activity. For example, a lumbar pathologic fracture may present with severe back and leg pain that is worse with sitting, standing, and walking. Taking a thorough history and understanding, the nature of the pain is critical to identifying pathologic fracture-related pain [44]. Table 16.2 describes the wide symptom-spectrum presented in the event of VCF.

Pain Associated with Spine Tumors

Neck or back pain is the dominant symptom accompanied with spinal column tumors. The difference in pain characteristics are related to the various causes of pain (Table 16.2). Mechanical pain worsening with movements or axial loading (sitting or standing) and relieved in recumbency is indicative of the inability of the spine to cope with the mechanical stress at different positions. Biological pain is characterized by constant local intractable pain, with no change in pain during upright position, movement, or lying down. This pain is likely due to destruction of the periosteum by cancer. This type of biological bone pain is responsive to steroids and tends to vary during the day irrespective of activity or weight-bearing. Patients not on supplemental steroid therapy often complain of pain worse in the morning and night, which is consistent with the diurnal variation of endogenous adrenal steroid production.

Signs and Symptoms of VCF

Craniovertebral Junction: Occipital Condyle to C2

The craniovertebral junction (CVJ) , specifically C1 (atlas) and C2 (axis), is a rare site of metastases, but the symptoms can be severe, leading

Table 16.2 Symptoms of spinal metastasis and pathological VCF

Spinal level	Most common symptoms
C0-C2	Cervical and suboccipital neck pain Instability pain Occipital neuralgia (in case of C2 nerve involvement), occipital headache Cranial neuropathies: Cranial nerve involvement in case tumor progresses at skull base Cervical myelopathy Dysphagia Bulbar pathology Intracranial hypertension, somnolence – Hydrocephalus Respiratory suppression/respiratory arrest
C3-C6	Neck pain (mechanical, nonmechanical), occipital neuralgia Retro-auricular and/or retro-orbital region headache Upper extremity pain, radiculopathy: Paresthesias and sensory deficits, nerve root compression: Upper extremity tingling/weakness/spasticity Spinal cord compression: Loss of walking ability, quadriparesis/paraparesis, ataxia Spinal shock: Flaccidity, loss of sphincter tone, fecal incontinence, priapism, loss of bulbocavernosus reflex Neurogenic shock: Hypotension, paradoxical bradycardia, flushed/dry/warm peripheral skin, poikilothermia Autonomic dysfunction: Ileus, urinary retention or incontinence RLN and SLN dysfunctions: Hoarseness, swallow dysfunction Airway compromise due to retropharyngeal hematoma or prevertebral soft tissue edema
C7-T2	Mechanical pain Nonmechanical pain (neck, shoulder, arm) Paresthesias, lower extremity weakness Radiculopathy Paraparesis/quadriparesis, paraplegia Urinary incontinence Cervicobrachialgia
T3-T10	Low back pain Abdominal pain Somnolence – Hydrocephalus
T11-L5	Paraplegia Hip and pelvis pain Cauda equina syndrome Lower extremity paralysis

VCF, vertebral compression fracture; SLN and RLN, superior and recurrent laryngeal nerve

to devastating pain [45, 46]. Destruction of the bone at the CVJ by tumor may lead to atlantoaxial instability. The pain associated with this area is severe rotational pain [40, 47]. Patients may complain of pain with turning their head side to side. They may also complain of increased effort to keep their head up. Mechanical pain, occipital neuralgia, and retro-auricular and/or retro-orbital headaches occur rather than neurologic compromise due to the wide spinal canal of the upper cervical spine (Table 16.2) [40, 46, 48, 49]. In severe cases, spinal cord compression may occur as a result of C1–2 subluxation and/or epidural extension of tumor, but most often there is more neck pain than neurological symptoms in this region.

Fractures may involve the occipital condyle, lateral masses of C1, the facets between C1–2, and even the odontoid [46]. Fractures or lytic destruction involving the lateral masses of C1 can result in severe mechanical pain. Because of the location, the C2 nerve root also may be affected, either by direct compression or traction due to instability at that segment. Though this site is rare for metastases, surgeons should have a high index of suspicion when cancer patients present with neck pain that is worse with head turning.

Subaxial Cervical Spine: C3 to C6

In the subaxial cervical spine, the spinal canal diameter is narrower, so it is more likely that a neurological deficit or symptom will accompany neck pain [46]. In contrast with the CVJ, where the ligaments are complex and strong, in the subaxial spine, the only barrier between the posterior part of the anterior column and the spinal canal is the posterior longitudinal ligament. Depending on the severity of spinal cord or nerve root compression, neurological compromise can vary from upper extremity weakness or spasticity to ataxia, paraparesis, and quadriparesis (Table 16.2) [50]. Patients with symptoms in this region may also have pain with head and neck rotation, though they will likely have more pain with neck flexion and extension. Patients may have some relief of this mechanical neck pain with the use of an external orthosis such as a neck collar prior to evaluation by a spine surgeon. Because of the location in the mobile cervical spine and the proximity to the spinal cord and nerve roots, patients may present with a radiculopathy similar to what is seen in the degenerative spine patient. Unilateral or bilateral symptoms may be present depending on the nature and extent of vertebral column involvement.

In this region, a carefully performed neurologic examination complements the radiographic assessment of fracture and involvement of the cervical vertebrae. Surgeons need to look for signs of spinal cord compression in addition to specific nerve root distribution pain, weakness, and sensory changes.

Given the location and the regional anatomy, cement augmentation is often not feasible in the subaxial cervical spine. As such, these patients should be evaluated for consideration of spine surgery to decompress and stabilize the spine if the fracture is significant and cord compression is present.

Cervicothoracic: C7 to T2

The cervicothoracic junction (CTJ) refers to the C7, T1, and T2 levels. Spinal metastasis of the CTJ presents with mechanical instability and movement-related pain, most commonly in extension. The presence of the ribs and clavicles adds stability to this region, so symptoms may present later in the disease. Furthermore, VCF can lead to subsequent spinal canal narrowing, and spinal cord or spinal nerve injury as the spinal canal is narrower in the sub-cervical spine (Table 16.2) [51].

Thoracic and Lumbar Spine: T3 to L5

Most metastases and VCFs occur in the thoracic and lumbar spine, about 60% and 20%, respectively. The cumulative mechanical forces that are transmitted through the vertebrae cranially to caudally, combined with the inferior bone quality, make these VCFs more common. Thoracic vertebrae are more vulnerable to VCF because of the geometric and loading alignment. VCF-related instability manifests as pain in movement: in the thoracic and thoracolumbar spine, pain worsens in recumbency revealing an unstable kyphosis, whereas in the lumbar spine, pain exacerbates when standing or sitting. Additionally, pain can be accompanied by lower extremity neurologic deficits, ambulatory loss, or even paraplegia. Spinal cord compression is more common at the thoracic spine due to the narrower spinal canal (Table 16.2).

Radiographic Diagnosis of Pathological Fractures of the Spine

If a pathologic fracture is suspected, the patient will need diagnostic imaging. The evaluation may start with plain radiographs; however, MRI and/or CT provides the most comprehensive diagnostic imaging [21].

Although anteroposterior (and lateral) chest X-ray is included at most institutions, it has a low sensitivity for detecting fractures [52]. Vertebral body compression, an abnormal vertebral cortex or erosion, calcification (in osteoblastic metastasis), and former instrumentation are indicative of a fracture. When possible, a standing X-ray can reveal alterations of vertebral alignment, kyphosis, retropulsion, and abnormality [46, 53]. CT can provide precise three-dimensional assessment of the bone elements, cortex, and vertebral body anatomy [52]. Osteolytic and/or sclerotic areas, free air in the vertebral body, and paravertebral masses can be also detected. CT is the examination of choice when MRI is contraindicated.

MRI is the imaging of choice to evaluate the extent of epidural extension. The image quality is superior to CT when evaluating soft tissue and the spinal cord. It also provides greater detail in the bone marrow. MRI reveals more detailed lesion delineation, allowing assessment of the degree of bone marrow involvement, spinal cord compression, and epidural and paraspinal extension, as well as determining the presence of other lesions and lesion vascularity [54]. T1 and T2 short-tau inversion recovery (STIR) sequence with fat suppression is specific for spine fractures, and T2 sequence are most useful for this purpose [55].

Certain signs are associated with common pathologies (Table 16.3), but none is specific for one type of VCF [54, 55]. Usually, a difference in signal intensity and morphology of the bone marrow and elements compared with the adjacent vertebra will reveal the VCF. The hematogenous spread of metastatic cells via Batson's venous plexus can distribute metastases throughout the spine [44, 56]. Thus, the finding of a VCF at the cervical spine at first presentation likely represents malignancy [40]. According to Tomoyuki Takigawa et al., certain MRI findings are associated with metastasis: posterior element involvement, pedicle involvement, and posterior wall diffuse protrusion were the findings with the highest sensitivity and specificity. If these three MRI features are detected together, there is 99.3% probability of malignancy [55]. Also, the existence of additional abnormal findings such as trabecular lesions, lytic osseous destruction, complete replacement/involvement of the vertebral body, compression of the entire vertebral body, diffuse posterior vertebral body convexity, end plate involvement, disc involvement, cortical destruction, rounded or diffuse alterations in bone marrow density, complete replacement of

Table 16.3 Radiographical signs for spine metastasis diagnosis

VCF type	Imaging method	Sign	Description
Malignant	X-ray	Owl sign	Destroyed pedicle due to lytic lesion
	CT		Lytic osseous destruction, particularly of the anterolateral and/or posterior vertebral body cortices, of cancellous bone or the pedicles
	MRI		Complete replacement normal bone marrow, pedicle/posterior elements/intervertebral disk involvement
	MRI/CT		Retropulsed fracture fragment, epidural mass
			Additional non-characteristic lesions, paraspinal mass larger than 5 mm, epidural mass, diffuse convexity of posterior vertebral border
	DWI-MRI		Enhancement heterogeneity (SIR>0.8)
Benign osteoporotic	CT	Intravertebral vacuum phenomenon, intravertebral air	Intravertebral vacuum cleft in osteoporotic fractures
		Band-like sign	Bone marrow edema
			Visualization of distinct fracture lines (as opposed to destruction, diffuse vertebral sclerosis, or an intravertebral vacuum cleft)
	MRI	Fluid-like sign	Presence of fluid signal adjacent vertebrae to the VCF level
	CE MRI	See-through sign	Osteoporotic
	MRI/CT		Coexistence of previously healed VCF
			Focal posterior vertebral border convexity
			Posterior/posterior-superior bone fragment of the vertebral body into the spinal canal

CT, computed tomography; MRI, magnetic resonance imaging; DW-MRI, diffusion-weighted MRI; SIR, spinal intensity ratio; CE MRI, contrast-enhanced MRI; VCF, vertebral compression fracture normal bone marrow, lesion with low density signal (hypointense) on T1 and STIR whereas high density signal (hyperintense) on T2 to normal bone marrow due to edema, paravertebral mass (attention in confusion with hematoma in benign VCF), epidural mass, and spinal cord band sign are highly associated with pathologic nature of the VCF [54].

In contrast, posterior focal vertebral body convexity, band-like edema area and "fluid sign" are associated with benign/osteoporotic fractures. Wang Mi Liu et al. proved that MRI imaging is an accurate, specific, and sensitive method in diagnosing pedicle involvement. The current technology with diffusion-weighted MRI and CT-PET scan for fracture differentiation has no clear use in excluding malignancy, which is the highest priority [52].

Furthermore, whole spine imaging is advised for detection of additional lesions. Due to the wide heterogeneity in image characteristics, if needed, biopsy confirmation of the underlying process is recommended [52]. This is particularly important if there is a solitary lesion for which the diagnosis is unclear. Though rare, a primary spinal column tumor such as chordoma or chondrosarcoma may present in this way. Because the treatment goals for tumors like this are different from that of metastatic lesions, it is critical to know what the diagnosis is before deciding upon any specific therapy, whether radiation, cement augmentation, or surgery. If in doubt, get the biopsy.

Assessment of Spine Stability in Cancer: SINS (Spinal Instability Neoplastic Score)

Concept of SINS

Determining whether a metastatic spinal lesion is unstable has historically been subjective and inexact. It often relied on clinical experience and surgical intuition [5, 57]. Given the need to quantify such instability and to have a standard nomenclature for identification and classification, the Spine Oncology Study Group (SOSG) introduced the Spinal Instability Neoplastic Score (SINS) [38]. Spinal instability in metastatic spine disease has different considerations than traumatic spinal injuries and as such requires a more specific classification. The SOSG defined spine metastatic instability as [38] *"loss of spinal integrity as a result of a neoplastic process that is associated with movement related pain, symptomatic or progressive deformity, and/or neural compromise under physiologic loads."*

SINS is also a communication tool among physicians to help diagnose and systematize clinical decision-making on referrals and management (Table 16.4) [38]. SINS represents a scoring algorithm based on clinical and imaging criteria. It organizes the evaluation process and represents specific spine-based criteria to aid in surgical decision-making. Each of the six criteria is

Table 16.4 The SINS algorithm

Elements of SINS		Score
A. Location		
Junctional (occiput-C2, C7–T2, T11–L1, L5–S1)		3
Mobile spine (C3–C6, L2–L4)		2
Semirigid (T3–T10)		1
Rigid (S2–S5)		0
B. Pain relief with recumbency and/or pain with movement/loading of the spine.		
Yes		3
No (occasional pain but not mechanical)		1
Pain-free lesion		0
C. Bone lesion		
Lytic		2
Mixed (lytic/blastic)		1
Blastic		0
D. Radiographic spinal alignment		
Subluxation/translation present		4
De novo deformity (kyphosis/scoliosis)		2
Normal alignment		0
E. Vertebral body collapse		
>50% collapse		3
<50% collapse		2
No collapse with 50% body involved		1
None of the above		0
F. Posterolateral involvement of the spinal elements (facet, pedicle, or CV joint fracture or replacement with tumor)		
Bilateral		3
Unilateral		1
None of the above		0
0–6: Stable	7–12: Potentially unstable	13–18: Unstable

independently assessed and scored to be summed to a total score out of 18; the higher the score, the more unstable the spine and the stronger is the indication for stabilization. Specifically, 0–6 indicates stability, 7–12 is an intermediate score, and a score higher than 13 indicates instability and the need for surgical consultation [38].

SINS in Clinical Practice

Since it was introduced, the utility of SINS as a decision-making tool has been investigated among various specialties (radiologist, radiation oncologists, spine surgeons) for initial assessment and surgical consultation [58–60]. Despite the limitations, SINS is an effective way of referring patients to surgery regardless of the evaluating physician (Table 16.5) [38, 61]. According to the scoring system, pathologic fractures generate the highest scores, based on pain, spinal alignment, and vertebral body collapse (Table 16.4) [38].

Several studies have separately tested the six criteria in order to spot any potential source of intra- or interobserver variability [62]. The quality of the bone lesion was the criterion with the widest variability in intraobserver characterization [58, 63, 64]. Experience of the assessor and medical specialty seem to play a major role in the accurate assessment. More importantly though, SINS was found to be suitable in detecting an unstable or potentially unstable spine since observers rated almost all unstable cases correctly which was the main initial objective of SINS [38]. Referrals among specialties were facilitated especially for the type of patient with a solitary metastasis where there is a need to decide on surgical consultation [59].

Table 16.5 SINS advantages and limitations

Advantages	Limitations
Clinical guide for predicting stability	Cases with multifocal involvement or noncontinuous lesions, primary spinal tumors, intradural or epidural tumors
Easy to use	Neurological and functional status of the patient is not scored
Comprehensive and focused (entire spine)	Normal findings are not defined, e.g., bone quality, vertebral alignment
Facilitates communication and referrals (surgeon, radiation, oncology)	Does not take into consideration the primary tumor, which implicates the prognosis
Guides treatment	Presence of former surgical procedure is not included (e.g., laminectomies, fusion)
–	C1 and C2 levels are not assessed comprehensively
–	Limited predictability: progression of the stability is not assessed

Versteeg et al. in an international study evaluated the effect of the introduction of SINS by calculating the mean and median score of patients with spine metastasis who were treated with radiotherapy or surgery. SINS resulted in a decrease of the mean score in both groups, with less patients meeting the surgical criteria and more patients being treated conservatively [65]. This reflected that only patients who will be benefited by surgical stabilization were candidates for surgery. Recent studies have questioned the role of SINS in predicting and assessing VCFs after SRS (Table 16.1) [27, 28, 33, 37]. Accordingly, Cunha et al. and Sahgal et al. supported that three of the SINS criteria, bone quality, vertebral alignment, and vertebral body compression, were predictive factors of post-SRS VCF [27, 28]. Huisman et al. showed that a higher SINS prior to SRS was indicative for VCF during postradiation period [66]. These findings confirm that SRS does not offer spine stability and supports that a higher pre-SRS SINS should alert the surgeons of impending instability or VCF; thus, patients may be benefited by a stabilizing surgery prior to SRS.

It is important to mention that SINS has limitations as presented on Table 16.5, which are a possible source of discord in management. The score assesses instability only and does not offer predictive treatment recommendation regarding survival or even complications. Cases of multifocal involvement, neurological and functional status, primary tumor histology, former surgical treatment, and the time interval for surgical intervention remain to be elucidated. It is a decision-making tool, one of many, to help the oncology provider assess and understand the nature of metastases affecting the spine.

Surgical Management of Common Pathologies

Surgeons should focus on the decision-making process, thoughtfully selecting patients that may benefit from surgery from spinal metastasis [67]. Each treatment is patient-specific, with a consideration of the criteria discussed above in addition to the patient's desires and expectations. It is essential to take into consideration that these patients are for the most part already at an end-stage of their disease and that their condition can significantly deteriorate as a result of surgery. The various classification systems such as the Tokuhashi and Tomita scores stratify patients based on the severity of their underlying medical condition [68].

The preoperative evaluation should include MRI, CT, spinal angiography, and possible embolization for hypervascular tumor such as renal cell carcinoma, hepatocellular carcinoma, and follicular thyroid carcinoma. Direct laryngoscopy for vocal cord (VC) and swallowing function assessment prior to an anterior cervical approach, recurrent (RLN) and superior laryngeal nerve (SLN) integrity, and brachial plexus functional evaluation can be very helpful though not always needed [2, 40, 47, 48, 57, 69, 70].

Each patient is unique and requires personalized treatment based on the level(s) of the lesion, the extent of involvement and the histology of the primary tumor [34, 40, 71, 72]. The decision of surgical approach (anterior, lateral, or posterior) depends not only on surgical experience but the patient's condition, anatomical characteristics, the anticipated morbidity and complications, and the feasibility of the intended approach [43, 72].

When the decision is made for surgery for a pathologic fracture, it needs to consider the needs for biomechanical reconstruction, stabilization, and neurologic decompression. Surgical stabilization needs to be rigid as the construct needs to be able to weather subsequent therapies like chemotherapy and radiation (Table 16.6).

Table 16.6 Indications and contraindications of spine surgery at the event of VCF

Indications	Contraindications
Mechanical stabilization – unstable fracture	Life expectancy less than 3–6 months
Neural tissue protection. Existence of a spinal cord or nerve compression (myelopathy, radiculopathy)	Patient not adequate for surgery – surgery contraindications
Palliative for pain	Uncomplicated spinal metastasis, stable spinal fracture, normal alignment
Stop further progression	Poor patient oncological status (extensive visceral metastatic disease)
Surgical excision with wide margins offers the only chance of cure	Multiple lesions, not enough healthy tissue to insert the screws
Radioresistant tumor	Lack of experience
Separation surgery	–
Biopsy, controversial radiographical image	–

The decision of technique and approach is determined by a number of factors such as the spine level(s) and the columns affected, the complexity of the reconstruction, and the technique with which the surgeon is best acquainted. Intraoperatively, somatosensory evoked potentials and motor evoked potential monitoring is advised but is not required [73, 74]. In cases where prolonged survival is expected, the safest approach with the most durable effect is considered more appropriate so that the patient may resume or start systemic therapies once recovered from surgery. Admittedly, the prognostication aspect of identifying which patients will survive long enough to benefit from surgery continues to be a major challenge.

Less invasive approaches as an alternate to surgery, such as vertebroplasty and kyphoplasty, are effective in carefully selected patients [75]. These techniques are discussed elsewhere in this textbook. Offering return to ambulation and pain alleviation, these techniques potentially reduce adverse outcomes associated with surgery [75].

Surgical Considerations: Cervical Spine and Cervicothoracic Junction

The neck has the unique role of holding the load of the head and hosting numerous vital structures while preserving flexibility and mobility [76]. Metastasis at the upper cervical spine is the rarest with a lower than 1% incidence, whereas metastasis in the sub-cervical spine is more common [77, 78]. Surgical stabilization is often chosen and well tolerated – anterior, posterior, or a combination of approaches are frequently used, depending on the elements involved and the number of vertebrae affected.

The CVJ allows for extension, flexion, lateral bending, and rotation of the head while protecting vital anatomical structures such as the spinal cord and the vertebral arteries [48]. The atlas and axis are mostly supported by the ligamentous structures and the neck muscles [78, 79]. The transverse ligament of C1 is clinically significant as it holds the dens and the lateral articular masses of C1 and C2. Biomechanically, forces are transmitted from the occipital condyles to the C1 and C2 lateral masses [80]. Metastases occur mainly at the anterior and anterolateral elements including the condyles and lateral masses of C1. Fractures or minimal subluxations that do not affect the alignment of the vertebra can be treated with radiotherapy only [48, 81]. A general rule is proposed that a subluxation greater than 5 mm or 3.5 mm of subluxation with an 11° angulation are indicative of instability [46, 48, 76, 78, 82]. Further indications for surgery are spinal cord compression, postradiation instability, or an inability to tolerate conservative treatment. Interestingly, SINS characterizes metastasis at CVJ with a maximum score, but C1 and C2 cannot be evaluated completely as the rest of the cervical vertebra as "vertebral body collapse" and "element involvement" may not adequately be assessed based on the CVJ biomechanics.

Vertebroplasty and Kyphoplasty

The current state of clinical practice does not support with evidence on the use of cement augmentation in this region. An open surgical approach is preferred in this region for mechanical instability. There are only case series and case reports published; patients with limited life expectancy where an open surgical intervention is contraindicated can potentially benefit from cement augmentation [49, 84, 85]. Carza Ramos et al. in his systematic review and meta-analysis reported 6 studies of level IV evidence where vertebroplasty or kyphoplasty were used in cervical spine (mainly C2) metastasis with satisfactory results [84, 86, 87]. However, its use in pathologic fractures in this region is limited.

Surgical Stabilization Techniques

Surgical CVJ stabilization is typically performed through a posterior midline approach. Open anterior and anterolateral (lateral extrapharyngeal with/without mandibular osteotomy) approaches through parapharyngeal, retropharyngeal, and prevertebral anatomical spaces, where vital vessels (internal jugular vein, VA, and common carotid arteries), nerves (lingual, marginal mandibular, vagal, RLN and SLN, hypoglossal, spinal accessory), and the submandibular gland exist, are associated with high complication rates [48, 78, 80]. As such, in the metastatic patient, anterior approaches to this region are hard to justify given the approach-related morbidity and the limited reconstruction and stabilization options from an anterior approach. Thus, limited exposure and increased morbidity made open anterior approaches less applicable and not as widely used. Transoral and transpalatopharyngeal approaches are associated with certain postoperative complications such as dysphagia and infection.

The approach through a posterior midline incision is usually sufficient to meet the goals of decompression and stabilization [76, 78, 88]. Spinal cord decompression is easily achieved through laminectomy [5, 48, 78]. Anterior stabilization techniques with odontoid screws do not provide stable constructs in the context of metastatic spinal disease due to altered anatomy and inferior bone quality [46, 83, 89].

Due to structural superiority, conventional rod-screw systems allow for rigid fixation at occiput and the posterior cervical spine. Typically, constructs may entail fixation with an occipital plate with extension to the subaxial cervical spine. Likewise, fixation may be at C1–2 or any other combination of levels for instability in this region [5, 48, 76, 78, 90]. CVJ fixation using an occipital plate and pedicle screws with rods offer the most durable and reliable outcome, with limited complications [88, 91]. Occipital plates with combination of screws at the midline keel of the suboccipital bone and lateral screws 10–18 mm diameter offer the greatest strength and the least injury risk of transverse sinus and torcula [78, 90]. Careful pedicle screw insertion at cervical vertebrae can be performed under navigation to decrease iatrogenic damage of the neural structures and the VA, especially at the C2 isthmus [9, 88]. The lateral masses of the cervical vertebrae are typically used for fixation, but in cases where the lateral masses have been destroyed, the cervical pedicles are an effective backup fixation strategy.

The lateral masses of C1 and the pars/pedicle of C2 are excellent points of fixation if not involved by tumor [92]. Special attention is required to position the rods in a way that maximizes cervical lordosis and does not create an iatrogenic deformity. Case 1 is a representative case of a C2 metastasis (Figs. 16.1 and 16.2).

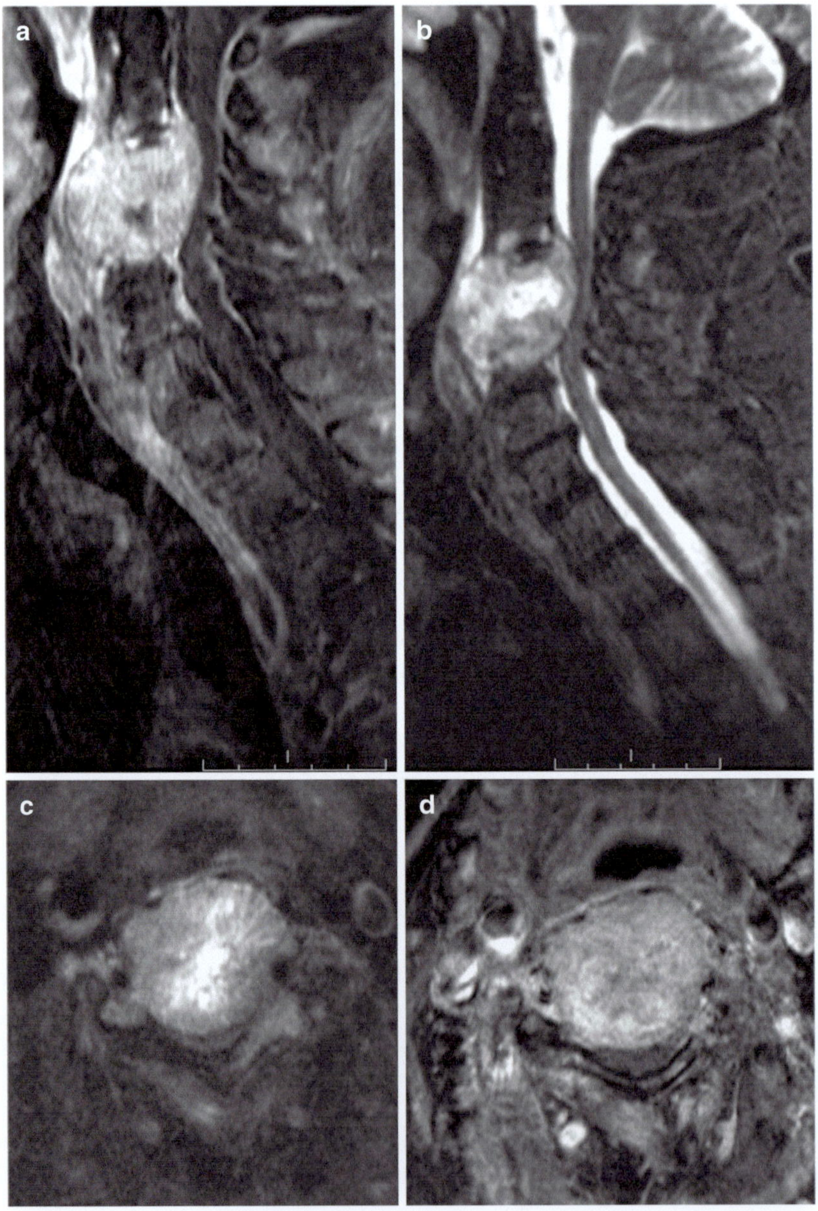

Fig. 16.1 Case 1: patient with lung Ca presents with neck pain quadriparesis. Cervical MRI reveals compression and fracture at C3,4,5. T1 and T2 sequences (**a**, **b**) sagittal images show the lytic lesion destroying the vertebral body of C3 to C5 vertebrae. Axial images (**c**) and (**d**) show severe spinal cord compression

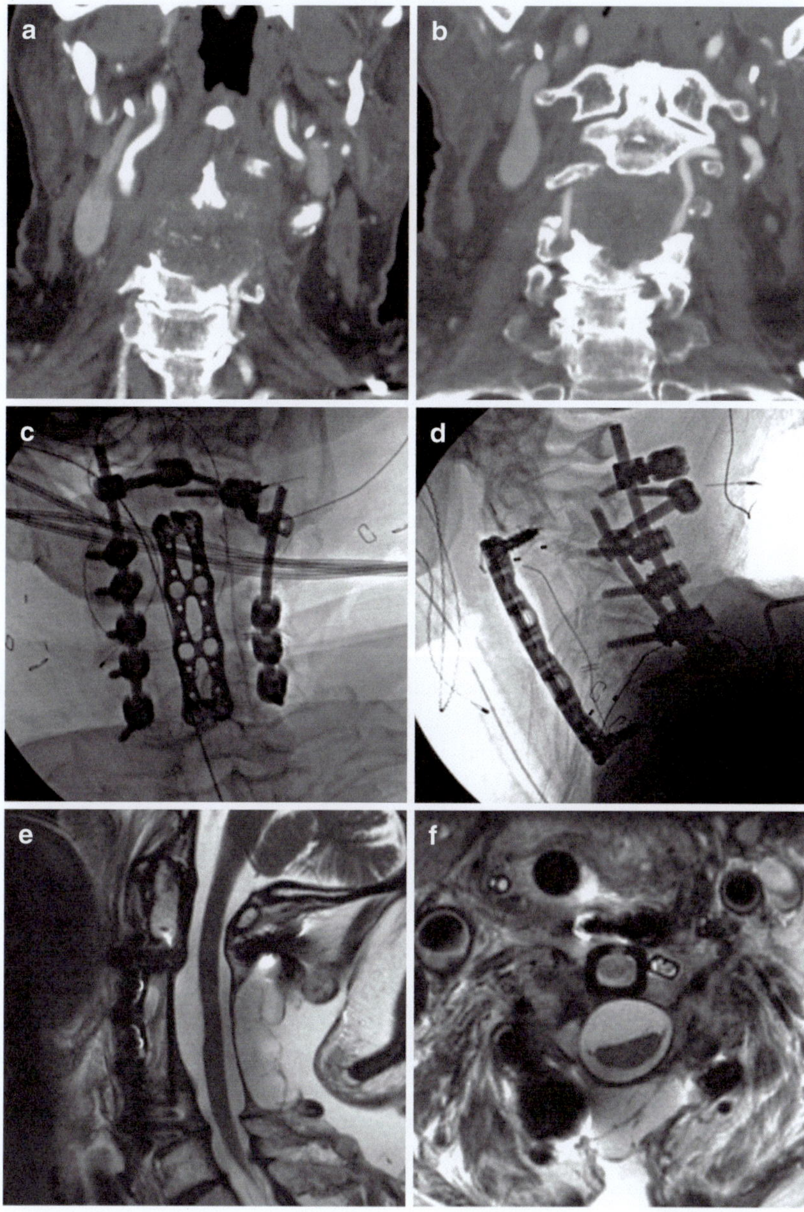

Fig. 16.2 Case 1 (continued): combined anterior-posterior approach. (**a**, **b**) *Preop coronal CT images show the extensive bone destruction. Anterior column was stabilized with C3 to C7 screw-plate system along with posterior fusion* (**c** and **d**). *Successful spinal alignment with spinal cord decompression* (**e** and **f**)

In the subaxial spine, anterior approaches allow for direct access from C3 to T1. Much of this depends on the patient's anatomy. The benefit of an anterior approach is the ability to resect the affected vertebral body(s), decompress the spinal cord and nerves, and reconstruct and stabilize the spine [5, 9, 76]. The anterior approach is familiar to most surgeons and is a facile technique with direct access to the vertebral body(s).

For single-level lesions, a corpectomy can be performed and reconstructed with a wide variety of implants and devices [2, 5, 40, 43, 93–96]. Stand-alone implants (polyetheretherketone cages, titanium cages, carbon fiber cages, expandable cages, bone grafts) without additional mechanical support tend to dislocate, so anterior screws and plates are used to supplement the anterior column reconstruction [2, 9, 40, 43, 96]. Due to poor bone quality and the possibility of hardware loosening and pullout, a consideration for supplemental fixation or an additional posterior approach should be considered [2, 43].

Posterior approaches are preferred in cases of multiple-level disease, posterior element involvement (lamina(e) and/or facet joints), high-grade epidural compression, and where extensive instrumentation is needed; see *Case 1* below [2, 5, 76, 95]. A combination of approaches is considered in multiple-level cases where a single approach cannot provide sufficient three-column reconstruction [2, 43, 76]. Posterior instrumentation can be performed at a second stage [97].

Metastasis at the cervicothoracic junction represents about 10% of spinal metastases; see *Case 2* [57, 72, 98–100]. Here, the cervical lordosis transitions to thoracic kyphosis. Anterior and transthoracic approaches include the supraclavicular approach (with/without median sternotomy), the left anterolateral cervical exposure, the transmanubrium osteotomy, a transsternal approach, the transmanubrial–transclavicular approach, the trap-door approach, and an anterolateral thoracotomy; these are usually performed in cases of primary tumors of the posterior mediastinum, anterior element disease with/without spinal cord compression, or where en block excisions should be performed [57, 101, 102]. T1 and T2 are located at the posterior part of superior mediastinum, so these approaches are performed with the aid of the thoracic surgeon [98]. For metastatic lesions, a corpectomy is performed with additional reconstruction using cement and Steinmann pins, plates with mesh, cage, autologous iliac crest grafts, and rib or fibula allografts [57, 101, 102].

Posterior approaches are associated with less morbidity and the ability to perform multilevel decompression and stabilization effectively [57, 72]. The open posterior approach is the workhorse for the spine surgeon [57, 76]. The posterior approach may include laminectomy, facetectomy, pedicle drilling, and costotransversectomy. Through a single posterior approach, stabilization and decompression can be performed. In the upper thoracic spine, anterior vertebral body intralesional resection along with anterior column reconstruction with cages, bone grafts, and cement with Steinmann pins can be performed without performing a thoracotomy [57, 98, 100–105] (Fig. 16.3).

Thoracic and Lumbar Spine: T3–L5

Thoracic and lumbar spine metastases are more common than cervical and CTJ. Approximately 60% and 20% occur at the thoracic and lumbar spine, respectively; their larger magnitude is accused for this high rate. Constant progress is achieved in surgical techniques, as cancer patients cannot undertake complex surgical approaches.

Cement augmentation is used in the thoracic and lumbar spines. Due to its limitations described in Table 16.7, it is indicated in specific cases. The procedure includes image-guided, unilateral or bilateral, percutaneous, transpedicular, or parapedicular approach, or when done intraoperatively, under direct visualization during open surgery [106]. Depending on the vertebral integrity (end plates, vertebral discs, and posterior wall), vertebral augmentation can successfully provide stability with minimal and subclinical cement extravasation into the paravertebral soft tissue or the spinal canal [107, 108].

Anterior approaches can be effective in treating thoracic and lumbar pathologic fractures (Case 3, Figs. 16.4 and 16.5). A combination of anterior with posterior or lateral approaches can also be used. A variety of implants for vertebral body reconstruction can be used such as static or expandable cages (see Case 4 at Figs. 16.6 and 16.7) or PMMA [74, 110–113]. Cages have been reported to be successfully applied to one-, two-, or three-level thoracolumbar tumors after corpectomy [112, 114].

A limitation of cages is that the superior and inferior end plates need to be intact to be able to mechanically support the cage in the intended orientation. Cage subsidence is an issue [113]. There is no clear superiority of any type of cage reconstruction strategy versus cement [115]. Various bone grafts (iliac crest, rib, fibula, femoral shaft, vascularized fibular bone graft) can also be used [116]. Spinal fusion with two levels above and

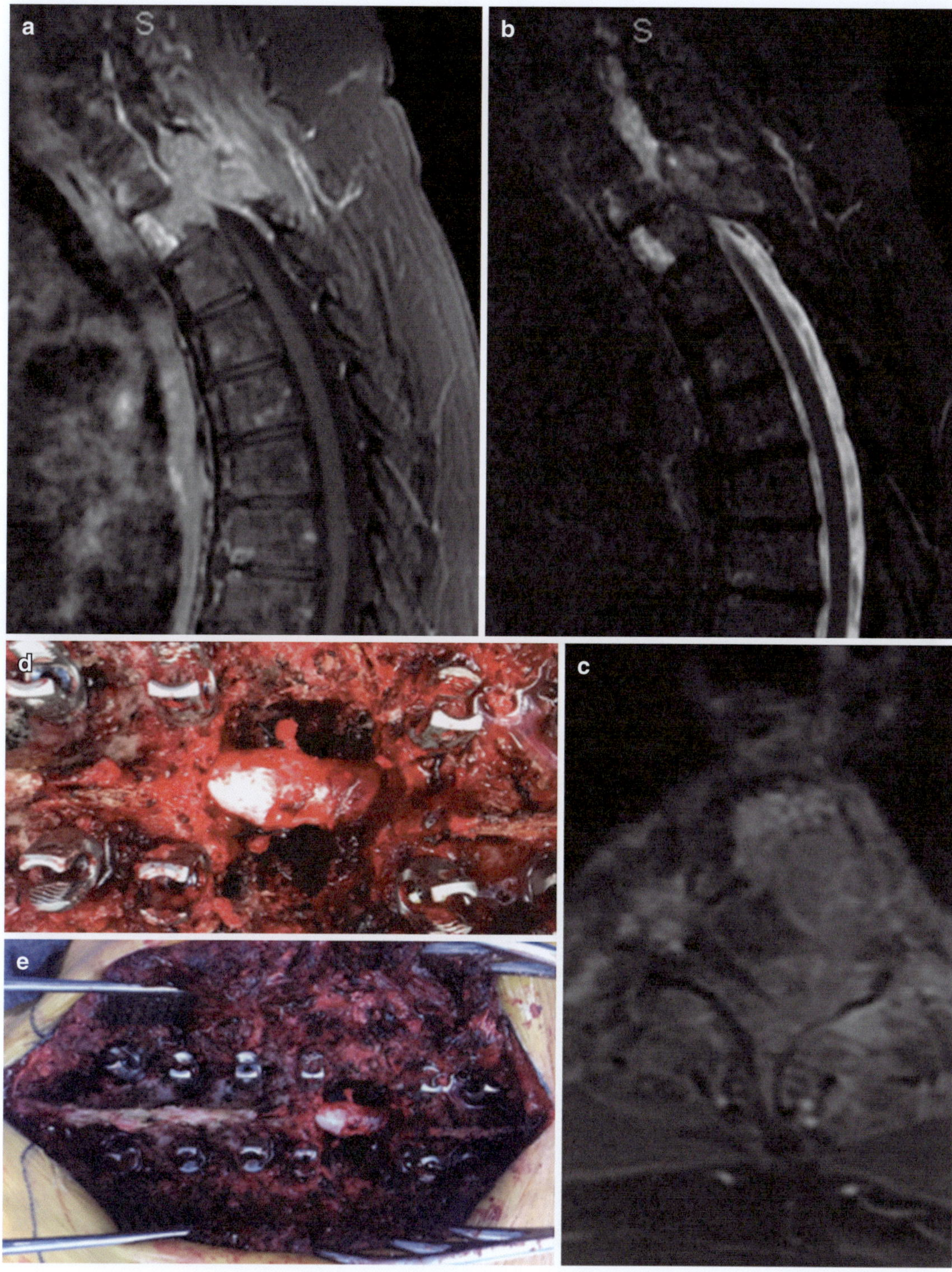

Fig. 16.3 Case 2: 64-year-old female patient with non-small cell lung cancer (EGFR+), who had undergone prior conventional radiotherapy to a lung lesion and 30Gy to spine for a T2 metastasis. (**a–c**) *Show* MRI *images of a mixed lesion involving the posterior elements and surrounding soft tissue, causing vertebral body subluxation as well as spinal cord compression. Posterior approach t*hrough a midline posterior incision *was performed. Spinal cord decompression was performed* (**d**) *C7-T6 stabilization*

Table 16.7 Indications and contraindications of vertebroplasty and kyphoplasty

Indications	Contraindications	Complications
Ideal for thoracic single-level lesions where only anterior elements are affected and the posterior or lateral elements are not affected	Multiple lesions	Pain or hematoma at needle-entry site
Ideal for compression pathological fractures with less than 1/3 compression	Not available in all levels of spine (lumbar, cervical)	Pedicle fracture
Less than 50% spinal canal compromise	Metastases with close proximity to important neurovascular structures	Infection
Combined with radiosurgery as primary treatment for metastatic vertebra collapse	Ineffective in cases with insufficient vertebral cortex or severely comminuted vertebral bodies	Spinal nerve or spinal cord injury
Treatment of choice in cases of multiple myeloma patients where the bone quality is not good enough to hold an instrumentation or vertebra hemangiomas	More complex patterns with instability and deformity, such as vertebral fractures with posterior elements involvement (higher risk of cement extravasation)	Cement leakage and migration (into the spinal canal, venous system – pulmonary, cardiac embolism)
Cases where open surgery is not indicated: less operation time than open surgery	Extended spinal cord compression (>50%)	Kyphoplasty needs general anesthesia
Vertebroplasty can be performed under sedation or local anesthesia for patients who cannot undertake general anesthesia	Complete or greater than 70% vertebral collapse (difficult for vertebral access)	–
Axial spine pain	Sclerotic lesions/solid tumors	–
–	Failure of former therapies	–
–	Lack of orthopedic and neurosurgical support	–

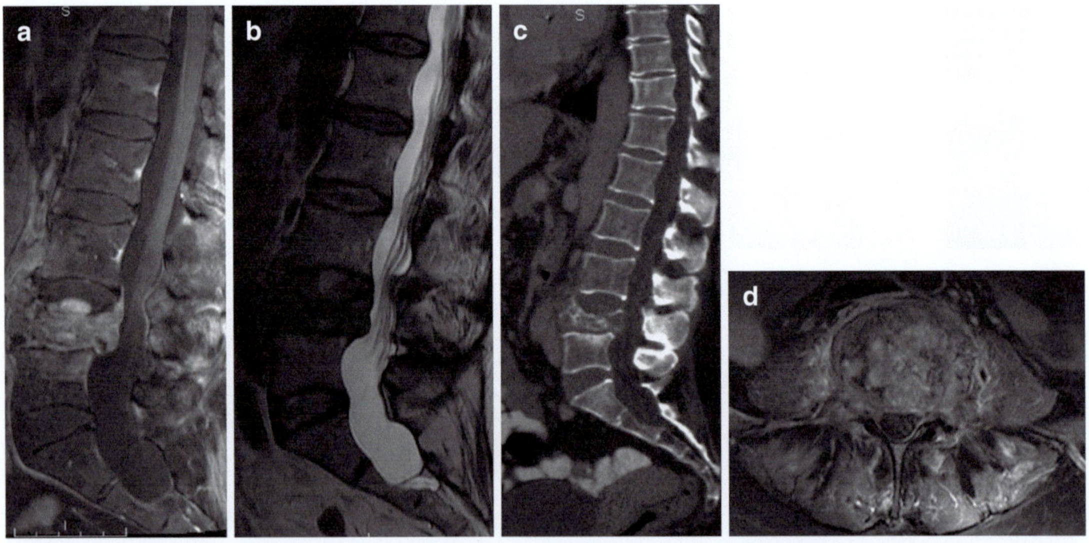

Fig. 16.4 Case 3: female 47-year-old patient with breast Ca presents with severe back and left leg pain worse with standing. She is unable to ambulate. MRI and CT reveal a L4 pathologic VCF with spinal canal compromise and both L4 nerve root compression (**a**–**d**). SINS: 13

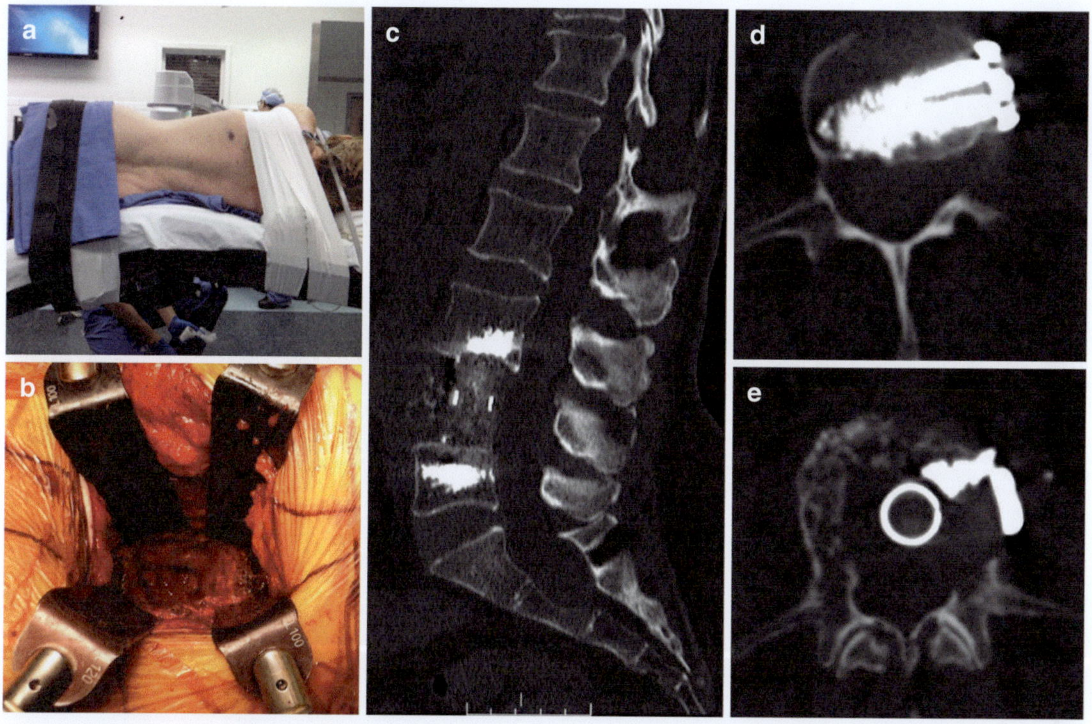

Fig. 16.5 Case 3 (continued): Minimally invasive anterolateral, retroperitoneal approach. Lateral position (**a**, **b**). Lateral vertebral body plate-screw system extending from L3 to L5 along with cage stabilization as presented at **c**–**e**

below the first and the last vertebra involved is a safe and common practice [113].

Posterior instrumentation provides rigid support and allows for correction of any kyphosis or deformity [5]. Various rod systems can be used to increase the rigidity of the construct (see Case 4, Figs. 16.6 and 16.7) [57]. The correct location of pedicle screws can be effectively assessed by X-ray or CT. Laboratory, cadaveric, and clinical studies have enlightened the correct technique and appropriate instrument selection at each case, although, detailed interpretation is beyond the objective of this chapter [117].

Depending on the spinal level and the local anatomy, devastating complications can occur, as presented in Table 16.8. Open surgeries are associated with complications related to patient comorbidities and surgery itself. In general, posterior approaches in the thoracic and lumbar spines are associated with less complications than anterior approaches as they do not include manipulation of intrathoracic or intraabdominal organs. Patients are living longer with a greater burden of systemic disease, so the morbidity of operative intervention should be taken into consideration so that the most durable reconstruction is performed [98].

New Techniques for Stabilization: Fenestrated Pedicle Screws

The inferior bone quality along with the need for more solid instrumentation led to the introduction of fenestrated pedicle screws (FPSs) [118]. Initially, FPSs were used for osteoporotic bone [118–120]. The design of these new screws allows for insertion of bone cement deep into the vertebral body through the cannulated core of the screws [118, 121, 122]. FPSs have holes along the shaft of the screw allowing cement injection into the vertebra to prevent loosening at the screw-bone interface. Cement-augmented FPSs have greater pullout strength than other

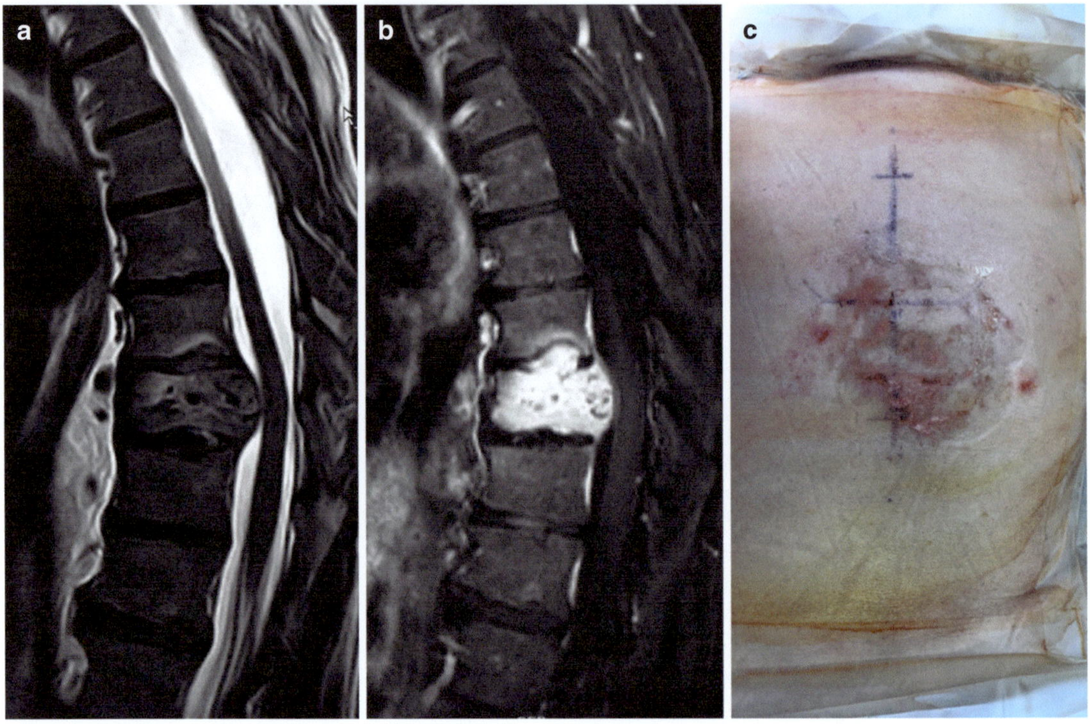

Fig. 16.6 Case 4: 49-year-old patient with a PMH of nephrectomy due to RCC presents with 3-month history of severe back pain and is unable to stand or ambulate. Muscle strength at both legs 5/5. MRI reveals a T10 VCF with cord compression (**a**, **b**). External 30Gy conventional radiotherapy was given with no pain relief and severe skin irritation (**c**), SINS: 12

screws (50–250% in osteoporotic bone) and provide more structural stability in patients with inferior bone quality, such as patients with cancer, osteopenia, revision cases, or VCFs where anatomic integrity of the spine, vertebral body, or pedicle may be suboptimal [125]. Using this technology, shorter constructs may be performed, and fusion levels may be reduced; furthermore, there is a lower degree of instrumentation failure following cement augmentation [109, 120, 123]. In cases of multilevel instrumentation, it is advisable to use cement-secured screws at both the cranial and caudal ends of the construct, intentionally skipping the intermediate levels to reduce cement toxicity [109, 120]. Although the volume of cement injected into the vertebral body is more targeted than during cement augmentation, cement extravasation is also present during this type of instrumentation in up to 39% [109]. Additionally, the indications for when to use cement-augmented screws are unclear; their use depends on the surgeon's preference and judgment since the long-term efficacy of this application has yet to be clarified.

Minimally Invasive Surgery Approaches

For cancer patients, minimally invasive surgery (MIS) may be an option (Case 5, Figs. 16.8 and 16.9) [124–138]. Although high-level evidence comparing MIS to conventional open surgery does not exist, MIS may have certain advantages such as reduced operative times, less intraoperative blood loss, less postoperative complications, and a quicker time to postoperative radiation [131, 139–148].

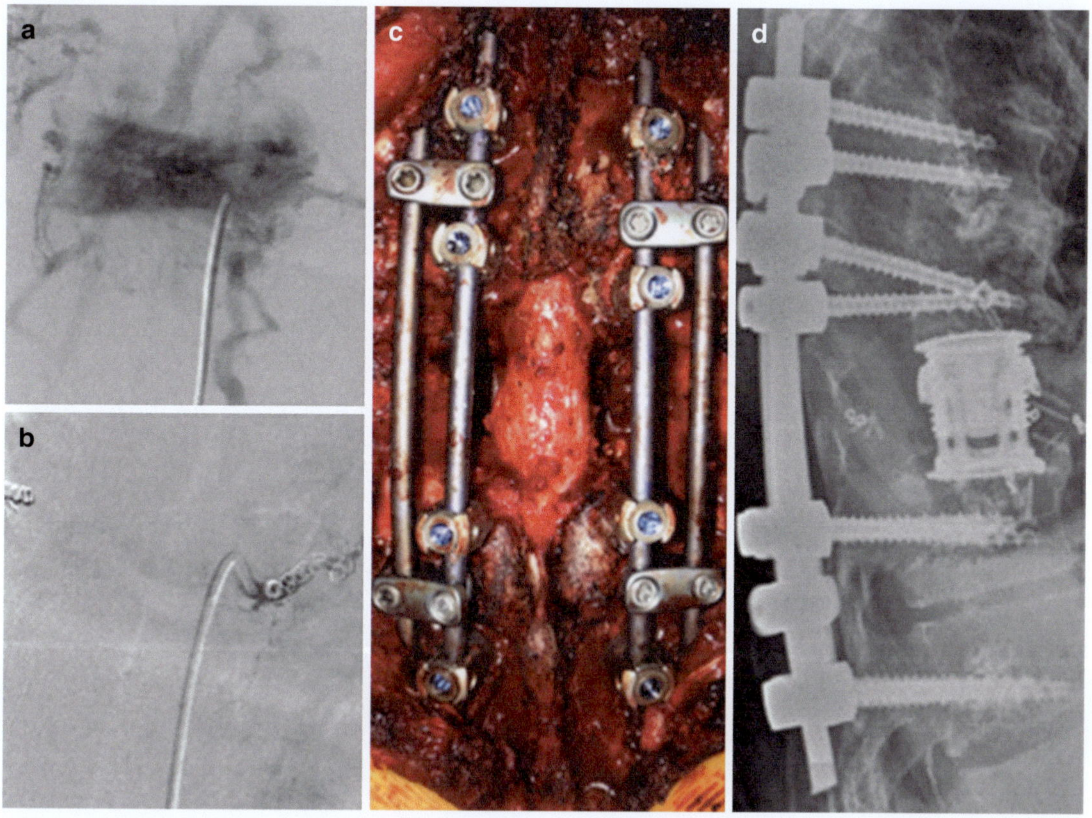

Fig. 16.7 Case 4 (continued): preoperative tumor arterial embolization was performed to reduce intraoperative bleeding (**a**, **b**). Posterior approach through midline incision. T10 vertebrectomy was performed with anterior column reconstruction using expandable cage and posterior column support with a T8-T12 double-rod construct (**c**, **d**)

Table 16.8 Reported surgical complications at pathological VCFs' surgery

Spine level	Approach	Complications (at specific levels)
C0-C2	Anterior [standard anterior, anterolateral (lateral extrapharyngeal with/without mandibular osteotomy), transoral, extrapharyngeal]	Dysphagia, esophageal injury Palatal dysfunction Retropharyngeal hematoma Increased risk of postoperative infections Pharyngeal wound failure/break Lower cranial neuropathies
	Posterior or Posterolateral	Atlantoaxial screw dislocation, rod break, implant failure, pseudarthrosis Pedicle fracture Adjacent segment degeneration VA injury from muscle dissection or screw placement Subdural hematoma from screws placed in the occipital bone Dizziness, chronic headache Increased tone of paraspinal and neck muscles
C3-C6	Anterior (transverse cervical incision)	RLN and SLN palsy Internal sensory branch of SLN injury: cough reflex impairment, swallowing problems, vocal cord paralysis Hypoglossal nerve injury
	Posterior, posterolateral	Analyzed below at general complications
	Combined (anterior/posterior)	Combination of anterior posterior

(continued)

Table 16.8 (continued)

Spine level	Approach	Complications (at specific levels)
C7-T2	Anterior [transthoracic (trap-door, manubrial osteotomy, trans-upper-sternal, sternotomy), low cervical, standard anterolateral cervical (with/without extension), Smith-Robinson approach with/without manubriotomy	Unilateral RLN injury (mild dysphagia and dysphonia with vocal cord palsy), bilateral RLN injury (bilateral vocal cord paralysis) Dysphagia Dysphonia Horner syndrome Respiratory muscles function impairment Myoskeletal stability impairment, weakness, deformity Mediastinitis Large vessel injury
	Posterior/posterolateral (Costotransversectomy, lateral thoracotomy, posterolateral thoracotomy lateral extracavitary)	(Analyzed below at general complications)
T3-L5	Anterior/anterolateral [standard open or mini-open anterior approach, thoracic endoscopy, transpleural approach combined with a diaphragmatic split (at or proximal to L1), mini-open extraperitoneal approach (lesions of L2 or below)]	Aorta rupture – Hemothorax Retroperitoneal hematoma Progressive kyphosis Transient intercostal neuralgia Postoperative atelectasis, pneumothorax, and pleural effusion Pleural exudate
	Posterior [transcavitary, transpedicular, or a lateral extracavitary, retroperitoneal, MIS percutaneous SRSI with VAT, percutaneous transpedicular coblation corpectomy with closed fracture reduction or cavity-coblation combined with VAT	(Analyzed below at general complications)
General complications	Hardware dislocation, misplaced screw/hook Fever, bacteremia, meningitis, pneumonia, urinary tract infection Deep vein thrombosis, pulmonary embolism, fat embolisms, hypoxia Myocardial infraction, stroke Wound dehiscence, deep or superficial infection, wound seroma Retroperitoneal hemorrhage Acute epidural hematoma, bleeding ulcer Cement emboli Dural tear, SCF leakage Pseudomeningocele Adjacent vertebral bodies subluxations Tumor recurrence Death	

Data on the table refer to the reported techniques used for VCF cases only. RLN and SLN: recurrent laryngeal nerve and superior laryngeal nerve

Conclusion and Expert Opinion

The operative management of pathologic fractures requires careful planning and consideration of the oncologic as well as spine-specific treatment goals. Scoring systems such as SINS and NOMS are helpful decision-making tools when caring for these challenging patients. Advances in oncology improve our ability to treat these patients, help prolong life expectancy, and improve patients' quality of life [104, 105, 136, 149, 150].

Patients with metastatic spinal disease and VCF are high-risk patients. They have limited recovery potential and have many comorbidities; they are frequently malnourished and deconditioned. Treatment outcome is largely determined

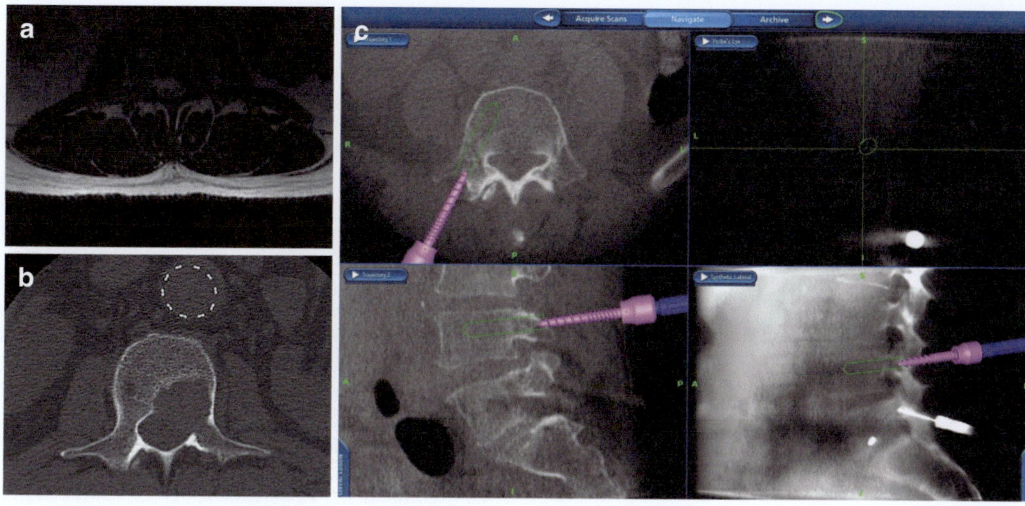

Fig. 16.8 Case 5: patient with PMH of RCC presents with L2 VCF (**a**). Patient complained about mechanical pain mainly at standing position. (**b**). Axial pre-operative CT demonstrates a lytic lesion within the left posterior vertebral body wall extending into the left pedicle. A posterior approach with MIS technique was performed, with computer-assisted navigation (**c**)

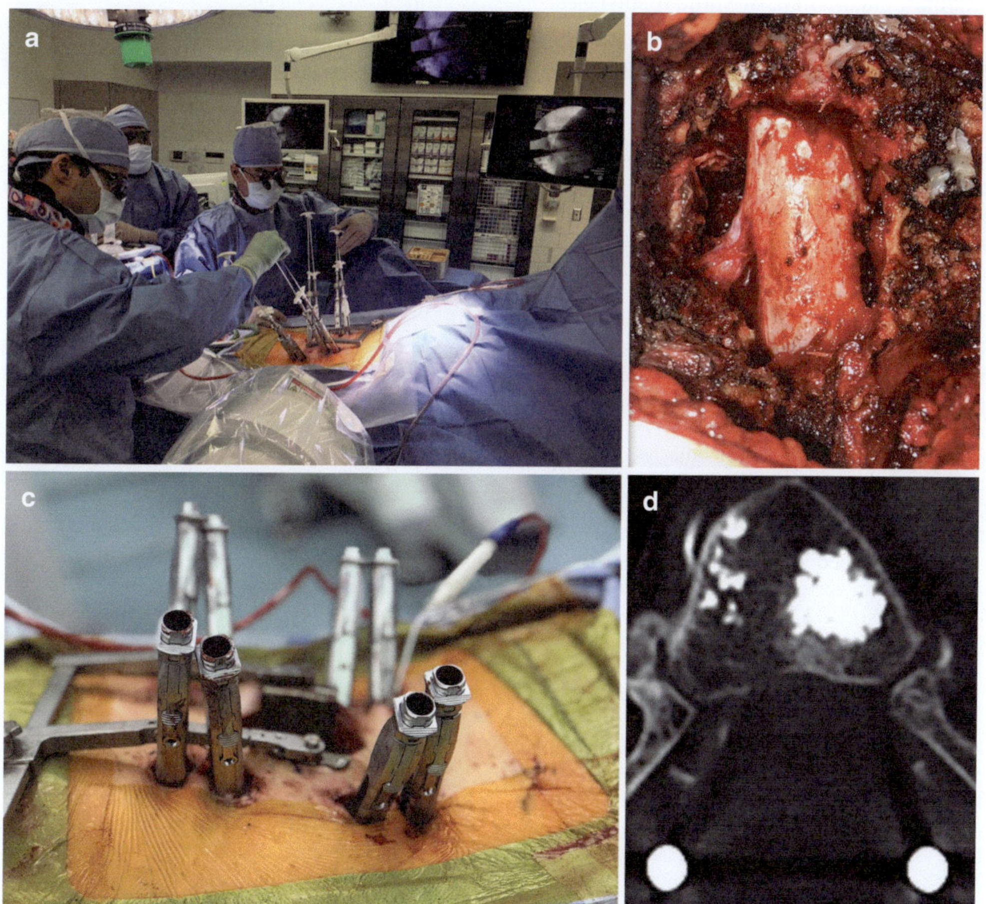

Fig. 16.9 Case 5 (continued): T12-L4 fusion (**a** and 16.9**c**). Tumor resection and neural decompression were performed (**b**). For maximum screw strength, percutaneous cement-augmented fenestrated pedicle screws were used (**d**)

by their disease status, and the spine surgeon's role in their overall care is quite small. However, the morbidity of surgical intervention may affect patient survival in a negative way if complications are not well tolerated and may lead to a decline in function.

Ultimately, spine surgery should be tailored to the individual; there are multiple options for decompression and stabilization. Oftentimes, the best option is to perform the surgery that the surgeon is most comfortable with, taking into consideration the regional anatomical nuances and the patient's expectations for recovery. As interventions become less invasive, the timing and threshold for intervention may also change [151, 152].

In conclusion, surgical decision-making should be done carefully, as the surgical treatment of pathological compression fractures is only one component of the multidisciplinary and multimodal management of spine metastases.

References

1. Siegel RL, Miller KD, Jemal A. Cancer statistics, 2018. CA Cancer J Clin. 2018;68(1):7–30.
2. Bilsky MH, Boakye M, Collignon F, Kraus D, Boland P. Operative management of metastatic and malignant primary subaxial cervical tumors. J Neurosurg Spine. 2005;2(3):256–64.
3. Weber MH, Burch S, Buckley J, Schmidt MH, Fehlings MG, Vrionis FD, et al. Instability and impending instability of the thoracolumbar spine in patients with spinal metastases: a systematic review. Int J Oncol. 2011;38(1):5–12.
4. Du Bois M, Donceel P. Outcome and cost of spinal fractures and spinal tumors. Eur Spine J. 2010;19(Suppl 1):S74–8.
5. Oda I, Abumi K, Ito M, Kotani Y, et al. Palliative spinal reconstruction using cervical pedicle screws for metastatic lesions of the spine: a retrospective analysis of 32 cases. Spine (Phila Pa 1976). 2006;31(13):1439–44.
6. Yao A, Sarkiss CA, Ladner TR, 3rd Jenkins AL. Contemporary spinal oncology treatment paradigms and outcomes for metastatic tumors to the spine: a systematic review of breast, prostate, renal, and lung metastases. J Clin Neurosci. 2017;41:11–23. Available from: http://dx.doi.org/10.1016/j.jocn.2017.04.004.
7. Rose PS, Laufer I, Boland PJ, Hanover A, Bilsky MH, Yamada J, et al. Risk of fracture after single fraction image-guided intensity-modulated radiation therapy to spinal metastases. J Clin Oncol. 2009;27(30):5075–9.
8. Saad F, Lipton A, Cook R, Chen Y, Smith M, Coleman R. Pathologic fractures correlate with reduced survival in patients with malignant bone disease. Cancer. 2007;110(8):1860–7.
9. Vazifehdan F, Karantzoulis VG, Igoumenou VG. Surgical treatment for metastases of the cervical spine. Eur J Orthop Surg Traumatol. 2017;27(6):763–75.
10. Huo M, Sahgal A, Pryor D, Redmond K, Lo S, Foote M. Stereotactic spine radiosurgery: review of safety and efficacy with respect to dose and fractionation. Surg Neurol Int. 2017;8:30.
11. Myrehaug S, Sahgal A, Hayashi M, Levivier M, Ma L, Martinez R, et al. Reirradiation spine stereotactic body radiation therapy for spinal metastases: systematic review. J Neurosurg Spine. 2017;27(4):428–35.
12. Redmond KJ, Robertson S, Lo SS, Soltys SG, Ryu S, McNutt T, et al. Consensus contouring guidelines for postoperative stereotactic body radiation therapy for metastatic solid tumor malignancies to the spine. Int J Radiat Oncol Biol Phys. 2017;97(1):64–74. Available from: http://dx.doi.org/10.1016/j.ijrobp.2016.09.014.
13. Sahgal A, Whyne CM, Ma L, Larson DA, Fehlings MG. Vertebral compression fracture after stereotactic body radiotherapy for spinal metastases. Lancet Oncol. 2013;14(8):e310–20. https://doi.org/10.1016/S1470-2045(13)70101-3.
14. Reynders K, Illidge T, Siva S, Chang JY, De Ruysscher D. The abscopal effect of local radiotherapy: using immunotherapy to make a rare event clinically relevant. Cancer Treat Rev. 2015;41(6):503–10. Available from: http://linkinghub.elsevier.com/retrieve/pii/S0305737215000560.
15. Puvanesarajah V, Lo SL, Aygun N, Liauw JA, Jusué-torres I, Lina IA, et al. Prognostic factors associated with pain palliation after spine stereotactic body radiation therapy. J Neurosurg Spine. 2015;23(5):620–9.
16. Smith VA, Lentsch EJ. Life-threatening cervical spine collapse as a result of postradiation osteonecrosis-case report and review of the literature. Head Neck. 2013;35(5):E142–6.
17. Whyne CM. Biomechanics of metastatic disease in the vertebral column. Neurol Res. 2014;36:493–501.
18. Al-Omair A, Smith R, Kiehl T-R, Lao L, Yu E, Massicotte EM, et al. Radiation-induced vertebral compression fracture following spine stereotactic radiosurgery: clinicopathological correlation. J Neurosurg Spine. 2013;18:430–5.
19. Chow E, Harris K, Fan G, Tsao M, Sze WM. Palliative radiotherapy trials for bone metastases: a systematic review. J Clin Oncol. 2007;25(11):1423–36. Available from: http://www.ncbi.nlm.nih.gov/pubmed/17416863.
20. Cox BW, Spratt DE, Lovelock M, Bilsky MH, Lis E, Ryu S, et al. International Spine Radiosurgery Consortium consensus guidelines for target volume

definition in spinal stereotactic radiosurgery. Int J Radiat Oncol Biol Phys. 2012;83(5):e597–605. https://doi.org/10.1016/j.ijrobp.2012.03.009.
21. Jawad MS, Fahim DK, Gerszten PC, Flickinger JC, Sahgal A, Grills IS, et al. Vertebral compression fractures after stereotactic body radiation therapy: a large, multi-institutional, multinational evaluation. J Neurosurg Spine. 2016;24:928–36.
22. Thibault I, Al-Omair A, Masucci GL, Masson-Côté L, Lochray F, Korol R, et al. Spine stereotactic body radiotherapy for renal cell cancer spinal metastases: analysis of outcomes and risk of vertebral compression fracture. J Neurosurg Spine. 2014;21:711–8.
23. Barzilai O, DiStefano N, Lis E, Yamada Y, Lovelock DM, Fontanella AN, et al. Safety and utility of kyphoplasty prior to spine stereotactic radiosurgery for metastatic tumors: a clinical and dosimetric analysis. J Neurosurg Spine. 2018;28(1):72–8. Available from: http://thejns.org/doi/10.3171/2017.5.SPINE1746.
24. Sung S-H, Chang U-K. Evaluation of Risk Factors for Vertebral Compression Fracture after Stereotactic Radiosurgery in Spinal Tumor Patients. Korean J Spine. 2014;11(3):103. Available from: http://www.ncbi.nlm.nih.gov/pubmed/25346753.
25. Guckenberger M, Mantel F, Gerszten PC, Flickinger JC, Sahgal A, Létourneau D, et al. Safety and efficacy of stereotactic body radiotherapy as primary treatment for vertebral metastases: a multi-institutional analysis. Radiat Oncol. 2014;9(1):226. Available from: http://ro-journal.biomedcentral.com/articles/10.1186/s13014-014-0226-2.
26. Boehling NS, Grosshans DR, Allen PK, McAleer MF, Burton AW, Azeem S, et al. Vertebral compression fracture risk after stereotactic body radiotherapy for spinal metastases. J Neurosurg Spine. 2013;31(27):5–8.
27. Sahgal A, Atenafu EG, Chao S, Al-Omair A, Boehling N, Balagamwala EH, et al. Vertebral compression fracture after spine stereotactic body radiotherapy: a multi-institutional analysis with a focus on radiation dose and the spinal instability neoplastic score. J Clin Oncol. 2013;31:3426.
28. Cunha MVR, Al-Omair A, Atenafu EG, Masucci GL, Letourneau D, Korol R, et al. Vertebral compression fracture (VCF) after spine stereotactic body radiation therapy (SBRT): analysis of predictive factors. Radiat Oncol Biol. 2012;84(3):e343–9. Available from: http://dx.doi.org/10.1016/j.ijrobp.2012.04.034.
29. Germano IM, Carai A, Pawha P, Blacksburg S, Lo YC, Green S. Clinical outcome of vertebral compression fracture after single fraction spine radiosurgery for spinal metastases. Clin Exp Metastasis. 2016;33(2):143–9.
30. Roesch J, Cho JBC, Fahim DK, Gerszten PC, Flickinger JC, Grills IS, et al. Risk for surgical complications after previous stereotactic body radiotherapy of the spine. Radiat Oncol. 2017;12(1):153.
31. Virk MS, Han JE, Reiner AS, Mclaughlin LA, Sciubba DM, Lis E, et al. Frequency of symptomatic vertebral body compression fractures requiring intervention following single-fraction stereotactic radiosurgery for spinal metastases. Neurosurg Focus. 2017;42:1–8.
32. Boyce-Fappiano D, Elibe E, Schultz L, Ryu S, Siddiqui MS, Chetty I, et al. Analysis of the factors contributing to vertebral compression fractures after spine stereotactic radiosurgery. Int J Radiat Oncol Biol Phys. 2017;97(2):236–45. Available from: http://dx.doi.org/10.1016/j.ijrobp.2016.09.007.
33. Lee SH, Tatsui CE, Ghia AJ, Amini B, Li J, Zavarella SM, et al. Can the spinal instability neoplastic score prior to spinal radiosurgery predict compression fractures following stereotactic spinal radiosurgery for metastatic spinal tumor? a post hoc analysis of prospective phase II single-institution trials. J Neurooncol. 2016;126(3):509–17.
34. Massicotte E, Foote M, Reddy R, Sahgal A. Minimal access spine surgery (MASS) for decompression and stabilization performed as an out-patient procedure for metastatic spinal tumours followed by spine stereotactic body radiotherapy (SBRT): first report of technique and preliminary outcomes. Technol Cancer Res Treat. 2012;11(1):15–25.
35. Thibault I, Atenafu EG, Chang E, Chao S, Ameen A-O, Zhou S, et al. Risk of vertebral compression fracture specific to osteolytic renal cell carcinoma spinal metastases after stereotactic body radiotherapy: A multi-institutional study. J Radiosurg SBRT. 2015;3(4):297–305. Available from: http://www.ncbi.nlm.nih.gov/pubmed/29296412.
36. Thibault I, Whyne CM, Zhou S, Campbell M, Atenafu EG, Myrehaug S, et al. Volume of lytic vertebral body metastatic disease quantified using computed tomography based image-segmentation predicts fracture risk following spine stereotactic body radiotherapy. Int J Radiat Oncol Biol Phys. 2017;97(1):75–81.
37. Lam T-C, Uno H, Krishnan M, Lutz S, Groff M, Cheney M, Balboni T. Adverse outcomes after palliative radiation therapy for uncomplicated spine metastases: role of spinal instability and single-fraction radiation therapy. Int J Radiat Oncol Biol Phys. 2015;93(2):373–81.
38. Fisher CG, Dipaola CP, Ryken TC, Bilsky MH, Shaffrey CI, Berven SH, et al. A novel classification system for spinal instability in neoplastic disease: An evidence-based approach and expert consensus from the spine oncology study group. Spine (Phila Pa 1976). 2010;35(22):E1221–9.
39. Gerszten PC, Germanwala A, Burton SA, Welch WC, Ozhasoglu C, Vogel WJ. Combination kyphoplasty and spinal radiosurgery: a new treatment paradigm for pathological fractures. J Neurosurg Spine. 2005;3(4):296–301.
40. Mesfin A, Buchowski JM, Gokaslan ZL, Bird JE. Management of metastatic cervical spine tumors. J Am Acad Orthop Surg. 2015;23(1):38–46.

41. Bilsky MH, Laufer I, Fourney DR, Groff M, Schmidt MH, Varga PP, et al. Reliability analysis of the epidural spinal cord compression scale. J Neurosurg Spine. 2010;13(3):324–8.
42. Laufer I, Rubin DG, Lis E, Cox BW, Stubblefield MD, Yamada Y, et al. The NOMS framework: approach to the treatment of spinal metastatic tumors. Oncologist. 2013;18(6):744–51.
43. Sayama CM, Schmidt MH, Bisson EF. Cervical spine metastases: techniques for anterior reconstruction and stabilization. Neurosurg Rev. 2012;35(4):463–75.
44. Dammers R, Bijvoet HWC, Driesse MJ, Avezaat CCJ. Occurrence of malignant vertebral fractures in an emergency room setting. Emerg Med J. 2007;24(10):707–9.
45. Mummaneni PV, Lu DC, Dhall SS, Mummaneni VP, Chou D. C1 lateral mass fixation: a comparison of constructs. Neurosurgery. 2010;66(3 Suppl):153–60.
46. Bilsky MH, Shannon FJ, Sheppard S, Prabhu V, Boland PJ. Diagnosis and management of a metastatic tumor in the atlantoaxial spine. Spine (Phila Pa 1976). 2002;27(10):1062–9.
47. Fung KY, Law SW. Management of malignant atlanto-axial tumours. J Orthop Surg (Hong Kong). 2005;13(3):232–9.
48. Moulding HD, Bilsky MH. Metastases to the craniovertebral junction. Neurosurgery. 2010;66(3 Suppl):113–8.
49. Zwolak P, Kröber M. Acute neck pain caused by atlanto-axial instability secondary to pathologic fracture involving odontoid process and C2 vertebral body: treatment with radiofrequency thermoablation, cement augmentation and odontoid screw fixation. Arch Orthop Trauma Surg. 2015;135(9):1211–5.
50. Wind JJ, Ammerman JM. Pathologic cervical burst fracture presenting with airway compromise. South Med J. 2010;103(6):551–3.
51. Samanci Y, Togay HS, Yakar R, Kabukcuoglu F, Celik SE. Acute hydrocephalus due to a primary malignant peripheral nerve sheath tumor of the cervicothoracic junction: A case report and review of the literature. Neurochirurgie. 2017;63(2):91–5.
52. Shah LM, Salzman KL. Imaging of spinal metastatic disease. Int J Surg Oncol. 2011;2011:769753.
53. Hunter A, McGreevy J, Linden J. Pathologic C-spine fracture with low risk mechanism and normal physical exam. Am J Emerg Med. 2017;35(9):1383.e1–2.
54. Thawait SK, Marcus MA, Morrison WB, Klufas RA, Eng J, Carrino JA. Research synthesis: what is the diagnostic performance of magnetic resonance imaging to discriminate benign from malignant vertebral compression fractures? Systematic review and meta-analysis. Spine (Phila Pa 1976). 2012;37(12):E736–44.
55. Jung HS, Jee WH, McCauley TR, Ha KY, Choi KH. Discrimination of metastatic from acute osteoporotic compression spinal fractures with MR imaging. Radiographics. 2003;23(1):179–87.
56. Maccauro G, Spinelli MS, Mauro S, Perisano C, Graci C, Rosa MA. Physiopathology of spine metastasis. Int J Surg Oncol. 2011;2011:107969.
57. Placantonakis DG, Laufer I, Wang JC, Beria JS, Boland P, Bilsky M. Posterior stabilization strategies following resection of cervicothoracic junction tumors: review of 90 consecutive cases. J Neurosurg Spine. 2008;9:111–9.
58. Fisher CG, Schouten R, Versteeg AL, Boriani S, Pal Varga P, Rhines LD, et al. Reliability of the Spinal Instability Neoplastic Score (SINS) among radiation oncologists: an assessment of instability secondary to spinal metastases. Radiat Oncol. 2014;9:1–7. Available from: http://www.ro-journal.com/content/9/1/69.
59. Fisher CG, Versteeg AL, Schouten R, Boriani S, Varga PP, Rhines LD, et al. Reliability of the spinal instability neoplastic scale among radiologists: An assessment of instability secondary to spinal metastases. Am J Roentgenol. 2014;203:869.
60. Versteeg AL, van der Velden JM, Verkooijen HM, van Vulpen M, Oner FC, Fisher CG, et al. The Effect of introducing the spinal instability neoplastic score in routine clinical practice for patients with spinal metastases. Oncologist. 2016;21(1):95–101.
61. Arana E, Kovacs FM, Royuela A, Asenjo B, Pérez-Ramírez Ú, Zamora J, et al. Spine Instability Neoplastic Score: agreement across different medical and surgical specialties. Spine J. 2016;16(5):591–9. Available from: http://dx.doi.org/10.1016/j.spinee.2015.10.006.
62. Fourney DR, Frangou EM, Ryken TC, DiPaola CP, Shaffrey CI, Berven SH, et al. Spinal instability neoplastic score: an analysis of reliability and validity from the spine oncology study group. J Clin Oncol. 2011;29(22):3072–7.
63. Fox S, Spiess M, Hnenny L, Fourney DR. Spinal Instability Neoplastic Score (SINS): reliability among spine fellows and resident physicians in orthopedic surgery and neurosurgery. Global Spine J. 2017;7(8):744–8.
64. Gallizia E, Apicella G, Cena T, Di Genesio Pagliuca M, Deantonio L, Krengli M. The spine instability neoplastic score (SINS) in the assessment of response to radiotherapy for bone metastases. Clin Transl Oncol. 2017;19(11):1382–7.
65. Versteeg AL, Verlaan JJ, Sahgal A, Mendel E, Quraishi NA, Fourney DR, et al. The Spinal Instability Neoplastic Score: impact on oncologic decision-making. Spine (Phila Pa 1976). 2016;41(Suppl 20):S231–7.
66. Huisman M, Van Der Velden JM, Van Vulpen M, Van Den Bosch MAAJ, Chow E, Öner FC, et al. Spinal instability as defined by the spinal instability neoplastic score is associated with radiotherapy failure in metastatic spinal disease. Spine J. 2014;14(12):2835–40.
67. Shah AN, Pietrobon R, Richardson WJ, Myers BS. Patterns of tumor spread and risk of fracture

and epidural impingement in metastatic vertebrae. J Spinal Disord Tech. 2003;16(1):83–9.
68. Aoude A, Amiot LP. A comparison of the modified Tokuhashi and Tomita scores in determining prognosis for patients afflicted with spinal metastasis. Can J Surg. 2014;57(3):188–93.
69. Bilsky MH, Laufer I. Burch S. Shifting paradigms in the treatment of metastatic spine disease. 2009;34(22):101–7.
70. Patchell RA, Tibbs PA, Regine WF, Payne R, Saris S, Kryscio RJ, et al. Direct decompressive surgical resection in the treatment of spinal cord compression caused by metastatic cancer: a randomised trial. Lancet. 2005;366(9486):643–8.
71. Dabravolski D, Eßer J, Lahm A, Merk H. Surgical treatment of tumours and metastases of the spine by minimally invasive cavity-coblation method. J Orthop Surg. 2017;25(1):2309499016684505.
72. Li Z, Long H, Guo R, Xu J, Wang X, Cheng X, et al. Surgical treatment indications and outcomes in patients with spinal metastases in the cervicothoracic junction (CTJ). J Orthop Surg Res. 2018;13(1):1–9.
73. Schnake KJ, Tropiano P, Berjano P, Lamartina C. Cervical spine surgical approaches and techniques. Eur Spine J. 2016;25(Suppl 4):486–7.
74. Jandial R, Kelly B, Chen MY. Posterior-only approach for lumbar vertebral column resection and expandable cage reconstruction for spinal metastases. J Neurosurg Spine. 2013;19(1):27–33.
75. Berenson J, Pflugmacher R, Jarzem P, Zonder J, Schechtman K, Tillman JB, et al. Balloon kyphoplasty versus non-surgical fracture management for treatment of painful vertebral body compression fractures in patients with cancer: a multicentre, randomised controlled trial. Lancet Oncol. 2011;12(3):225–35.
76. Fehlings MG, David KS, Vialle L, Vialle E, Setzer M, Vrionis FD. Decision making in the surgical treatment of cervical spine metastases. Spine (Phila Pa 1976). 2009;34(22 Suppl):S108–17.
77. Wang VY, Chou D. The cervicothoracic junction. Neurosurg Clin N Am. 2007;18(2):365–71.
78. Zuckerman SL, Kreines F, Powers A, Iorgulescu JB, Elder JB, Bilsky MH, et al. Stabilization of tumor-associated craniovertebral junction instability: indications, operative variables, and outcomes. Neurosurgery. 2017;81(2):251–8.
79. Roldan H, Ribas-Nijkerk JC, Perez-Orribo L, Garcia-Marin V. Stabilization of the cervicothoracic junction in tumoral cases with a hybrid less invasive-minimally invasive surgical technique: report of two cases. J Neurol Surg A Cent Eur Neurosurg. 2014;75(3):236–40.
80. Kawashima M, Tanriover N, Rhoton AL Jr, Ulm AJ, Matsushima T. Comparison of the far lateral and extreme lateral variants of the atlanto-occipital transarticular approach to anterior extradural lesions of the craniovertebral junction. Neurosurgery. 2003;53(3):662–75.
81. Azad TD, Esparza R, Chaudhary N, Chang SD. Stereotactic radiosurgery for metastasis to the craniovertebral junction preserves spine stability and offers symptomatic relief. J Neurosurg Spine. 2016;24(2):241–7.
82. Kirchner R, Himpe B, Schweder B, Jürgens C, Gille JJ, Faschingbauer M. Das klinische Outcome okzipitozervikaler Stabilisierungen bei Metastasen der oberen Halswirbelsäule: Eine konsekutive Fallserie mit systematischem Review der Literatur [The clinical outcome after occipitocervical fusion due to metastases of the upper cervical spine: a consecutive case series and a systematic review of the literature]. Z Orthop Unfall. 2014;152(4):358–65.
83. Shin H, Barrenechea IJ, Lesser J, Sen C, Perin NI. Occipitocervical fusion after resection of craniovertebral junction tumors. J Neurosurg Spine. 2006;4(2):137–44.
84. Sun G, Wang LJ, Jin P, Liu XW, Li M. Vertebroplasty for treatment of osteolytic metastases at C2 using an anterolateral approach. Pain Physician. 2013;16(4):E427–34.
85. Masala S, Anselmetti GC, Muto M, Mammucari M, Volpi T, Simonetti G. Percutaneous vertebroplasty relieves pain in metastatic cervical fractures. Clin Orthop Relat Res. 2011;469(3):715–22.
86. De la Garza-Ramos R, Benvenutti-Regato M, Caro-Osorio E. Vertebroplasty and kyphoplasty for cervical spine metastases: a systematic review and meta-analysis. Int J Spine Surg. 2016;10:7.
87. Monterumici DA, Narne S, Nena U, Sinigaglia R. Transoral kyphoplasty for tumors in C2. Spine J. 2007;7(6):666–70.
88. De Iure F, Donthineni R, Boriani S. Outcomes of C1 and C2 posterior screw fixation for upper cervical spine fusion. Eur Spine J. 2009;18(Suppl 1):2–6.
89. Ailon T, Torabi R, Fisher CG, Rhines LD, Clarke MJ, Bettegowda C, et al. Management of locally recurrent chordoma of the mobile spine and sacrum: a systematic review. Spine (Phila Pa 1976). 2016;41(Suppl 20):S193–8.
90. Fourney DR, York JE, Cohen ZR, Suki D, Rhines LD, Gokaslan ZL. Management of atlantoaxial metastases with posterior occipitocervical stabilization. J Neurosurg. 2003;98(2 Suppl):165–70.
91. Kast E, Mohr K, Richter HP, Börm W. Complications of transpedicular screw fixation in the cervical spine. Eur Spine J. 2006;15(3):327–34.
92. Yoshihara H, Passias PG, Errico TJ. Screw-related complications in the subaxial cervical spine with the use of lateral mass versus cervical pedicle screws. a systematic review. J Neurosurg Spine. 2013;19(5):614–23.
93. Ringel F, Reinke A, Stüer C, Meyer B, Stoffel M. Posterior C1-2 fusion with C1 lateral mass and C2 isthmic screws: accuracy of screw position, alignment and patient outcome. Acta Neurochir (Wien). 2012;154(2):305–12.

94. Caspar W, Pitzen T, Papavero L, Geisler FH, Johnson TA. Anterior cervical plating for the treatment of neoplasms in the cervical vertebrae. J Neurosurg. 1999;90(1 Suppl):27–34.
95. Eleraky M, Setzer M, Vrionis FD. Posterior transpedicular corpectomy for malignant cervical spine tumors. Eur Spine J. 2010;19(2):257–62.
96. Waschke A, Walter J, Duenisch P, Kalff R, Ewald C. Anterior cervical intercorporal fusion in patients with osteoporotic or tumorous fractures using a cement augmented cervical plate system. J Spinal Disord Tech. 2013;26(3):112–7.
97. Clarke MJ, Zadnik PL, Groves ML, Sciubba DM, Witham TF, Bydon A, et al. Fusion following lateral mass reconstruction in the cervical spine. J Neurosurg Spine. 2015;22(2):139–50.
98. Le H, Balabhadra R, Park J, Kim D. Surgical treatment of tumors involving the cervicothoracic junction. Neurosurg Focus. 2003;15(5):E3.
99. Bayoumi AB, Efe IE, Berk S, Kasper EM, Toktas ZO, Konya D. Posterior rigid instrumentation of C7: surgical considerations and biomechanics at the cervicothoracic junction. A review of the literature. World Neurosurg. 2018;111:216–26.
100. Salem KM, Fisher CG. Anterior column reconstruction with PMMA: an effective long-term alternative in spinal oncologic surgery. Eur Spine J. 2016;25(12):3916–22.
101. Pointillart V, Aurouer N, Gangnet N, Vital JM. Anterior approach to the cervicothoracic junction without sternotomy: a report of 37 cases. Spine (Phila Pa 1976). 2007;32(25):2875–9.
102. Pointillart V, Aurouer N, Gangnet N, Vital JM. Anterior approach to the cervicothoracic junction without sternotomy: a report of 37 cases. Spine (Phila Pa 1976). 2007;32(25):2875–9.
103. Mazel C, Hoffmann E, Antonietti P, Grunenwald D, Henry M, Williams J. Posterior cervicothoracic instrumentation in spine tumors. Spine (Phila Pa 1976). 2004;29(11):1246–53.
104. De Ruiter GC, Nogarede CO, Wolfs JF, Arts MP. Quality of life after different surgical procedures for the treatment of spinal metastases: results of a single-center prospective case series. Neurosurg Focus. 2017;42(1):E17.
105. Guzik G. Quality of life of patients after surgical treatment of cervical spine metastases. BMC Musculoskelet Disord. 2016;17(1):1–6. Available from: http://dx.doi.org/10.1186/s12891-016-1175-8.
106. Bae JW, Gwak HS, Kim S, Joo J, Shin SH, Yoo H, et al. Percutaneous vertebroplasty for patients with metastatic compression fractures of the thoracolumbar spine: clinical and radiological factors affecting functional outcomes. Spine J. 2016;16:355.
107. Papanastassiou ID, Phillips FM, Van Meirhaeghe J, Berenson JR, Andersson GBJ, Chung G, et al. Comparing effects of kyphoplasty, vertebroplasty, and non-surgical management in a systematic review of randomized and non-randomized controlled studies. Eur Spine J. 2012;21(9):1826–43.
108. McGirt MJ, Parker SL, Wolinsky JP, Witham TF, Bydon A, Gokaslan ZL. Vertebroplasty and kyphoplasty for the treatment of vertebral compression fractures: an evidenced-based review of the literature. Spine J. 2009;9(6):501–8.
109. Frankel BM, Jones T, Wang C. Segmental polymethylmethacrylate-augmented pedicle screw fixation in patients with bone softening caused by osteoporosis and metastatic tumor involvement: A clinical evaluation. Neurosurgery. 2007;61:531.
110. Knoeller SM, Huwert O, Wolter T. Single stage corpectomy and instrumentation in the treatment of pathological fractures in the lumbar spine. Int Orthop. 2012;36(1):111–7.
111. De Ruiter GC, Lobatto DJ, Wolfs JF, Peul WC, Arts MP. Reconstruction with expandable cages after single- and multilevel corpectomies for spinal metastases: a prospective case series of 60 patients. Spine J. 2014;14(9):2085–93.
112. Viswanathan A, Abd-El-Barr MM, Doppenberg E, Suki D, Gokaslan Z, Mendel E, et al. Initial experience with the use of an expandable titanium cage as a vertebral body replacement in patients with tumors of the spinal column: A report of 95 patients. Eur Spine J. 2012;21:84.
113. Wang JC, Boland P, Mitra N, Yamada Y, Lis E, Stubblefield M, et al. Single-stage posterolateral transpedicular approach for resection of epidural metastatic spine tumors involving the vertebral body with circumferential reconstruction: results in 140 patients. Invited submission from the Joint Section Meeting on Disorders of the Spine and Peripheral Nerves, March 2004. J Neurosurg Spine. 2004;1(3):287–98.
114. Arts MP, Peul WC. Vertebral body replacement systems with expandable cages in the treatment of various spinal pathologies: a prospectively followed case series of 60 patients. Neurosurgery. 2008;63:537.
115. Eleraky M, Papanastassiou I, Tran ND, Dakwar E, Vrionis FD. Comparison of polymethylmethacrylate versus expandable cage in anterior vertebral column reconstruction after posterior extracavitary corpectomy in lumbar and thoraco-lumbar metastatic spine tumors. Eur Spine J. 2011;20(8):1363–70.
116. Yanamadala V, Rozman PA, Kumar JI, Schwab JH, Lee SG, Hornicek FJ, et al. Vascularized fibular strut autografts in spinal reconstruction after resection of vertebral chordoma or chondrosarcoma: a retrospective series. Neurosurgery. 2017;81:156.
117. Stamatopoulos T, Yanamadala V, Shin JH. Use of cadaveric models in simulation training in spinal procedures. In 2018 [cited 2018 Jul 6]. p. 119–30. Available from: http://link.springer.com/10.1007/978-3-319-75583-0_9.
118. Soo Jang J, Lee SH, Rhee HC, Lee SH. Polymethylmethacrylate-augmented screw fixation for stabilization in metastatic spinal tumors Technical note. J Neurosurg Spine. 2002;96:131.

119. Amendola L, Gasbarrini A, Fosco M, Simoes CE, Terzi S, De Iure F, et al. Fenestrated pedicle screws for cement-augmented purchase in patients with bone softening: A review of 21 cases. J Orthop Traumatol. 2011;12:193.
120. Moussazadeh N, Rubin DG, McLaughlin L, Lis E, Bilsky MH, Laufer I. Short-segment percutaneous pedicle screw fixation with cement augmentation for tumor-induced spinal instability. Spine J. 2015;15(7):1609–17.
121. Renner SM, Lim TH, Kim WJ, Katolik L, An HS, Andersson GB. Augmentation of pedicle screw fixation strength using an injectable calcium phosphate cement as a function of injection timing and method. Spine (Phila Pa 1976). 2004;29(11):E212–6.
122. Özkan N, Sandalcioglu IE, Petr O, Kurniawan A, Dammann P, Schlamann M, et al. Minimally invasive transpedicular dorsal stabilization of the thoracolumbar and lumbar spine using the minimal access nontraumatic insertion system (MANTIS): preliminary clinical results in 52 patients. J Neurol Surgery, Part A Cent Eur Neurosurg. 2012;73(6):369–76.
123. Harel R, Doron O, Knoller N. Minimally invasive spine metastatic tumor resection and stabilization: new technology yield improved outcome. Biomed Res Int. 2015;2015:948373.
124. Hansen-Algenstaedt N, Knight R, Beyerlein J, Gessler R, Wiesner L, Schaefer C. Minimal-invasive stabilization and circumferential spinal cord decompression in metastatic epidural spinal cord compression (MESCC). Eur Spine J. 2013;22:2142.
125. Shea TM, Laun J, Gonzalez-Blohm SA, Doulgeris JJ, Lee WE, Aghayev K, et al. Designs and techniques that improve the pullout strength of pedicle screws in osteoporotic vertebrae: current status. Biomed Res Int. 2014;2014:748393.
126. Pennington Z, Ahmed AK, Molina CA, Ehresman J, Laufer I, Sciubba DM. Minimally invasive versus conventional spine surgery for vertebral metastases: a systematic review of the evidence. Ann Transl Med. 2018;6(6):103.
127. Donnelly DJ, Abd-El-Barr MM, Lu Y. Minimally invasive muscle sparing posterior-only approach for lumbar circumferential decompression and stabilization to treat spine metastasis - technical report. World Neurosurg. 2015;84(5):1484–90.
128. Smith ZA, Li Z, Chen NF, Raphael D, Khoo LT. Minimally invasive lateral extracavitary corpectomy: cadaveric evaluation model and report of 3 clinical cases. J Neurosurg Spine. 2012;16(5):463–70.
129. Le Huec JC, Lesprit E, Guibaud JP, Gangnet N, Aunoble S. Minimally invasive endoscopic approach to the cervicothoracic junction for vertebral metastases: report of two cases. Eur Spine J. 2001;10(5):421–6.
130. Park MS, Deukmedjian AR, Uribe JS. Minimally invasive anterolateral corpectomy for spinal tumors. Neurosurg Clin N Am. 2014;25(2):317–25.
131. Sulaiman OAR, Garces J, Mathkour M, Scullen T, Jones RB, Arrington T, et al. Mini-open thoracolumbar corpectomy: perioperative outcomes and hospital cost analysis compared with open corpectomy. World Neurosurg. 2017;99:295.
132. Zuckerman SL, Laufer I, Sahgal A, Yamada YJ, Schmidt MH, Chou D, et al. When less is more: the indications for MIS techniques and separation surgery in metastatic spine disease. Spine (Phila Pa 1976). 2016;41(Suppl 20):S246–53.
133. Archavlis E, Papadopoulos N, Ulrich P. Corpectomy in destructive thoracolumbar spine disease: cost-effectiveness of 3 different techniques and implications for cost reduction of delivered care. Spine (Phila Pa 1976). 2015;40(7):E433–8.
134. Archavlis E, Schwandt E, Kosterhon M, Gutenberg A, Ulrich P, Nimer A, et al. A modified microsurgical endoscopic-assisted transpedicular corpectomy of the thoracic spine based on virtual 3-dimensional planning. World Neurosurg. 2016;91:424–33. Available from: http://dx.doi.org/10.1016/j.wneu.2016.04.043.
135. Gerszten PC, Monaco EA. Complete percutaneous treatment of vertebral body tumors causing spinal canal compromise using a transpedicular cavitation, cement augmentation, and radiosurgical technique. Neurosurg Focus. 2009;27(6):E9.
136. Bernard F, Lemée JM, Lucas O, Menei P. Postoperative quality-of-life assessment in patients with spine metastases treated with long-segment pedicle-screw fixation. J Neurosurg Spine. 2017;26(6):725–35.
137. Zairi F, Arikat A, Allaoui M, Marinho P, Assaker R. Minimally invasive decompression and stabilization for the management of thoracolumbar spine metastasis. J Neurosurg Spine. 2012;17(1):19–23.
138. Hariri O, Takayanagi A, Miulli DE, Siddiqi J, Vrionis F. Minimally invasive surgical techniques for management of painful metastatic and primary spinal tumors. Cureus. 2017;9(3):e1114.
139. Park HY, Lee SH, Park SJ, Kim ES, Lee CS, Eoh W. Minimally invasive option using percutaneous pedicle screw for instability of metastasis involving thoracolumbar and lumbar spine: a case series in a single center. J Korean Neurosurg Soc. 2015;57(2):100.
140. Kim P, Kim SW. Bone cement-augmented percutaneous screw fixation for malignant spinal metastases: is it feasible? J Korean Neurosurg Soc. 2017;60(2):189–94.
141. Mobbs RJ, Park A, Maharaj M, Phan K. Outcomes of percutaneous pedicle screw fixation for spinal trauma and tumours. J Clin Neurosci. 2016;23:88–94.
142. Schizas C, Kosmopoulos V. Percutaneous surgical treatment of chance fractures using cannulated pedicle screws. Report of two cases. J Neurosurg Spine. 2007;7(1):71–4.
143. Tancioni F, Navarria P, Pessina F, Marcheselli S, Rognone E, Mancosu P, et al. Early surgical experience with minimally invasive percutaneous approach for patients with metastatic epidural spinal cord compression (MESCC) to poor prognoses. Ann Surg Oncol. 2012;19:294.

144. Kumar N, Zaw AS, Reyes MR, Malhotra R, Wu PH, Makandura MC, et al. Versatility of percutaneous pedicular screw fixation in metastatic spine tumor surgery: a prospective analysis. Ann Surg Oncol. 2015;22(5):1604–11.
145. Tancioni F, Navarria P, Pessina F, Marcheselli S, Rognone E, Mancosu P, et al. Early surgical experience with minimally invasive percutaneous approach for patients with metastatic epidural spinal cord compression (MESCC) to poor prognoses. Ann Surg Oncol. 2012;19(1):294–300.
146. Versteeg AL, Verlaan JJ, de Baat P, Jiya TU, Stadhouder A, Diekerhof CH, et al. Complications after percutaneous pedicle screw fixation for the treatment of unstable spinal metastases. Ann Surg Oncol. 2016;23(7):2343–9.
147. Kwan MK, Lee CK, Chan CY. Minimally invasive spinal stabilization using fluoroscopic-guided percutaneous screws as a form of palliative surgery in patients with spinal metastasis. Asian Spine J. 2016;10(1):99–110.
148. Sawakami K, Yamazaki A, Ishikawa S, Ito T, Watanabe K, Endo N. Polymethylmethacrylate augmentation of pedicle screws increases the initial fixation in osteoporotic spine patients. J Spinal Disord Tech. 2012;25(2):E28–35.
149. Ibrahim A, Crockard A, Antonietti P, Boriani S, Bünger C, Gasbarrini A, et al. Does spinal surgery improve the quality of life for those with extradural (spinal) osseous metastases? An international multicenter prospective observational study of 223 patients. Invited submission from the Joint Section Meeting on Disorders of the Spine and Peripheral Nerves, March 2007. J Neurosurg Spine. 2008;8(3):271–8.
150. Moliterno J, Veselis CA, Hershey MA, Lis E, Laufer I, Bilsky MH. Improvement in pain after lumbar surgery in cancer patients with mechanical radiculopathy. Spine J. 2014;14(10):2434–9.
151. Lee RS, Batke J, Weir L, Dea N, Fisher CG. Timing of surgery and radiotherapy in the management of metastatic spine disease: expert opinion. J Spine Surg. 2018;4(2):368–73.
152. Itshayek E, Yamada J, Bilsky M, Schmidt M, Shaffrey C, Gerszten P, et al. Timing of surgery and radiotherapy in the management of metastatic spine disease: a systematic review. Int J Oncol. 2010;36(3):533–44.

Osteoporotic Vertebral Compression Fractures Adjacent to Previous Spinal Fusion

17

Peter G. Passias, Rivka C. Ihejirika-Lomedico, Hesham Saleh, Max Egers, Avery E. Brown, Haddy Alas, Katherine E. Pierce, Cole Bortz, and Yael Ihejirika

Evaluation

Introduction

Recent improvements in surgical technique and instrumentation have enabled surgeons to address adult spinal deformity and other degenerative spine conditions in increasingly high-risk populations, including the elderly, frail, and osteoporotic patients [1–3]. A number of reports show consistent and durable correction of sagittal spinal alignment through the use of rigid fusion constructs; however, increased construct rigidity is often associated with greater mechanical stress, facet loading, and motion in adjacent segments [4–6]. Increased biomechanical load in segments adjacent to previous fusions can result in structural failure, often times manifesting in the form of vertebral body fracture or proximal junctional fracture. For elderly patients and patients with osteoporosis, proximal junctional fracture is of particular concern, since it may lead to severe pain, exacerbation of spinal deformity, mechanical instability, neurologic compromise, and an increased risk of reoperation. Given the growing population of patients eligible for spine surgery and the rising prevalence of osteoporosis in patients undergoing instrumented spinal fusion, a thorough understanding of the diagnosis and management of osteoporotic vertebral compression fracture (VCF) adjacent to previous spinal fusions is increasingly pertinent [7].

Mechanisms of Proximal Junctional Fracture

(a) *Biomechanical*

While the pathogenesis of VCF adjacent to a previous fusion has not been explicitly investigated in osteoporotic patient populations, a number of studies have explored the mechanisms of proximal junctional fracture in elderly patients with a history of multilevel thoracolumbar fusion. A common theme linking these mechanistic analyses of VCF appears to be a disparity between compressive forces on the anterior column and tensile forces in the posterior column [8, 9].

In a case series of 12 patients who underwent surgery between 2008 and 2015 for degenerative spine pathologies, Faundez et al. identified 6 cases of proximal junctional fracture [9]. In this series of patients, a key driver of vertebral failure appeared to be abnormal postoperative curve harmony, as assessed by increased upper

P. G. Passias (✉) · R. C. Ihejirika-Lomedico
H. Saleh · M. Egers · A. E. Brown · H. Alas
K. E. Pierce · C. Bortz · Y. Ihejirika
Department of Orthopedic Surgery, NYU Langone Orthopedic Hospital, NYU Langone Medical Center, New York, NY, USA
e-mail: Rivka.Ihejirika-Lomedico@nyulangone.org; hesham.saleh@nyumc.org; haddy.alas@downstate.edu

A. E. Razi, S. H. Hershman (eds.), *Vertebral Compression Fractures in Osteoporotic and Pathologic Bone*, https://doi.org/10.1007/978-3-030-33861-9_17

lumbar lordosis (as defined by the lordosis above the lumbar apex) and decreased lower lumbar lordosis (lordosis below the lumbar apex). While all patients in this case series showed successful restoration of global lumbar lordosis (L1-S1), the researchers hypothesized that failure to restore lordosis below the lumbar apex drove anterior sagittal compensation, in turn causing junctional failure and subsequent proximal junctional collapse.

(b) *Cellular level:* changes in bone mineral density in adjacent segments following surgery.

Bogdanffy et al. evaluated changes in bone mineral density in adjacent segments after L4-S1 instrumented fusion [10]. There were significant decreases in bone mineral density above fused segments, perhaps due to immobilization or altered mechanics associated with fusion. These changes persisted through 6 months of follow-up. Furthermore, it was found that trabecular bone is more susceptible than cortical bone, due to higher metabolic activity. Succinctly, long lumbar instrumented fusions can lead to loss of bone mineral density; when segments adjacent to the fusion are rigid, the environment is ripe for compression fractures.

Risk Factors for VCF

DeWald et al. assessed the effect on outcomes of long fusion constructs in patients with osteoporosis [11]. Forty seven patients over 65 years underwent a minimum five-level fusion. Two developed early postoperative compression fractures adjacent to the construct, and one developed a late VCF adjacent to the fusion. These results suggest that long fusions, especially those in the lumbar spine extending into the lower thoracic spine, place osteoporotic patients at higher risk of VCF.

Etebar et al. conducted a retrospective analysis of 125 fusion patients from a single surgeon [12]. Of the 125 women, 31 were postmenopausal. Eighteen patients developed adjacent segment disease (ASD), 15 of whom were postmenopausal women. VCF was responsible for 28% of the ASD cases in this series. The authors concluded that the risk for post-fusion VCF/ASD in general is higher in postmenopausal women.

Medical Management

Management of osteoporotic VCF adjacent to a prior spinal fusion (VCF-ASF) is a result of many different processes, frequently requiring a multidisciplinary approach to management of these injuries. Typically, the primary complaint of patients after sustaining a VCF is pain. The degree of pain and resultant disability is frequently worse in patients with a kyphotic deformity associated with vertebral height loss, compensatory lumbar hyperlordosis, postural change, and sagittal imbalance. In those without significant deformity, disability, or neurologic compromise, pharmacological pain management and rehabilitation are the mainstays of care.

Traditional pain medications including acetaminophen, nonsteroidal anti-inflammatories, and opiates are commonly used for treating acute pain in this setting. While not traditionally indicated for the treatment of VCF, anticonvulsants, antidepressants, and muscle relaxant medication may provide therapeutic benefits in carefully selected patients. Anticonvulsants such as gabapentin and pregabalin are primarily used in treatment of radiating nerve pain and require increasing dosage over several weeks to achieve clinical efficacy. In cases where patients have persistent localizable nerve irritation, these medications may be a useful adjunct [13]. Cyclobenzaprine, a nonaddictive muscle relaxant, has been shown to improve sleep and reduce chronic back pain in a number of studies. Its use may be considered in VCF patients with combined unremitting back pain and insomnia. Despite an unfavorable side-effect profile, tricyclic antidepressants such as amitriptyline may provide pain relief in patients with chronic back pain and should be considered as a third-line agent [14]. There is no literature to support the use of oral steroids in this group of patients, and prolonged steroid use may worsen outcomes [15].

There are no rigorous studies regarding bracing for the treatment of pain in patients with VCF-ASF; in our clinical experience, bracing in this subset of patients offers no substantial benefit. As an early adjunct to oral pain medication, short-term bed rest, physical therapy, and bracing may provide comfort, but prolonged use may lead to muscle atrophy and should be avoided.

Despite evidence that VCF-ASF patients on average have a higher BMD than VCF patients with no prior spine surgery, McAfee's work demonstrating that spinal rigidity can lead to osteoporosis in adjacent vertebrae supports the idea that addressing bone density is imperative for medical management and is a necessity prior to surgical intervention [16, 17]. Treating osteoporosis involves medication and rehabilitation to either stop bone loss, enhance bone mass, or both. Anti-resorptive agents help to stem bone loss and include bisphosphonates, selective estrogen receptor modulators (SERM), RANK ligand inhibitors, and calcitonin. Anabolic agents such as teriparatide and abaloparatide are increasing in popularity for VCF prophylaxis. Addressing osteoporosis may help reduce recurrent VCF, thereby reducing pain and the subsequent need for revision surgery.

Frailty, defined as an increased susceptibility to injury, should be addressed in all patients with regular exercise and nutrition. While calcium and vitamin D are important regulators of bone formation, many patients do not receive adequate amounts in their diet. Supplementation to ensure 1200 mg of calcium and 1000 IU of vitamin D intake daily from all sources is recommended.

Bisphosphonates act as inhibitors of the HMG-CoA reductase pathway and have been used to prevent osteoporosis for over 40 years. They diminish osteoclast activity resulting in diminished bone resorption. These drugs are approved for the prevention and treatment of osteoporosis with intermittent administration and can reduce VCFs by up to 70% [18].

Studies have shown that teriparatide, a recombinant human parathyroid hormone, improves bone quality and density while preventing proximal junctional kyphosis and reducing screw pullout after posterior spinal fusion in osteoporotic patients [19, 20]. Furthermore, teriparatide has been useful in treating back pain after osteoporotic vertebral compression fractures (OVCF) [21]. In a randomized double-blind study by Hadji et al., teriparatide was compared to risedronate for the treatment of patients with OVCF. After 6 months of treatment, roughly 60% of patients in both groups had more than a 30% reduction in back pain. Those who were treated with teriparatide had significantly fewer vertebral compression fractures and increased BMD in the lumbar spine and femoral neck compared to those who received risedronate. Since numerous studies have shown the superiority of teriparatide over bisphosphonates in the treatment and prevention of VCF, serious consideration should be given to starting this medication when poor bone density is discovered [22–24].

The available literature regarding the management of vertebral compression fractures does not differentiate between isolated fractures and those associated with spinal fusion. The goals of medical management include diagnosis, pain control, functional optimization, and the prevention of future fractures [25]. According to the World Health Organization, a T-score below −2.5 is diagnostic for osteoporosis; however, in the absence of trauma, a vertebral compression fracture is pathognomonic for osteoporosis regardless of the T-score [26]. Patients with a T-score between −1 and −2.5 have osteopenia, and should also be started on preventive medications, as will be discussed further.

Pain control following vertebral compression fractures allows for early mobilization, which helps to prevent bone loss, pressure ulcers, and deep vein thromboses [1]. NSAIDs or Tylenol are usually the mainstay of treatment [27]. NSAIDs have been suggested to inhibit bone healing, but this has not been shown in clinical studies [28]. Gastrointestinal bleeding and ulcers are potential side effects of NSAIDs and should be used cautiously, particularly in the elderly population. Opioids may also be used in the acute setting. These medications are generally well-tolerated when used appropriately, but side effects include decreased gastrointestinal motility, urinary retention, and decreased respiratory drive [29].

Muscle relaxants are most effective in preventing paravertebral muscle spasms within the first 2 weeks of injury; however, they are associated with drowsiness and dizziness [30]. Despite their widespread use in the acute setting, the AAOS reports that there is a lack of adequate data for the use of complementary medicine, opioids, and other analgesics and thus designates an "inconclusive recommendation" for these treatment options [28]. On the other hand, the AAOS gives a recommendation of moderate strength to calcitonin, a PTH antagonist [31]. When started within 5 days of injury and continued for a total of 4 weeks, calcitonin has been shown to decrease pain. Perhaps more impressive, it has been shown to decrease pain even 3 months from the time of the initial injury.

Physical therapy is an important means of promoting early mobilization following compression fractures. Its main purposes are to strengthen the patient's axial musculature and to improve his/her proprioception to help decrease the risk of future falls [32]. For example, strengthening the erector spinae muscles improves posture and lumbar lordosis, thus addressing some back pain and kyphosis often associated with vertebral compression fractures [29]. The Spinal Proprioception Extension Exercise Dynamic (SPEED) program is an example of a 4-week exercise regimen that has been shown to improve back pain, reduce the risk of fall, and increase the overall level of physical activity of patients. [30] Most importantly, physical therapy should be performed in an observed setting by qualified professionals to maximize its benefits and ensure safety.

There is a paucity of literature regarding the effectiveness of bracing for vertebral compression fractures. Some studies have shown that while spinal orthoses may improve posture and promote pain relief, they may also cause muscular atrophy and skin breakdown when used improperly [25]. When utilized, braces should ideally be lightweight and easy to apply, especially for elderly patients [27]. Because of the heterogenous conclusions in the literature, the AAOS gives an "inconclusive recommendation" for bracing in patients with vertebral compression fractures [28].

The prevention of further fractures is a primary objective of medical management for vertebral compression injuries. Ibandronate, a nitrogen-containing bisphosphonate, has been shown to significantly decrease new symptomatic fractures 3 years from the initial injury, without notable adverse effects [28]. Strontium ranelate also helps prevent vertebral compression fractures by increasing bone formation and density, while reducing bone resorption [31]. Aside from medications, activity modifications also help promote bone health and, thus, help to prevent compression fractures. Smoking cessation is highly recommended, as smoking accelerates bone loss.i Lastly, targeted exercise therapy improves patients' overall bone health and proprioception skills, thus decreasing the risk of falls and consequent compression fractures [30].

Surgical Management

As management of patients with osteoporosis and adjacent segment VCF is often wrought with complications, literature is scant regarding the surgical management of this subgroup. The three main surgical options are vertebroplasty, kyphoplasty, and/or extension of the fusion construct to include the level of injury and correct deformity. Unfortunately, after maximizing medical management, many of these patients will continue to have significant back pain. Pain and moderate degrees of deformity may be addressed through minimally invasive surgical procedure such as kyphoplasty or vertebroplasty.

A case-control study by Ahn and Lee suggests that treatment of a VCF-ASF with vertebroplasty has similar results to those treated for VCF without prior spinal surgery [16]. They compared the results of nine patients who underwent vertebroplasty with PMMA cement for VCF-ASF to control VCF patients and found that those with VCF-ASF had a reduction in their visual analog score (VAS) from 8.1 to 3.2 and a satisfaction rate of 88.9%, both of which were not significantly different than the control group. There were no complications after vertebroplasty in the VCF-ASF group [33]. A case series by Wu et al. demonstrated an improvement of up to 70% in the kyphotic angle of adjacent segment VCF when treated with vertebroplasty [34].

In the case of significant kyphotic deformity, traumatic unstable fracture, or neurological compromise revision surgery, extending the fusion may be necessary. The literature discussing the management of VCF-ASF in this situation is limited to case reports, and there is no consensus on best practice [35–37]. Despite this, it is important to recognize that outcomes are at least in part related to the degree of sagittal imbalance. Deformity correction should address sagittal alignment through the judicious use of osteotomies as with primary adult spinal deformity.

Technical pearls for managing these fractures can be gleaned from the literature on kyphosis management in the non-fractured patient. Much controversy exists regarding single versus multiple stage correction for kyphotic VCF. In a retrospective study with 184 patients undergoing vertebral column resection, Gum et al. demonstrated no difference in complications associated with multistaged versus single-staged procedure; however other studies have demonstrated increased complications following staged procedures [38]. A retrospective analysis of ten patients with kyphotic VCF showed a reduction of pain and minimal complications at long-term follow-up after treatment with single-staged posterolateral vertebrectomy [39]. Some authors prefer a multistaged approached as it allows for cement augmentation prior to screw placement [40]. While the goal of cement augmentation is to increase the pullout strength of the construct, evidence is lacking [41]. Lastly, when performing a three-column osteotomy, outcomes have been shown to be superior with the use of a 3- and 4-rod constructs versus 2-rod constructs with respect to rod breakage and the need for revision for pseudoarthrosis [42].

In the setting of VCF-ASF, surgical intervention should also aim to address the modulus mismatch between the mobile and immobile spinal segments in addition to addressing the pain and deformity. In long fusions, prophylactic kyphoplasty or vertebroplasty of the level above the upper instrumented vertebra may prevent the formation of a new VCF in vulnerable patients [43, 44].

Considerations

Advances in surgical technique and instrumentation have enabled surgeons to treat symptomatic adult spinal deformity in high-risk populations such as elderly and osteoporotic patients that previously had more limited treatment options [45]. Unfortunately, in doing so, it has unveiled additional complications including adjacent segment disease. The rigid instrumentation which facilitates the correction and maintenance of spinal alignment brings with it increased loading in adjacent segments, which can lead to adjacent level pathology and mechanical. In osteoporotic patients, diminished bone quality in the vertebral bodies proximal to a fusion subjects the vertebrae to increased loads which can lead to OVCF.

Management of OVCF requires a multidisciplinary approach and involves preoperative and postoperative interventions to address the underlying osteoporosis, pain, and frailty. Pharmacologic treatments of the osteoporosis and pain are the mainstays of treatment. Physical therapy is also an effective treatment with the goal of strengthening axial musculature to improve posture and lumbar lordosis as well as improving proprioception and decreasing fall risk. There is also evidence to support the efficacy of physical therapy in treating pain and increasing the overall activity of OVCF patients. In circumstances where the osteoporotic adjacent segment fracture manifests with significant structural failure, deformity, and clinical symptoms such as neurologic compromise, additional surgical intervention is warranted. Surgical options include minimally invasive techniques like kyphoplasty or vertebroplasty when the pain and deformity are moderate. In more severe cases, revision surgery with proximal extension of the instrumentation and fusion may be necessary, along with the cautious and judicious use of osteotomies when kyphotic deformity is present, since osteotomies in patients with osteoporosis have been shown to have significant complications [46]. The high complication rate of this revision surgery has led to extensive debate over multiple technical aspects of the procedure including whether to perform the correction in a single vs. multistaged fashion and the use of prophylactic vertebral cement augmentation of the proximal unfused vertebrae to prevent recurrent VCF. The literature concerning these points of contention is sparse, and further research is required to form definitive guidelines for the surgical treatment of OVCF leading to PJF.

Adjacent segment disease is a major cause of complication in spinal deformity surgery and is especially relevant in the osteoporotic population. OVCF in segments adjacent to previous spinal fusion exist on a spectrum with symptoms ranging from asymptomatic, benign PJK on one end to severe PJF on the other. As the population continues to age, further research will be required to better understand and improve the prevention and management of this condition.

References

1. Tomé-Bermejo F, Piñera AR, Alvarez-Galovich L. Osteoporosis and the management of spinal degenerative disease (I). Arch Bone Joint Surg. 2017;5:272–82.
2. Yagi M, Fujita N, Okada E, Tsuji O, Nagoshi N, Tsuji T, et al. Impact of frailty and comorbidities on surgical outcomes and complications in adult spinal disorders. Spine (Phila Pa 1976). 2018;22:1.
3. Challier V, Boissière L, Diebo BG, Lafage V, Lafage R, Castelain J-E, et al. The Dubousset functional test: introducing a new assessment to evaluate multimodal balance in the setting of adult spine deformity. Unpublished data. 2017.
4. Bastian L, Lange U, Knop C, Tusch G, Blauth M. Evaluation of the mobility of adjacent segments after posterior thoracolumbar fixation: a biomechanical study. Eur Spine J. 2001;10(4):295–300.
5. Chow DH, Luk KD, Evans JH, Leong JC. Effects of short anterior lumbar interbody fusion on biomechanics of neighboring unfused segments. Spine (Phila Pa 1976). 1996;21(5):549–55.
6. Park P, Garton HJ, Gala VC, Hoff JT, McGillicuddy JE. Adjacent segment disease after lumbar or lumbosacral fusion: review of the literature. Spine (Phila Pa 1976). 2004;29(17):1938–44.
7. Chin DK, Park JY, Yoon YS, Kuh SU, Jin BH, Kim KS, et al. Prevalence of osteoporosis in patients requiring spine surgery: incidence and significance of osteoporosis in spine disease. Osteoporos Int. 2007;18(9):1219–24.
8. Le Huec J-C, Richards J, Tsoupras A, Price R, Leglise A, Faundez AA. The mechanism in junctional failure of thoraco-lumbar fusions. Part I: biomechanical analysis of mechanisms responsible of vertebral overstress and description of the cervical inclination angle (CIA). Eur Spine J. 2018;27(Suppl 1):129–38.
9. Faundez AA, Richards J, Maxy P, Price R, Leglise A, Le Huec J-C. The mechanism in junctional failure of thoraco-lumbar fusions. Part II: analysis of a series of PJK after thoraco-lumbar fusion to determine parameters allowing to predict the risk of junctional breakdown. Eur Spine J. 2018;27(Suppl 1):139–48.
10. Bogdanffy GM, Ohnmeiss DD, Guyer RD. Early changes in bone mineral density above a combined anteroposterior L4-S1 lumbar spinal fusion. A clinical investigation. Spine (Phila Pa 1976). 1995;20(15):1674–8.
11. Quality PB, Dewald CJ, Stanley T. Instrumentation-related complications of multilevel fusions for adult spinal deformity patients over age 65: surgical considerations and treatment options in patients with poor bone quality. Spine (Phila Pa 1976). 2006;31(19 Suppl):S144–51.
12. Etebar S, Cahill DW. Risk factors for adjacent-segment failure following lumbar fixation with rigid instrumentation for degenerative instability. J Neurosurg. 1999;90(2 Suppl):163–9.
13. Lee SH, Kim ES, Sung JK, Park YM, Eoh W. Clinical and radiological comparison of treatment of atlantoaxial instability by posterior C1-C2 transarticular screw fixation or C1 lateral mass-C2 pedicle screw fixation. J Clin Neurosci. 2010;17(7):886–92.
14. Salerno SM, Browning R, Jackson JL. The effect of antidepressant treatment on chronic back pain: a meta-analysis. Arch Intern Med. 2002;162(1):19–24.
15. Deibert CP, Gandhoke GS, Paschel EE, Gerszten PC. A Longitudinal Cohort Investigation of the development of symptomatic adjacent level compression fractures following balloon-assisted kyphoplasty in a series of 726 patients. Pain Physician. 2016;19(8):E1167–72.
16. Ahn Y, Lee S-H. Vertebroplasty for adjacent vertebral fracture following lumbar interbody fusion. Br J Neurosurg. 2011;25(1):104–8.
17. Granville M, Berti A, Jacobson RE. Vertebral compression fractures after lumbar instrumentation. Cureus. 2017;9(9):–e1729.
18. Wang T, Zhang X, Bikle DD. Osteogenic differentiation of periosteal cells during fracture healing. J Cell Physiol. 2017;232(5):913–21.
19. Yagi M, Ohne H, Konomi T, Fujiyoshi K, Kaneko S, Komiyama T, et al. Teriparatide improves volumetric bone mineral density and fine bone structure in the UIV+1 vertebra, and reduces bone failure type PJK after surgery for adult spinal deformity. Osteoporos Int. 2016;27(12):3495–502.

20. Sato M, Sainoh T, Orita S, Yamauchi K, Aoki Y, Ishikawa T, et al. Posterior and anterior spinal fusion for the management of deformities in patients with Parkinson's disease. Case Rep Orthop. 2013;2013:140916.
21. Lyritis G, Marin F, Barker C, Pfeifer M, Farrerons J, Brixen K, et al. Back pain during different sequential treatment regimens of teriparatide: results from EUROFORS. Curr Med Res Opin. 2010;26(8):1799–807.
22. Seki S, Hirano N, Kawaguchi Y, Nakano M, Yasuda T, Suzuki K, et al. Teriparatide versus low-dose bisphosphonates before and after surgery for adult spinal deformity in female Japanese patients with osteoporosis. Eur Spine J. 2017;26(8):2121–7.
23. Hsu WK, Goldstein CL, Shamji MF, Cho SK, Arnold PM, Fehlings MG, et al. Novel osteobiologics and biomaterials in the treatment of spinal disorders. Neurosurgery. 2017;80(3):S100–7.
24. Inoue G, Takaso M, Miyagi M, Kamoda H, Ishikawa T, Nakazawa T, et al. Risk factors for L5-S1 disk height reduction after lumbar posterolateral floating fusion surgery. J Spinal Disord Tech. 2014;27(5):187–92.
25. McCarthy J, Davis A. Diagnosis and management of vertebral compression fractures. Am Fam Physician. 2016;94(1):44–50.
26. McGirt M, Wong MJ. Vertebral compression fractures: a review of current management and multimodal therapy. J Multidiscip Healthc. 2013;6:205.
27. Longo UG, Loppini M, Denaro L, Maffulli N, Denaro V. Osteoporotic vertebral fractures: current concepts of conservative care. Br Med Bull. 2012;102:171–89.
28. AAOS Guideline on The Treatment of Osteoporotic Spinal Compression Fractures Summary of Recommendations. https://www.aaos.org/research/guidelines/SCFsummary.pdf.
29. Hongo M, Miyakoshi N, Shimada Y, Sinaki M. Association of spinal curve deformity and back extensor strength in elderly women with osteoporosis in Japan and the United States. Osteoporos Int. 2012;23(3):1029–34.
30. Sinaki M. Exercise for patients with osteoporosis: management of vertebral compression fractures and trunk strengthening for fall prevention. PM R. 2012;4(11):882–8.
31. Spector TD, Calomme MR, Anderson SH, Clement G, Bevan L, Demeester N, et al. Choline-stabilized orthosilicic acid supplementation as an adjunct to Calcium/Vitamin D3 stimulates markers of bone formation in osteopenic females: a randomized, placebo-controlled trial. BMC Musculoskelet Disord. 2008;9(1):85.
32. Daly RM, Dalla Via J, Duckham RL, Fraser SF, Helge EW. Exercise for the prevention of osteoporosis in postmenopausal women: an evidence-based guide to the optimal prescription. Braz J Phys Ther. 2019;23(2):170.
33. Ahn J-S, Lee J-K, Kim B-K. Prognostic factors that affect the surgical outcome of the laminoplasty in cervical spondylotic myelopathy. Clin Orthop Surg. 2010;2(2):98–104.
34. Wu H, Pang Q, Jiang G. Medium-term effects of Dynesys dynamic stabilization versus posterior lumbar interbody fusion for treatment of multisegmental lumbar degenerative disease. J Int Med Res. 2017;45(5):1562–73.
35. Missori P, Ramieri A, Costanzo G, Peschillo S, Paolini S, Miscusi M, et al. Late vertebral body fracture after lumbar transpedicular fixation. J Neurosurg Spine. 2005;3(1):57–60.
36. Sorge O, Günther L, Strasser E, Gahr RH. Two times unlucky: treatment of repeated adjacent vertebral fractures following posterolateral interbody fusion. Arch Orthop Trauma Surg. 2006;126(5):346–9.
37. Cho K-J, Suk S-I, Park S-R, Kim J-H, Kim S-S, Lee T-J, et al. Short fusion versus long fusion for degenerative lumbar scoliosis. Eur Spine J. 2008;17(5):650–6.
38. Schwab FJ, Hawkinson N, Lafage V, Smith JS, Hart R, Mundis G, Burton DC, Line B, Akbarnia B, Boachie-Adjei O, Hostin R. Risk factors for major peri-operative complications in adult spinal deformity surgery: a multi-center review of 953 consecutive patients. Eur Spine J. 2012;21(12):2603–10.
39. Dreimann M, Hempfing A, Stangenberg M, Viezens L, Weiser L, Czorlich P, et al. Posterior vertebral column resection with 360-degree osteosynthesis in osteoporotic kyphotic deformity and spinal cord compression. Neurosurg Rev. 2018;41(1):221–8.
40. Behrbalk E, Uri O, Folman Y, Rickert M, Kaiser R, Boszczyk BM. Staged correction of severe thoracic kyphosis in patients with multilevel osteoporotic vertebral compression fractures. Glob Spine J. 2016;6(7):710–20.
41. Weiser L, Dreimann M, Huber G, Sellenschloh K, Püschel K, Morlock MM, et al. Cement augmentation *versus* extended dorsal instrumentation in the treatment of osteoporotic vertebral fractures. Bone Joint J. 2016;98–B(8):1099–105.
42. Hyun S-J, Lenke LG, Kim Y-C, Koester LA, Blanke KM. Comparison of standard 2-rod constructs to multiple-rod constructs for fixation across 3-column spinal osteotomies. Spine (Phila Pa 1976). 2014;39(22):1899–904.
43. Kebaish KM, Martin CT, O'Brien JR, LaMotta IE, Voros GD, Belkoff SM. Use of vertebroplasty to prevent proximal junctional fractures in adult deformity surgery: a biomechanical cadaveric study. Spine J. 2013;13(12):1897–903.
44. Nas ÖF, İnecikli MF, Hacıkurt K, Büyükkaya R, Özkaya G, Özkalemkaş F, et al. Effectiveness of percutaneous vertebroplasty in patients with multiple myeloma having vertebral pain. Diagn Interv Radiol. 2016;22(3):263–8.
45. Nguyen VH. Osteoporosis prevention and osteoporosis exercise in community-based public health programs. Osteoporos Sarcopenia. 2017;3(1):18–31.
46. Okuda S, Oda T, Yamasaki R, Haku T, Maeno T, Iwasaki M. Surgical outcomes of osteoporotic vertebral collapse: a retrospective study of anterior spinal fusion and pedicle subtraction osteotomy. Global Spine J. 2012;2(4):221–6.

Surgical Strategies in Osteoporotic Bone

18

Joseph M. Zavatsky and Robert A. McGuire Jr

Background

The US population is expected to grow by 9.5% between 2013 and 2025 based on data from the US Census Bureau, with the population age 65 and older projected to grow nearly 45% [1]. By 2050 the US population age 65 and older is projected to reach 89 million – more than double the 40.5 million elderly people in 2010 [2, 3]. The prevalence of adult scoliosis in the general population has been reported to be as high as 32% [4–7] and as high as 68% in the older population [8]. Using the current prevalence estimates, there are approximately 27.5 million elderly people with one form or another of spinal deformity, and with this high growth rate, the number of adults with spinal deformity would reach more than 60 million by 2050. Increasing age correlates with decreasing bone mineral density (BMD). Osteoporosis presents a unique challenge to surgeons attempting to instrument and fuse the spine, particularly in patients with the goal of surgery being to correct an already complex spinal deformity problem.

Generally, the surgical management of patients with adult spinal deformity (ASD) is considered for patients who have progressive deformity, neurologic compromise, and unrelenting pain. Patients usually present with pain and functional limitations that are not responsive to medical and interventional pain modalities including physical therapy, yoga, medications, and epidural steroid injections. The decision to pursue surgical treatment in patients with ASD is largely a factor of baseline disability. Once a patient is indicated for surgery, routine preoperative radiological imaging often includes standing full-length scoliosis AP and lateral X-rays, MRI, CT scan, and DEXA scan. Most insurance companies limit repeat DEXA scans to every 2 years; DEXA scans that are not up-to-date may overestimate a patient's current bone mineral density. Additionally, variations in the techniques used to obtain DEXA scans can affect the true T-score; T-scores obtained from a deformed spine may be artificially elevated.

DEXA (T-Score) Vs. Spinal Computed Tomography (Hounsfield Unit (HU))

Because bone mineral density (BMD) measurements at various sites differ in the relative amounts of cortical and trabecular bone that they assess, they also differ in their sensitivity for detecting osteopenia. Lateral spine dual-energy

J. M. Zavatsky (✉)
Spine and Scoliosis Specialists, Tampa, FL, USA

R. A. McGuire Jr
Department of Orthopaedic Surgery,
University of Mississippi Medical Center,
Jackson, MS, USA
e-mail: rmcguire@umc.edu

A. E. Razi, S. H. Hershman (eds.), *Vertebral Compression Fractures in Osteoporotic and Pathologic Bone*, https://doi.org/10.1007/978-3-030-33861-9_18

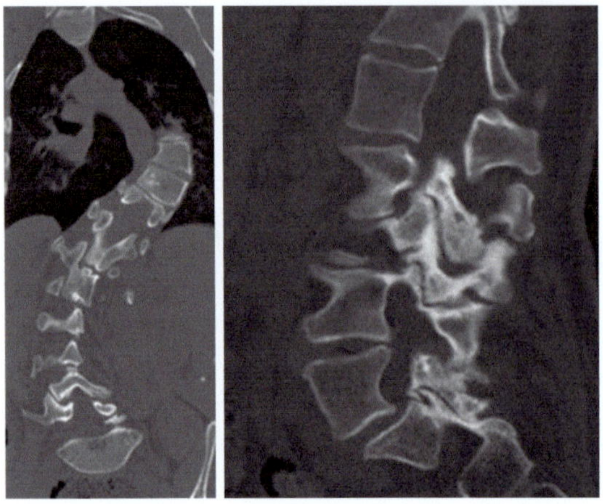

Fig. 18.1 Coronal and sagittal CT scan of adult scoliosis revealing sclerosis of a lumbar facet joints. AP DEXA scan would be falsely elevated due to the sclerosed facet joints comprised of primarily cortical bone

X-ray absorptiometry (DEXA) allows measurement of BMD of the vertebral bodies, which contain mainly trabecular bone. Typically, there is no contribution from the posterior vertebral elements, which consist of dense cortical bone (Fig. 18.1). Finkelstein et al. assessed the ability of DEXA to estimate trabecular bone mass and compared AP and lateral DEXA spine measurements with trabecular bone measurements by quantitative computed tomography (QCT) in 58 patients [9]. They compared AP vs. lateral spine DEXA measurements in three groups. Group 1 consisted of 300 women referred for routine bone densitometry, Group 2 contained 30 glucocorticoid-treated women, and Group 3 was made up of 44 women with vertebral compression fractures. The association between QCT and DXA measurements was stronger when DEXA measurements were made in the lateral ($r = 0.784$) or mid-lateral ($r = 0.823$) projection than in the AP ($r = 0.571$) projection. Additionally, the association of BMD with age was stronger when DEXA measurements were made in the lateral ($r = 0.536$) or mid-lateral ($r = 0.536$) projection than in the AP ($r = 0.382$) projection. The declines in BMD with age for AP, lateral, and mid-lateral DEXA measurements were 0.48%, 0.60%, and 0.88% per year, respectively. In the women referred for routine densitometry, lateral DEXA measurements were significantly ($P < 0.05$) more abnormal than AP measurements obtained from young women. This was also true in the women treated with glucocorticoids and in women with vertebral compression fractures. Lateral DEXA often detected osteopenia in patients whose AP DEXA was normal. The authors concluded that lateral DEXA measurements identify patients with osteopenia more often than AP DEXA measurements, probably because lateral DEXA more accurately estimates trabecular bone mass (Fig. 18.1).

Insurance companies often limit how frequently a repeat DEXA scan can be performed. Additionally, there are inconsistencies in the T-scores depending upon the technique used (lateral vs. AP) to obtain the DEXA scan. Since many surgeons obtain a CT scan of the spine as part of the normal preoperative workup, the diagnostic efficacy of the Hounsfield unit (HU) in spine CT scans may provide a better alternative to the T-score obtained with DEXA scans; however this was refuted by Kohan et al. [10].

The dual-energy X-ray absorptiometry (DEXA) scan is an easy and cost-effective method of assessing bone mineral density (BMD). However, in patients with degenerative changes of the spine, overestimation of the T-score on DEXA scan can occur despite low BMD during pedicle screw placement in spine surgery. Choi assessed BMD using Hounsfield units (HU) from computed tomography (CT) and correlated these measurements with DEXA T-scores in patients with nondegenerative and degenerative spines [11]. This study included 80 nondegenerative and 30 degenerative patients who underwent DEXA and spine CT assessment. The HU value on the midbody axial images of CT and DEXA T-scores was measured from the L1–L4 vertebrae. In the nondegenerative group, HU values had a strong positive correlation with BMD and T-score, exhibiting correlation coefficients (r) greater than 0.7. BMD assessed as +100 HU matched a T-score of −2.0, while +150 matched a T-score of −1.0, and + 200 HU matched T-scores of 0.0; these differences were significant ($P < 0.001$). In the degenerative group, there was a weak positive correlation with an r of approximately 0.4. The authors concluded that the HU values provide a meaningful assessment of BMD and have a strong correlation with T-score. However, in degenerative patients, the DEXA T-score tended to be higher than the actual BMD. BMD assessment using HU might be helpful in predicting real BMD in patients undergoing instrumented spinal surgery with degenerative changes of the spine. Accurate BMD assessment is even more critical in elderly patients who are undergoing large deformity correction surgery, as these patient's spines are often increasingly degenerated (Fig. 18.1) and BMD can be falsely elevated.

Bisphosphonates Vs. Teriparatide

Patients identified with low BMD should be considered for treatment for their low BMD prior to any instrumented spinal surgery to decrease the risk of hardware loosening or failure. Low BMD may be defined as having a lateral DEXA T-score of −1.0 to −2.5 or a spinal CT scan HU measurement of +150 to +90 (osteopenia) or a T-score of −2.5 or lower or HU measurement less than +90 (osteoporosis). Two of the most common medical treatments for osteoporosis are bisphosphonates and teriparatide.

Bisphosphonates are primary agents in the current pharmacological arsenal against osteoclast-mediated bone loss due to osteoporosis, Paget disease of the bone, malignancies metastatic to the bone, multiple myeloma, and hypercalcemia of malignancy. Like their natural analogue inorganic pyrophosphate (PPi), bisphosphonates have a very high affinity for bone mineral because they bind to hydroxyapatite crystals. Accordingly, bisphosphonate skeletal retention depends on the availability of hydroxyapatite-binding sites. Bisphosphonates are preferentially incorporated into sites of active bone remodeling, as commonly occurs in conditions characterized by accelerated skeletal turnover. In addition to their ability to inhibit calcification, bisphosphonates inhibit hydroxyapatite breakdown, thereby effectively suppressing bone resorption [12]. This fundamental property of bisphosphonates has led to their utility as clinical agents in the treatment of osteoporosis. More recently, it has been suggested that bisphosphonates also function to limit both osteoblast and osteocyte apoptosis [13, 14].

Teriparatide is a recombinant protein form of parathyroid hormone consisting of the first (N-terminus) 34 amino acids, which is the bioactive portion of the hormone. It is an effective anabolic (promoting bone formation) agent [15] used in the treatment of some forms of osteoporosis [16]. It is also occasionally used off-label to speed fracture healing, promote spinal fusion, decrease the risk of spinal hardware loosening, and reduce the risk of proximal junction kyphosis in long instrumented spinal fusions. Teriparatide is identical to a portion of human parathyroid hormone (PTH), and intermittent use activates osteoblasts more than osteoclasts, leading to an overall increase in the bone.

There are data comparing the efficacy of bisphosphonates versus teriparatide in the treatment of osteoporosis, specifically in the lumbar spine, showing improved fusion rates with teriparatide administration, along with its positive effects on protecting spinal instrumentation.

Yuan et al. performed a meta-analysis to compare the efficacy of teriparatide and bisphosphonates for reducing vertebral fracture risk and improving bone mineral density (BMD) in the lumbar spine and femoral neck in postmenopausal women with osteoporosis [17]. Only randomized controlled trials that compared teriparatide and bisphosphonates for reducing vertebral fracture risk in postmenopausal women with osteoporosis were included. Results demonstrated that compared with bisphosphonates, teriparatide was associated with a reduction of the vertebral fracture risk (risk ratio (RR) = 0.57, 95% confidence interval (CI): 0.35, 0.93, $P = 0.024$). Furthermore, teriparatide therapy increased the mean percent change in BMD in the lumbar spine at 6 months, 12 months, and 18 months more than bisphosphonates did ($P < 0.05$), and only teriparatide was beneficial at increasing the mean percent change in BMD in the femoral neck at 18 months ($P < 0.05$). There was no significant difference between teriparatide and bisphosphonates in terms of adverse events.

Ohtori and colleagues published the first study examining teriparatide in the context of spinal fusion [18] – the study was a prospective trial of 57 women with osteoporosis undergoing elective posterior spinal fusion (PSF) in the setting of degenerative spondylolisthesis. The women were divided into a teriparatide group and a bisphosphonate group prior to undergoing a 1–2 level instrumented posterolateral fusion (PSF) with local bone graft. Teriparatide was maintained for 10 months total, starting 2 months before the operation. Although pain scores were not different between the groups, the teriparatide group achieved bony union in 82% of patients versus 68% in the bisphosphonate group, with union achieved an average of 2 months earlier in the teriparatide group ($P < 0.05$).

Ohtori followed up their original study and investigated the rates of pedicle screw loosening in a prospective study of 62 osteoporotic women with degenerative spondylolisthesis undergoing decompression and 1–2 level instrumented PSF [19]. There were three patient cohorts (teriparatide, bisphosphonates, and a control group without pharmacologic treatment), and the patients were assessed radiographically, clinically, and by computed tomography (CT) at 12 months. Therapies were started 2 months before surgery and maintained for a total of 12 months. The incidence of pedicle screw loosening was 7–13% in the teriparatide group, which was significantly lower than the bisphosphonate and control groups, 13–26% and 15–25%, respectively ($P < 0.05$). The authors hypothesized that one of the mechanisms in which teriparatide improves fusion rates may be by enhancing implant fixation.

The impact of teriparatide on spine surgery is particularly relevant in the setting of adult spinal deformity surgery, where the prevalence of osteoporosis-related complications approaches 33% [20]. Kaliya-Perumal investigated teriparatide use in multilevel PSF for lumbar degenerative pathologies (average 4.5 levels) [21]. The retrospective study of 62 patients involved a teriparatide group starting daily therapy on postoperative day 1 and a control group receiving no therapy. In total, 66% of teriparatide patients showed solid fusion at 1 year versus only 50% of controls, but this was not statistically significant ($P = 0.20$). However, there was a significantly higher rate of radiographic screw loosening in the control group (24% vs. 13%; $P = 0.001$). The improved screw fixation and fusion trends with teriparatide seen with one- or two-level fusions also seem to apply to multilevel fusions. Yagi and colleagues investigated the impact of teriparatide on proximal junctional kyphosis (PJK) in multilevel fusions for osteopenic and osteoporotic adult spinal deformity patients [22]. In their prospective comparative study, patients who started daily teriparatide immediately after surgery were compared to controls not receiving therapy; patients were followed for 2 years. Six months postoperatively, the teriparatide group achieved a statistically significant increase in both BMD and bone mineral content of the vertebrae above the construct, as well as an increase in hip BMD as compared to the control group ($P < 0.05$). They observed increases in both the thickness and number of trabeculae in the vertebrae, as well as a general improvement in the bone volume-to-tissue ratio. Unsurprisingly, the teriparatide group had a significantly lower rate of PJK at 2-year follow-up, 4.6% compared with 15.2% in the control group, ($P = 0.02$).

Surgical Techniques to Augment Spinal Instrumentation

In addition to the medical management of patients with osteoporosis undergoing instrumented spinal fusion surgery, there are multiple techniques available to the surgeon intraoperatively that can be utilized to decrease the rate of instrumentation loosening and hardware failure.

Choosing the optimal pedicle screws diameter and length can affect stiffness. Brantley and colleagues evaluated the effects of pedicle screw size, including diameter and length, on fixation stiffness in osteoporotic and non-osteoporotic vertebrae in vitro [23] using fresh-frozen human spines. Bone mineral densities were determined using dual-energy radiograph absorptiometry; this was followed by non-destructive mechanical testing of the specimens instrumented with pedicle screws using a loading technique that more closely mimicked loading of pedicle screws in vivo. The results revealed that in non-osteoporotic bone, screw size had a significant effect on fixation stiffness, but the effect of penetration depth (length) depended on pedicle fill (diameter) and vice versa. In non-osteoporotic bone, the use of longer screws increased fixation stiffness if the screws filled up the pedicle by 70% or more. The use of wider screws increased the fixation stiffness if the penetration depth was 80% or more (Fig. 18.2). In the osteoporotic specimens, increased fill did not increase stiffness for any length screw. However, increased length may have increased the stiffness somewhat, independent of percent fill. The authors concluded that the success of posterior stabilization of the spine using pedicle screws can be enhanced in non-osteoporotic bone by selecting the largest clinically acceptable pedicle screw, in both length and diameter, but did caution about overfilling the pedicle and resultant pedicle fracture. In general, one parameter is not always more significant than the other because of their noted interdependence. Unfortunately, optimizing pedicle screw size seems to be less effective in osteoporotic bone. In 1994, the authors suggested that additional studies evaluating alternative instrumentation techniques, including inserting pedicle screws at greater angles and augmenting screws with bone cement, warranted further investigation (see Fig. 18.2).

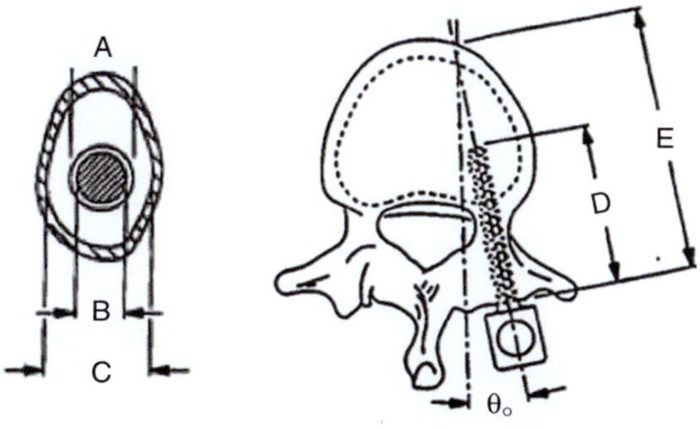

Fig. 18.2 Pedicle screw diameter should fill up the pedicle 70% or more to increase pullout strength (A/C × 100≥70%). Pedicle screw penetration depth should be at least 80% or greater to increase pullout strength (D/E × 100≥80%)

More recent pedicle screw insertion techniques, including the cortical bone trajectory (CBT) technique, have attracted some attention recently; some biomechanical studies have demonstrated a superior fixation capacity of screws placed using the CBT. In addition to demonstrating superior fixation strength, CBT screws can be inserted using less invasive techniques for lumbar instrumentation, thus minimizing soft-tissue dissection. However, until recently, there was little consensus on the selection of screw size, and no biomechanical study elucidated the most suitable screw size for CBT.

Matsukawa and colleagues evaluated the effect of screw size on fixation strength in an attempt to identify the ideal screw size for optimal fixation using CBT [24]. In their study, they evaluated a total of 720 CBT screws with various diameters (4.5–6.5 mm) and lengths (25–40 mm) in simulations of 20 different lumbar vertebrae (mean age: 62.1 ± 20.0 years, 8 males and 12 females) using a finite element (FE) method. First, the fixation strength of a single screw was evaluated by measuring the axial pullout strength. Then, vertebral fixation strength of a paired-screw construct was examined by applying forces simulating flexion, extension, lateral bending, and axial rotation to the vertebra. And lastly, the equivalent stress value of the bone-screw interface was calculated. The results demonstrated that larger-diameter screws increased the pullout strength and vertebral fixation strength and decreased the equivalent stress around the screws. However, there were no statistically significant differences between 5.5 and 6.5 mm screws. The screw diameter was a factor more strongly affecting the fixation strength of CBT than the screw fit within the pedicle (percent fill). Longer screws significantly increased the pullout strength and vertebral fixation strength in axial rotation. The amount of screw length within the vertebral body (percent length) was more important than the actual screw length, contributing to the vertebral fixation strength and distribution of stress loaded to the vertebra. The authors concluded that the fixation strength of CBT screws varied depending on screw size.

Contrary to previous studies that demonstrated that longer screws improved fixation only if the screws were inserted deep enough to engage the anterior vertebral cortex [25, 26], Matsukawa's study on CBT showed that the effects of both diameter and length are equivalent even if the screws did not penetrate the anterior cortex. This could be theoretically explained by the variations in bone density in the vertebral body. Traditional trajectory pedicle screws pass through the pedicle and are directed toward the central portions of the vertebral body with lower density bone. However, CBT screws are directed toward the peripheral portions of the vertebral body with higher density bone (Fig. 18.3). Additionally, CBT screw fixation relies mainly on the denser cortical bone between the pars interarticularis and the inferior part of the pedicle. In addition to screw diameter and length, BMD was also a predictive factor of pullout strength. Among these factors, BMD most strongly affected the fixation strength of CBT screws, which is consistent with the results of previous biomechanical studies [27, 28]. In the present study, the equation demonstrated that a 0.1 g/cm^2 decrease in femoral neck BMD corresponded to a 100 N decrease in pullout strength. Ultimately, the authors felt that the ideal screw size for CBT is a diameter larger than 5.5 mm, and length longer than 35 mm, and the screw should be placed sufficiently deep into the vertebral body (see Fig. 18.3).

Surgeons are faced with persistent challenges in spine surgery to improve pedicle screw fixation in patients with poor bone quality. Additional fixation techniques have been described in an attempt to augment pedicle screw fixation in the face of an osteoporotic spine; augmenting pedicle screws with cement appears to be a promising approach. Elder and colleagues performed a systematic review of the literature to assess the previous biomechanical studies on pedicle screw augmentation with cement augmentation [29]. Their review found numerous studies that demonstrated that polymethylmethacrylate (PMMA) was an effective material for enhancing pedicle screw fixation in both osteoporosis and revision spine surgery models. Several other calcium ceramics also appeared promising. PMMA delivery through fenestrated screws appears to have some benefits, but pullout strength was similar to screw fixation when prefilling the pedicle screw pilot hole with cement with a solid screw. There were differences found in screw biomechanics with varying cement volume and curing time, and some benefits from a kyphoplasty approach over a vertebroplasty approach were noted. Additionally, in cadaveric models, cement-augmented pedicle screws were able to be removed, albeit at higher extraction torques, without catastrophic damage to the vertebral body. However, there is a risk of cement extravasation leading to potentially neurological or cardiovascular complications with cement use.

Burval and colleagues further evaluated pedicle screw pullout strength in osteoporotic bone utilizing two specific cement augmentation techniques, a kyphoplasty technique and a standard transpedicular prefilling augmentation technique [30]. Thirteen osteoporotic and 9 healthy human lumbar vertebrae were tested, and all specimens were instrumented with pedicle screws using a

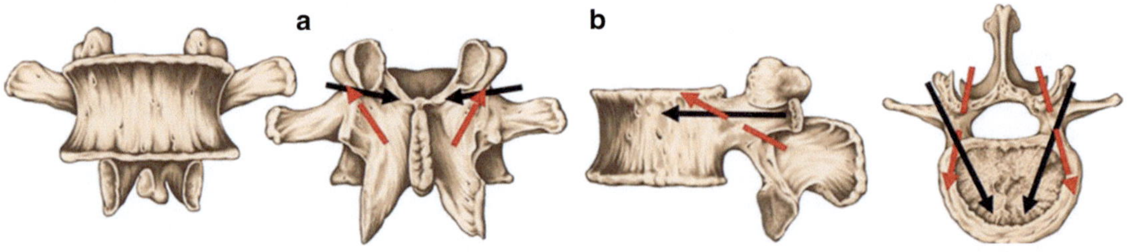

Fig. 18.3 AP and lateral views of the lumbar spine demonstrating traditional pedicle screw tracts (black arrows) and cortical bone trajectory tracts (red arrows)

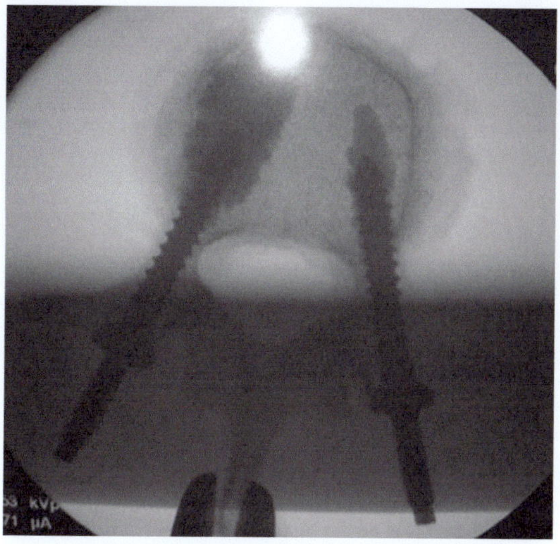

Fig. 18.4 Cement augmentation techniques of pedicle screws. On the left, a kyphoplasty-type cement technique; and on the right, a transpedicular prefilling cement technique

uniform technique. Osteoporotic pedicles were augmented with polymethylmethacrylate (PMMA) using either a kyphoplasty-type technique or a transpedicular prefilling augmentation technique (Fig. 18.4). Screws were tested in a paired testing array, randomly assigning the augmentation techniques to opposite sides of each vertebra. Pullout to failure was performed either primarily or after a 5000-cycle tangential fatigue conditioning exposure. After testing, following screw removal, specimens were cut in the axial plane through the center of the vertebral body to inspect the cement distribution. The study revealed that pedicle screws placed in osteoporotic vertebrae had higher pullout loads when augmented with the kyphoplasty technique compared to transpedicular prefill augmentation (1414 +/− 338 versus 756 +/− 300 N, respectively; P <0.001). An unpaired t-test showed that fatigued pedicle screws in osteoporotic vertebrae augmented by kyphoplasty showed higher pullout resistance than those placed in healthy control vertebrae ($P = 0.002$). Both kyphoplasty type augmentation ($P = 0.007$) and transpedicular prefill augmentation ($P = 0.02$) increased pullout loads compared to pedicle screws placed in non-augmented osteoporotic vertebrae when tested after fatigue cycling. The authors highlighted that pedicle screws augmented using the kyphoplasty technique had significantly greater pullout strength than those augmented with a vertebroplasty augmentation technique and those placed in healthy control vertebrae with no augmentation (see Fig. 18.4).

Pedicle screw augmentation with PMMA cement has been shown to significantly improve the fixation strength even in a severely osteoporotic spine. Costa and colleagues further evaluated the difference in pullout strength between five different cement augmentation techniques [31]. Uniform synthetic bone (Sawbones, Washington, USA) was used to simulate severe osteoporosis by providing a platform for each augmentation technique; polyaxial screws and acrylic cement (PMMA) at medium viscosity were used. Five groups were analyzed: (I) screw only without PMMA (control group), (II) retrograde cement prefilling of the tapped pedicle screw pilot hole, (III) cannulated and fenestrated screw with cement injection through perforations in the screw, (IV) injection using a standard trocar of PMMA (vertebroplasty) with retrograde prefilling of the tapped pilot hole, and (V) injection through a fenestrated trocar and retrograde prefilling of the tapped pilot hole (Fig. 18.5). Standard X-rays were taken in order to confirm cement distribution in each group. A total of 30 pedicle screws at full insertion were then tested for axial pullout failure using a mechanical testing machine. The results of pullout analysis revealed better resistance to pull out in all groups as compared to the control group without cement augmentation. In particular, the statistical analysis showed a difference between Group V ($P = 0.001$) and all other groups, suggesting better load resistance to axial forces when the distribution of the PMMA is uniform and elongated along the screw stem due to combining a fenestrated trocar and prefilling augmentation technique (see Fig. 18.5).

In addition to augmenting pedicle screws with cement, there are several other surgical techniques that can be utilized to increase construct stiffness, even in the face of osteoporosis.

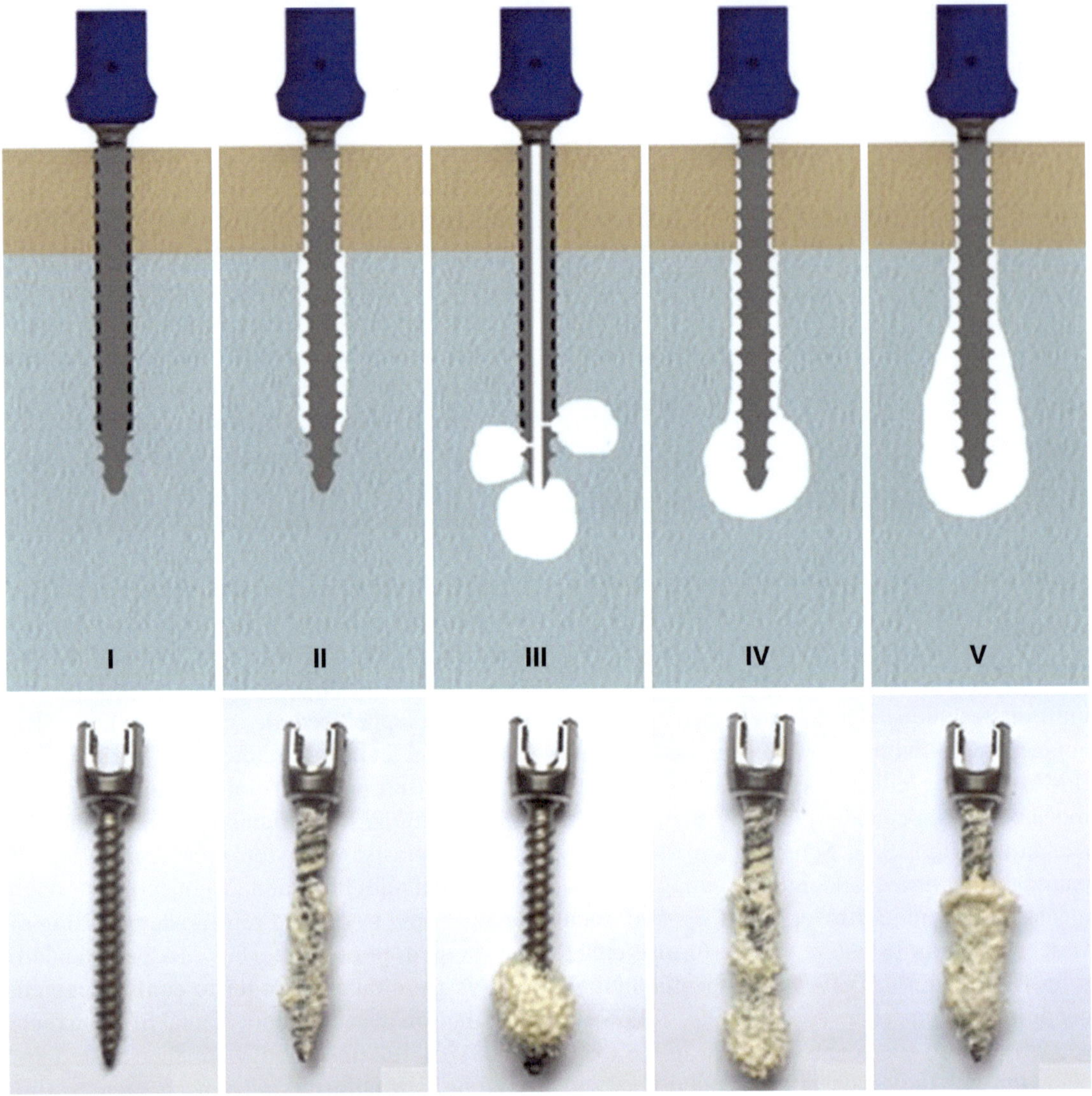

Fig. 18.5 Pedicle screw cement augmentation groups: (I) screw only without PMMA (control group), (II) retrograde cement prefilling of the tapped pedicle screw pilot hole, (III) cannulated and fenestrate screw with cement injection through perforations in the screw, (IV) injection using a standard trocar of PMMA (vertebroplasty) and retrograde prefilling of the tapped pilot hole, and (V) injection through a fenestrated trocar and retrograde prefilling of the tapped pilot hole

Specifically, in the thoracic spine, PMMA cement augmentation of pedicle screws is riskier secondary to the risk of cement extravasation into the thoracic spinal canal and the possibility of injuring the spinal cord. Paxinos and colleagues performed an in vitro biomechanical study on the thoracic spine comparing the pull-out strength and mechanism of failure of four posterior fixation thoracic constructs in relation to bone mineral density (BMD) [32]. A total of 80 vertebrae from 11 fresh-frozen thoracic spines (T2–12) were used. Based on the results from peripheral quantitative CT, specimens were divided into two groups – Group (A) osteopenic bone and Group (B) normal bone. They were then randomly assigned to one of four different instrumentation systems: pedicle screws, sub-laminar wires, lamina claw hooks, and pedicle

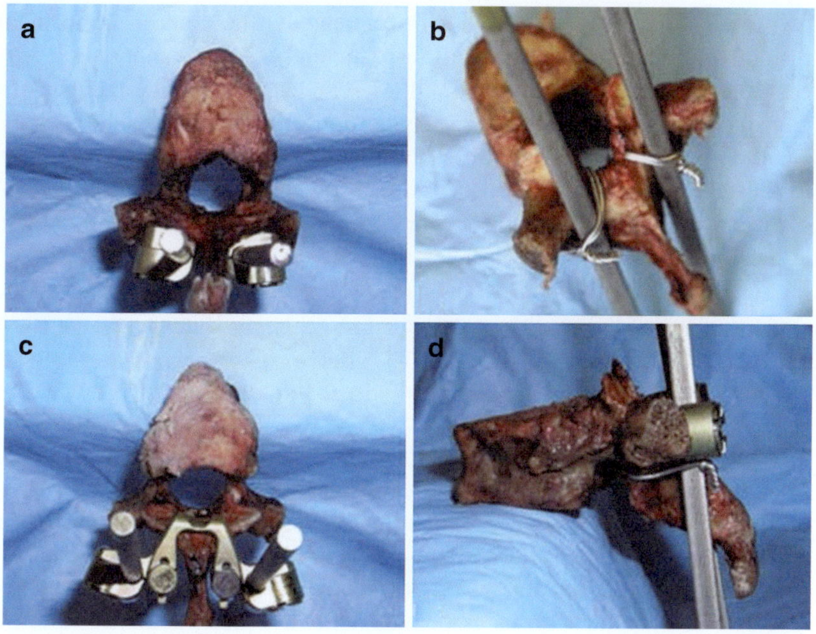

Fig. 18.6 Four different instrumentation constructs tested: (**a**) pedicle screws, (**b**) sublaminar wires, (**c**) lamina claw hooks, and (**d**) pedicle screws with sublaminar wires

screws with sublaminar wires (Fig. 18.6). The construct was completed with two titanium rods and two transverse connectors, creating a stable frame. The pullout force to failure perpendicular to the rods, as well as the pattern of fixation failure, was recorded. The mean pullout force in Group A (36 vertebrae) was 473.2 ± 179.2 N, and in Group B (44 vertebrae), the pullout force was 1414.5 ± 554.8 N. In Group A, no significant difference in pullout strength was identified among the different implant constructs ($P = 0.96$). In Group B, the hook system failed because of dislocation with significantly less force than the other three constructs (931.9 ± 345.1 N vs. an average of 1538.6 ± 532.7 N; $P = 0.02$). In the osteopenic group, larger screws demonstrated greater resistance to pullout ($P = 0.011$). The most common failure mechanism in both groups was through pedicle base fracture. As demonstrated in all the previous studies, bone quality is an important factor that influences stability of posterior implants in the thoracic spine, and fixation strength in the osteopenic group was one-fourth of the value measured in vertebrae with good bone quality, irrespective of the instrumentation used (see Fig. 18.6).

Proximal Junction Kyphosis (PJK)

Osteoporosis not only increases the risk of hardware loosening and failure at the primary site of instrumentation, but it can also increase the risk of complications to vertebra adjacent to the instrumentation in the form of vertebral fractures and resultant proximal junction kyphosis (PJK). Stiffness at the upper instrumented vertebra (UIV) can increase the stress at the adjacent vertebra (UIV + 1) immediately superior to the instrumented vertebra. In patients with osteoporosis, this junctional stress further increases the risk for vertebral fracture at the UIV + 1 and can result in PJK.

In 2008, Hart and colleagues reported on their series of patients treated with prophylactic vertebral augmentation above instrumented lumbar fusions and analyzed the costs associated with prophylactic vertebroplasty vs. kyphoplasty vs. revision instrumented fusion [33]. In a retrospective chart review and cost analysis, all female patients older than 60 years undergoing extended lumbar fusions were reviewed to establish the incidence of proximal junctional acute collapse. Cost estimates for two-level vertebroplasty, two-level kyphoplasty, and revision instrumented fusion were calculated using billing data and cost-to-charge ratios. They reviewed 28 female patients older than 60 years of age who underwent lumbar fusions from L5 or S1 extending up to the thoracolumbar junction (T9–L2). Fifteen of the 28 patients had prophylactic vertebroplasty at the level cranial to the fused segment. Acute proximal junctional collapse requiring revision surgery occurred in 2 of the 13 patients (15.3%) treated without prophylactic vertebroplasty. None of the 15 patients undergoing prophylactic cement augmentation experienced PJK. Assuming a 15% decrease in the incidence of acute proximal junctional collapse, the estimated cost to prevent a single acute proximal junctional collapse was $46,240 using vertebroplasty and $82,172 using kyphoplasty. Cost analysis revealed the inpatient costs associated with a revision instrumented fusion averaged $77,432. This data supports that prophylactic vertebral cement augmentation for the prevention of proximal junctional acute collapse is a cost-effective intervention in elderly female patients undergoing long lumbar fusions.

Kebaish was one of the first to perform a biomechanical study evaluating the effectiveness of prophylactic vertebral augmentation in reducing the incidence of vertebral compression fractures at the proximal junction after a long spinal fusion in a cadaveric model [34]. In his study, 18 cadaveric spine specimens were divided into 3 groups of 6 spines each: a control group, a group treated with one-level prophylactic vertebroplasty at the upper instrumented vertebra (UIV), and a group treated with two-level prophylactic vertebroplasty at the upper instrumented vertebra (UIV) and the supra-adjacent vertebra (UIV + 1). All spines were instrumented with pedicle screws and rods from L5 to T10. Using eccentric axial loading, the specimens were compressed until failure. Failure was defined as a precipitous decrease in load with increasing compression. The effect of augmentation on load to failure was checked using linear regression, and the effect of augmentation on the incidence of adjacent fractures was checked using logistic regression. They identified fractures in 12 of 18 specimens: 5 in the control group, 6 in the one-level cemented group, and only 1 in the two-level cemented group. The number of fractures in the UIV + 1 group was significantly less ($P = 0.021$) than that in the UIV or control groups. Prophylactic vertebroplasty at the UIV and UIV + 1 levels reduced the incidence of junctional fractures after long posterior spinal instrumentation in this axially loaded cadaveric model.

Raman and Kebaish performed a follow-up clinical study evaluating the long-term radiographic and clinical outcomes and the incidence of PJK and proximal junctional failure (PJF) after prophylactic vertebroplasty for long-segment thoracolumbar posterior spinal fusion (PSF) at a 5-year follow-up time point [35]. A prospective cohort of 39 patients, 87% of whom were female, who underwent two-level prophylactic vertebroplasty at the UIV and UIV + 1 at the time of index surgery were included. Clinical outcomes were assessed using the SRS-22 and SF-36 questionnaires and the Oswestry Disability Index (ODI) . Radiographic parameters including PJK angle, and coronal and sagittal alignment, were calculated along with relevant perioperative complications and revision rates. Of the 41 patients who received two-level prophylactic vertebroplasty at the UIV and UIV + 1 during the index PSF, 39 (95%) completed 5-year follow-up (average: 67.6 months). Proximal junctional kyphosis was defined as a change in the PJK angle ≥10° between the immediate postoperative and final follow-up radiographs. Proximal junctional failure (PJF) was defined as an acute proximal junctional fracture, fixation failure, or kyphosis requiring extension of the fusion within the first 6 months postoperatively. Thirty-nine patients with a mean age of 65.6 (41–87) years were included in this study. Of the 39 patients, 11 developed PJK (28.2% –7.7% at 2 years, 20.5% between 2 and 5 years), and 5.1% developed acute PJF. Two of the 11 PJK patients required revision for progressive worsening of their PJK. There were no proximal junctional fractures. There was no significant difference in the preoperative, immediate postoperative, and final follow-up measurements of thoracic kyphosis, lumbar lordosis, and coronal or sagittal alignment between patients who developed PJK, PJF, or neither (P >0.05). There was no significant difference in ODI, SRS-22, or SF-36 scores between those with and without PJK or PJF (P >0.05). This clinical long-term follow-up study demonstrates that prophylactic vertebroplasty may minimize the risk for junctional failure in the early postoperative period. However, it does not appear to decrease the incidence of PJK at 5 years.

Expanding upon the research performed by Kebaish, where prophylactic vertebral cement augmentation at the UIV and UIV + 1 decreased the incidence of proximal junctional vertebral fractures above long instrumented fusion constructs, Zavatsky and colleagues evaluated if a tapered dose of vertebral cement at the UIV, UIV + 1, and UIV +2 would further reduce the rate of fractures at the proximal junction in a cadaveric model following T10-pelvis instrumentation [36]. In a cadaveric study, 15 ligamentous, osteoporotic T6-pelvis specimens with screw and rod constructs from T10-S1 were divided equally into 3 groups: Group (1) no cement, Group (2) 4 cc of cement (2 cc through each pedicle) in T10 (UIV) and 4 cc in T9 (UIV + 1), and Group (3) 4 cc of cement in T10 (UIV), 3 cc total in T9 (UIV + 1), and 2 cc in T8 (UIV +2) (Fig. 18.7). The pelvis and T6 vertebra were potted, and compression was applied 10 mm anterior to the center of T6 using an MTS actuator; the maximum load to failure was measured in newtons (N). The spines were evaluated using fluoroscopy and CT. The data demonstrated a significant reduction in fractures in Group 3 vs. 2 and 1 (0 vs. 5 vs. 5, P = 0.0019, respectively). Posterior ligamentous rupture occurred in four specimens in Group 3, three in Group 2, and one in Group 1. There was no statistically significant difference in specimen DEXA values (P = 0.71), and there was no hardware failure in any group. Finite element analysis (FEA) was also performed and mirrored the cadaveric data; the maximum load to failure increased from Groups 1 to 3. Endplate stresses were reduced in Group 3 vs. Groups 2 and 1. In both cadaveric and FEA models, tapering the dose of cement in the UIV, UIV + 1, and UIV + 2 (Group 3) decreased endplate stresses, increased the load required for failure, and significantly reduced vertebral fractures above long instrumented constructs. The authors detailed that this technique may protect the spine from PJK due to fracture but may increase the risk of posterior ligamentous stress and failure, but further clinical validation was warranted (see Fig. 18.7).

Current Recommended Management

Before scheduling a surgical patient for elective instrumented spinal fusion for either their degenerative spinal conditions or deformity, a lateral DEXA scan of the spine (T-score) or a spinal CT scan (Hounsfield Units (HU)) should be obtained to more accurately assess the patient's bone mineral density (BMD). Patients with any T-score of less than −2.5, HU less than +90, or history of

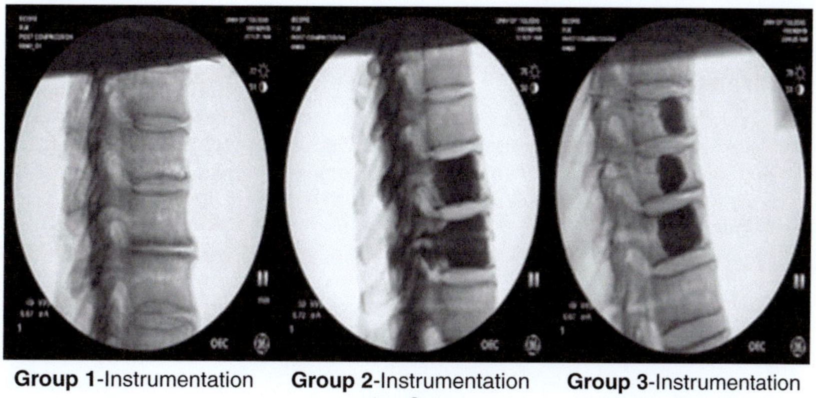

Fig. 18.7 Three cement configuration groups: Group (1) no cement (control), Group (2) 4 cc of cement (2 cc through each pedicle) in T10 (UIV) and 4 cc in T9 (UIV + 1), and tapered cement Group (3) 4 cc of cement in T10 (UIV), 3 cc total in T9 (UIV + 1), and 2 cc in T8 (UIV +2)

fragility fracture (especially of the hip or spine) should be referred to endocrinology for initiation of anabolic therapy. This referral should be done as early as possible, as the insurance company approval process for these medications can be challenging and lengthy. It is clear that anabolics have the potential to improve fusion rates, strengthen implant fixation, and reduce junctional complications for women with postmenopausal osteoporosis undergoing posterior spinal fusion.

On the basis of the available evidence, there appears to be multiple techniques that surgeons can utilize intraoperatively to enhance spinal instrumentation and decrease the risk of loosening and hardware failure in the osteoporotic spine. These surgical techniques include using the largest diameter and length pedicle screws possible. Whether it's a traditional tract or cortical bone trajectory (CBT) pedicle screw, cortical fixation can improve construct stiffness and decrease the risk of pullout. Augmenting spinal instrumentation with sublaminar wires or PMMA cement also decreases the risk of fixation failure. Injecting PMMA cement through a fenestrated trocar and performing retrograde prefilling of the tapped pedicle screw pilot hole result in the greatest pullout strength. Lastly, in addition to augmenting the pedicle screws with PMMA, prophylactic cement augmentation using a tapered dose of bone cement in the upper instrumented vertebra UIV (4 cc), the UIV +1 (3 cc), and the UIV + 2 (2 cc) may decrease the risk of proximal supra-adjacent vertebral fractures, PJK, and revision surgery.

References

1. United States Census Bureau. 2012 US Census Bureau. Available at: http://www.census.gov/population/projections/data/national/2012.html. Accessed 27 Aug 2014.
2. Jacobs LA, Kent M, Lee M, et al. America's aging population. Popul Bull. 2011;66:2e16.
3. Grayson VK, Velkoff VA. The next four decades, the older population in the United States: 2010 to 2050. In: Current population reports. Washington, D.C.: United States Census Bureau; 2010. p. 25e1138.
4. Carter OD, Haynes SG. Prevalence rates for scoliosis in US adults: results from the first National Health and Nutrition Examination Survey. Int J Epidemiol. 1987;16:537e44.
5. Francis RS. Scoliosis screening of 3,000 college-aged women. The Utah Study–phase 2. Phys Ther. 1988;68:1513e6.
6. Kostuik JP, Bentivoglio J. The incidence of low-back pain in adult scoliosis. Spine (Phila Pa 1976). 1981;6:268e73.
7. Perennou D, Marcelli C, Herisson C, et al. Adult lumbar scoliosis. Epidemiologic aspects in a low-back pain population. Spine (Phila Pa 1976). 1994;19:123e8.
8. Schwab F, Dubey A, Gamez L, et al. Adult scoliosis: prevalence, SF-36, and nutritional parameters in an elderly volunteer population. Spine (Phila Pa 1976). 2005;30:1082e5.
9. Finkelstein JS, Cleary RL, Butler JP, Antonelli R, Mitlak BH, Deraska DJ, Zamora-Quezada JC, Neer RM. A comparison of lateral versus anterior-posterior spine dual energy x-ray absorptiometry for the diagnosis of osteopenia. J Clin Endocrinol Metabol. 1994;78(3):724–30.
10. Kohan E, Nemani V, Hershman SH, Kang D, Kelly MP. Lumbar computed tomography scans are not appropriate surrogates for bone mineral density scans in primary adult spinal deformity. Neurosurg Focus. 2017;43(6):E4.
11. Choi MK, Kim SM, Lim JK. Diagnostic efficacy of Hounsfield units in spine CT for the assessment of real bone mineral density of degenerative spine: correlation study between T-scores determined by DEXA scan and Hounsfield units from CT. Acta Neurochir. 2016;158:1421.
12. Russell RG, Muhlbauer RC, Bisaz S, Williams DA, Fleisch H. The influence of pyrophosphate, condensed phosphates, phosphonates and other phosphate compounds on the dissolution of hydroxyapatite in vitro and on bone resorption induced by parathyroid hormone in tissue culture and in thyroparathyroidectomised rats. Calcif Tissue Res. 1970;6(3):183–96.
13. Plotkin LI, Weinstein RS, Parfitt AM, Roberson PK, Manolagas SC, Bellido T. Prevention of osteocyte and osteoblast apoptosis by bisphosphonates and calcitonin. J Clin Invest. 1999;104(10):1363–74.
14. Plotkin LI, Aguirre JI, Kousteni S, Manolagas SC, Bellido T. Bisphosphonates and estrogens inhibit osteocyte apoptosis via distinct molecular mechanisms downstream of extracellular signal-regulated kinase activation. J Biol Chem. 2005;280:7317–25. Epub 2004 Dec 6.
15. Riek AE, Towler DA. The pharmacological management of osteoporosis. Mo Med. 2011;108(2):118–23.
16. Saag KG, Shane E, Boonen S, et al. Teriparatide or alendronate in glucocorticoid-induced osteoporosis. N Engl J Med. 2007;357(20):2028–39.
17. Yuan F, Peng W, Yang C, Zheng J. Teriparatide versus bisphosphonates for the treatment of postmeno-

pausal osteoporosis: a meta-analysis. Int J Surg. 2019;66:1–11.
18. Ohtori S, Inoue G, Orita S, et al. Teriparatide accelerates lumbar posterolateral fusion in women with postmenopausal osteoporosis: prospective study. Spine. 2012;37:E1464–8.
19. Ohtori S, Inoue G, Orita S, et al. Comparison of teriparatide and bisphosphonate treatment to reduce pedicle screw loosening after lumbar spinal fusion surgery in postmenopausal women with osteoporosis from a bone quality perspective. Spine. 2013;38:E487–92.
20. Bjerke BT, Zarrabian M, Aleem IS, et al. Incidence of osteoporosis-related complications following posterior lumbar fusion. Global Spine J. 2018;8:563–9.
21. Kaliya-Perumal AK, Lu ML, Luo CA, et al. Retrospective radiological outcome analysis following teriparatide use in elderly patients undergoing multilevel instrumented lumbar fusion surgery. Medicine. 2017;96:e5996.
22. Yagi M, Ohne H, Konomi T, et al. Teriparatide improves volumetric bone mineral density and fine bone structure in the UIV+1 vertebra, and reduces bone failure type PJK after surgery for adult spinal deformity. Osteoporos Int. 2016;27:3495–502.
23. Brantley AG, Mayfield JK, Koeneman JB, Clarck KR. The effects of pedicle screw fit. An in vitro study. Spine. 1994;19(15):1752–8.
24. Matsukawa K, Yato Y, Imabayashi H, et al. Biomechanical evaluation of fixation strength among different sizes of pedicle screws using the cortical bone trajectory: what is the ideal screw size for optimal fixation? Acta Neurochir. 2016;158:465–71.
25. Karami KJ, Buckenmeyer LE, Kiapour AM, et al. Biomechanical evaluation of the pedicle screw insertion depth effect on screw stability under cyclic loading and subsequent pullout. J Spinal Disord Tech. 2014;28:E133. https://doi.org/10.1097/BSD.0000000000000178.
26. Zindrick MR, Wiltse LL, Widell EH, Thomas JC, Holland WR, Field BT, Spencer CW. A biomechanical study of intrapeduncular screw fixation in the lumbosacral spine. Clin Orthop. 1986;203:99–112.
27. Halvorson TL, Kelly LA, Thomas KA, et al. Effects of bone mineral density on pedicle screw fixation. Spine. 1994;19:2415–20.
28. Soshi S, Shiba R, Kondo H, Murota K. An experimental study on transpedicular screw fixation in relation to osteoporosis of the lumbar spine. Spine. 1991;16:1335–41.
29. Elder BD, Lo SF, Holes C, et al. The biomechanics of pedicle screw augmentation with cement. Spine J. 2015;15(6):1432–45.
30. Burval DJ, McLain RF, Milks R, Inceoglu S. Primary pedicle screw augmentation in osteoporotic lumbar vertebrae – biomechanical analysis of pedicle fixation strength. Spine. 2007;32(10):1077–83.
31. Costa F, Ortolina A, Galbusera F, et al. Pedicle screw cement augmentation. A mechanical pullout study on different cement augmentation techniques. Med Eng Phys. 2016;38(2):181–6.
32. Paxinos O, Tsitsopoulos PP, Zindrick MR, et al. Evaluation of pullout strength and failure mechanism of posterior instrumentation in normal and osteopenic thoracic vertebrae. Laboratory investigation. J Neurosurg Spine. 2010;13:469–76.
33. Hart RA, Prendergast MA, Roberts WG, et al. Proximal junctional acute collapse cranial to multilevel lumbar fusion: a cost analysis of prophylactic vertebral augmentation. Spine J. 2008;8:875–81.
34. Kebaish KM, Martin CT, O'Brien JR, et al. Use of vertebroplasty to prevent proximal junctional fractures in adult deformity surgery: a biomechanical cadaveric study. Spine J. 2013;13:1897–903.
35. Raman T, Miller E, Martin CT, Kebaish KM. The effect of prophylactic vertebroplasty on the incidence of proximal junctional kyphosis and proximal junctional failure following posterior spinal fusion in adult spinal deformity: a 5-year follow-up study. Spine J. 2017;17:1489–98.
36. Zavatsky J, Shah A, McGuire R, et al. Reduced rate of proximal junctional fractures above long-segment instrumented constructs utilizing a tapered dose of bone cement for prophylactic vertebroplasty, a biomechanical investigation. Global Spine J. 2017;6(1):s-0036-1582954. https://doi.org/10.1055/s-0036-1582954.

Sacral Insufficiency Fractures

19

Nicholas Shepard and Nirmal C. Tejwani

Key Points

1. SIF are increasingly recognized in elderly patients with atraumatic low back pain or following low-energy trauma.
2. A high degree of suspicion for SIF is needed given frequently negative initial workup and imaging.
3. Management of SIF consists of conservative therapies with emphasis on analgesia and early mobilization.
4. Operative therapy including screw fixation or sacroplasty may be indicated in patients with displaced fracture or with persistent intractable pain and morbidity.

Introduction

Sacral insufficiency fractures (SIF) are a common cause of low back pain in the elderly. First described by Lourie in 1982, SIF are increasingly recognized as a source of morbidity in older patients [1]. These fractures may occur spontaneously or following low-energy trauma in patients with risk factors such as osteoporosis, malignancy, or prior radiation. SIF can be classified as a type of stress fractures, in which repetitive loading exceeds the mechanical resistance of bone. The two primary types of stress fractures include insufficiency and fatigue fractures, which are differentiated based on underlying bone physiology and mechanism of injury. Specifically, an insufficiency fracture occurs when normal or physiologic stress is applied to abnormal bone with decreased elastic resistance. This differs from fatigue fractures, which result when abnormal stresses are applied to normal bone [2]. This strict classification of SIF is difficult, as they can occur when osteoporotic bone is subjected to minor trauma. Therefore, some authors have preferred to define these osteoporotic fractures as fragility fractures of the pelvis [3].

Incidence

The true incidence of SIF is difficult to estimate given its subtle presentation and diagnosis. Compared to other types of osteoporotic fractures, especially those involving the axial spine, the relative incidence is still low [4]. However, with an aging population, the prevalence of osteoporotic fractures including SIF is expected

N. Shepard
Department of Orthopedic Surgery, NYU Langone Orthopedic Hospital, NYU Langone Medical Center, New York, NY, USA
e-mail: Nicholas.shepard@nyumc.org

N. C. Tejwani (✉)
Department of Orthopedics, NYU Langone Orthopedic Hospital, NYU Langone Medical Center, New York, NY, USA
e-mail: Nirmal.Tejwani@nyumc.org

A. E. Razi, S. H. Hershman (eds.), *Vertebral Compression Fractures in Osteoporotic and Pathologic Bone*, https://doi.org/10.1007/978-3-030-33861-9_19

to increase over the next 20 years. The most frequent sites include fractures of the vertebra (27%), wrist (19%), hip (14%), pelvis (7%), and other locations (33%) [5].

With increasing awareness, SIF are being more commonly recognized and diagnosed with a reported incidence of 1% to 20% in at-risk populations [4, 6–9]. Early reports by Weber et al. noted an incidence of 1.8% in 1015 female patients older than 55 years admitted to their institution for low back pain [9]. This was lower than those rates reported by Hatzl-Griesenhofer et al. who found 102 sacral fractures on bone scintigraphy in elderly patients with acute-onset low back pain following incidental trauma with negative radiographs over a 2-year period [7]. In another single-center retrospective review of 1017 bone scans in patients over 70 years, 194 (19%) SIF were identified [8]. Recently, a review of 250 patients with atraumatic acute back pain presenting to the emergency room identified 11 (4.4%) sacral fractures diagnosed via CT or MRI [10].

SIF often go unrecognized due to nonspecific symptoms and negative initial imaging. A high level of suspicion is needed in high-risk patients, particularly elderly females with a preexisting history of osteoporosis or osteopenia. Given these difficulties, there is frequently a delay between clinical presentation and the use of appropriate sacral imaging that may identify previously missed or misdiagnosed SIF. Various reports have found an average delay in the accurate diagnosis of SIF between 24 and 55 days, emphasizing the need for a high index of suspicion during the initial evaluation [10, 11].

Anatomy and Biomechanics

The sacrum is a triangular or wedge-shaped bone formed by the fusion of five vertebral segments. Important articulations include the ilium along its lateral border, fifth lumbar vertebra along its cranial border and coccyx at its caudal extension. While there is no classification specific to SIF, the sacrum and associated fractures have been characterized by Denis and consists of three

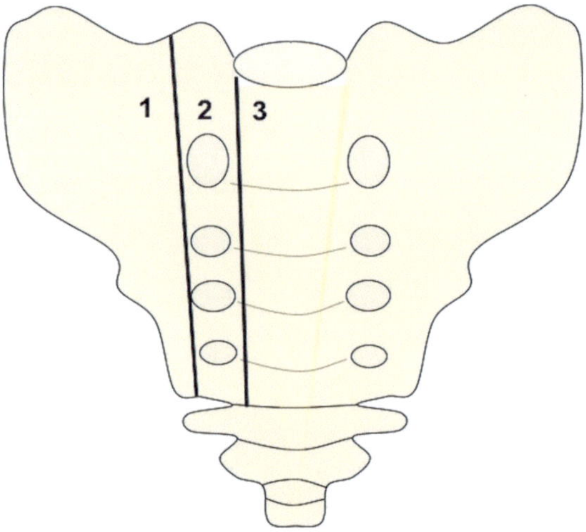

Fig. 19.1 Denis classification. Zone 1 falls lateral to sacral foramina. Zone 2 includes the sacral foramina without extension into the central canal. Zone 3 consists of the sacral body and central canal

zones (Fig. 19.1) [12]. Zone 1, which includes the sacral ala and falls lateral to the neural foramina, is the most common site for SIF [13]. Zone 2 includes the sacral foramina without extension into the spinal canal. Zone 3 involves the sacral body and central spinal canal. Given its relationship to the sacral nerve roots and central canal, SIF are rarely associated with neurologic symptoms, which differ from fractures in zones 2 and 3 that are commonly traumatic in nature and may have neurologic deficits on initial presentation [12, 14, 15].

SIF classically consist of an H-type fracture that runs vertically along both sacral ala and is connected by a horizontal component through the sacral body (Fig. 19.2) [1]. However, each of these segments may be absent, and instead an isolated unilateral or bilateral vertical fracture or unilateral vertical fracture with horizontal component may predominate. While bilateral fractures are thought to be most common, studies examining fracture morphology have failed to identify a predominant type [16, 17]. In one review of 102 SIF diagnosed with bone scan, only 19.6% exhibited typical H-type pattern versus 32.4% unilateral vertical, 6.9% bilateral vertical, 27.4% horizontal, and 13.7% half H-type fractures [7]. This differed from analysis of 85

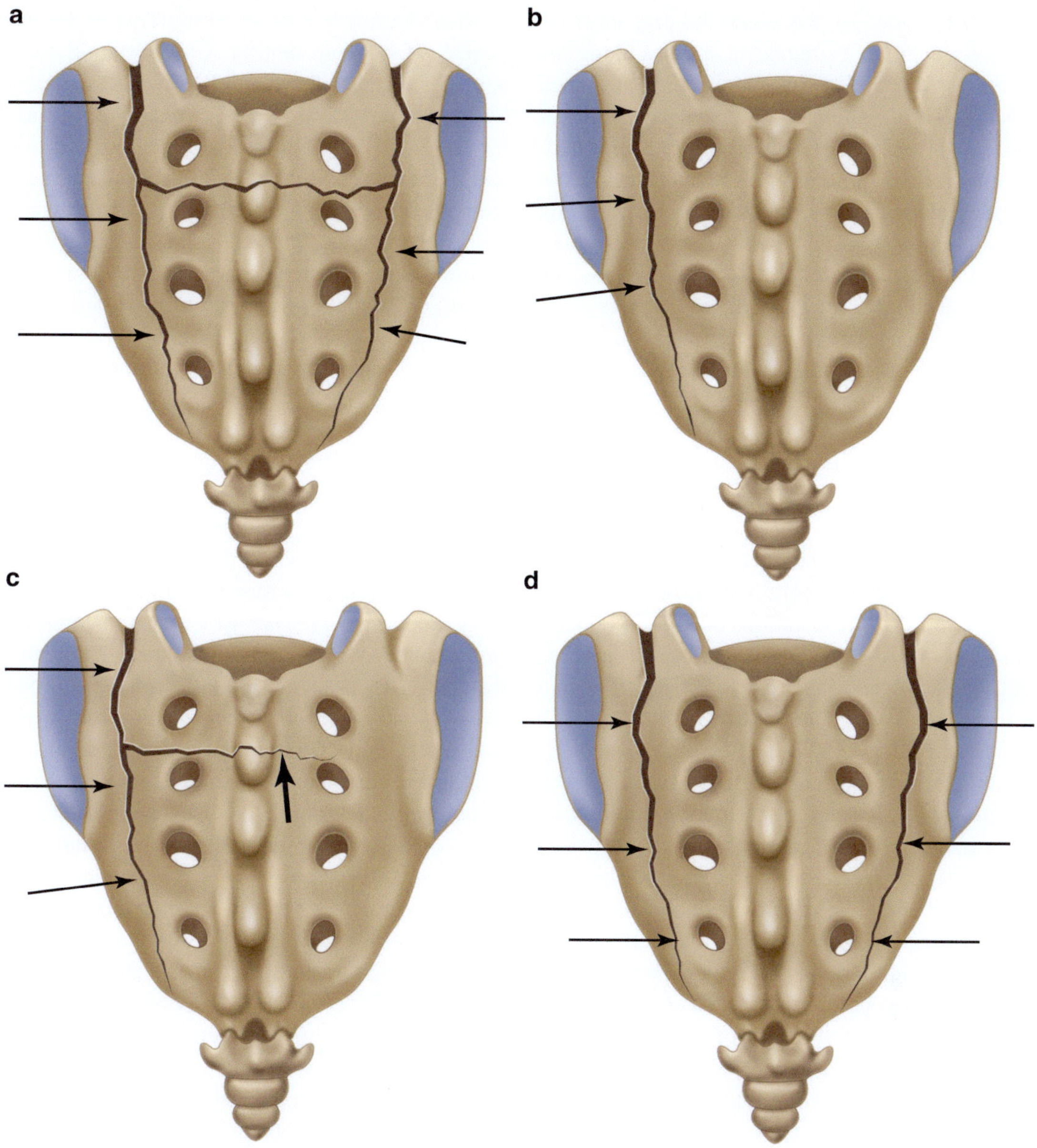

Fig. 19.2 Characteristic SIF fracture patterns (**a**) depict classical H-type fracture consisting of bilateral vertical fractures with horizontal segment, (**b**) unilateral vertical fracture, (**c**) unilateral vertical fracture with horizontal component, and (**d**) bilateral isolated vertical fractures

osteoporotic fractures, which had 61.2% H-type, 19.8% unilateral vertical only, 11.8% bilateral vertical only, and 8.2% unilateral vertical plus horizontal component [18].

Fracture morphology is likely related to the underlying osteoporosis, which preferentially affects trabecular rather than cortical bone. The ala, which has a high ratio of trabecular to cortical bone compared to the sacral body and neural foraminal region, is therefore particularly susceptible. As hypothesized by Cooper, when a bilateral vertical fracture occurs, the sagittal support provided by the sacral ala may be compromised leading to increased stresses along the central portion of the sacrum. With sustained axial stress in conjunction with natural lumbar lordosis, compression of the anterior sacral bodies may result in a horizontal fracture component [19]. Anatomic pelvic models of stress during ambulation support this theory and have demonstrated little to no transverse stress across the central portion of the sacrum if the sacrum is intact. A potential exception is patients with excessive lumbar lordosis, atypical stress patterns, or advanced osteoporosis [18].

Risk Factors

Multiple metabolic and mechanical risk factors have been associated with SIF (Table 19.1). The most common presentation occurs in elderly postmenopausal females with osteoporosis [2, 6, 20]. Age has been found to be a separate risk factor, with the average age of SIF ranging from 65 to 71 years old [13, 21, 22]. In their systematic review, Yoder et al. analyzed 101 cases of SIF and found that 75 patients were elderly females with an average age of 70.5 years, and 36 had a preexisting diagnosis of osteoporosis [21]. This was similar to the meta-analysis conducted by Finiels et al. who analyzed 493 SIF in the literature and 15 from the author's institution. They found that most fractures occurred in patients over 60 years of age and over two-thirds were insidious in onset without a history of trauma [22].

Other common risk factors involve processes that compromise the mechanical strength of bone. This includes metabolic conditions and medical therapy that either temporarily or permanently affect bone density. Corticosteroid therapy, which can lead to steroid-induced osteopenia with long-term use, is a well-established risk factor for SIF [21]. Similarly, rheumatoid arthritis and its treatment with long-term steroid suppression has been show to increase the risk for insufficiency fractures. These patients are also likely to have a mechanical component due to their impaired functional demand and resultant stress applied to the bone [23–26]. Additional causes of secondary osteoporosis reported in the literature include hyperparathyroidism [27], renal osteodystrophy [28], and Paget's disease [29]. Transplant patients including the liver, kidney, and lung are also at increased risk due to a combination of the required medical therapy and metabolic derangements that may result from solid-organ transplantation [30–32].

Tables 19.1 Metabolic and mechanical risk factors for SIF

SIF risk factors	
Osteoporosis	Radiation therapy
Rheumatoid arthritis	Corticosteroid therapy
Organ transplant (lung, liver, kidney)	Anorexia nervosa
Paget's disease	Prior spinal instrumentation
Renal osteodystrophy	

A history of pelvic irradiation is another important consideration in patients with potential SIF. Its association with impaired bone strength and insufficiency fractures in oncologic patients is well documented; however, delays in diagnosis often occur due to complicated symptomology and high suspicion for tumor recurrence or metastases [28, 33–36]. Ikushima et al. reviewed 158 patients with gynecologic malignancies who underwent pelvic irradiation and noted an 11.4% incidence of insufficiency fractures, the majority of which occurred within 12 months. In cases of SIF following irradiation, the typical symmetric bilateral vertical fracture pattern occurred, which can help to differentiate between SIF and metastases [36]. Blomile et al. noted even higher rates (89%) of insufficiency fractures in 18 patients with cervical cancer who underwent pelvic irradiation, 7 of whom were premenopausal [33]. Males are also at increased risk following radiation for conditions such as prostate cancer. One review of 134 males with prostate cancer who had pelvic radiation as part of their definitive treatment found a 6.8% 5-year incidence of SIF [35].

Prior spinal surgery and instrumentation may also impact the structural integrity of the spinal column and sacrum, thereby increasing the risk for sacral stress fractures especially in patients with preexisting osteoporosis. In these instances, the primary cause is due to the abnormal distribution of force along the spinal column and sacrum following fusion and instrumentation, which is more consistent with a fatigue-type fracture [37]. When noted, sacral stress fractures frequently occur at or the level below instrumentation and may be an isolated horizontal fracture [38]. The exact timing of presentation is variable but occurs on average 5 months following the index procedure [39]. Meredith et al. analyzed 394 patients who underwent spinopelvic fusion from L5-S1 and found 24 (6.1%) sacral fractures at a mean of 4.3 months. Females over 67 years who had instrumentation of three or more levels were at the highest risk [40].

Clinical Presentation and Evaluation

Patients with SIF often have a vague and nonspecific presentation, which makes it difficult to obtain the appropriate imaging and diagnosis. A thorough history is necessary to identify possible risk factors that may predispose to stress fractures and any history of trauma. The most common presenting symptoms are diffuse, intractable low back and buttock pain, though patients may also present with pelvic, hip, or groin discomfort with or without radiation to the thigh [9, 13, 21]. Tamaki et al. noted that low back pain (36.4%), gluteal pain (63.6%), and coxalgia (19.2%) were the most frequent complaints in patients with traumatic SIF presenting to the emergency room [10].

Antecedent trauma typically consists of a low-energy mechanism, e.g., a mechanical trip and fall from standing height or a seated position. Cadaveric studies have shown that as little force as 3200 ± 1200 N is required to reproduce SIF in an osteoporotic sacrum [41]. Minor trauma preceding the onset of symptoms may occur in only one-third of cases, as many SIF occur spontaneously with the acute onset of sudden pain that is exacerbated by weight-bearing and restricted functional mobility [22, 42]. Neurologic symptoms are rare and if present can be indicative of concomitant pathology of the central cord, lumbar spine, or pelvis. Case reports of SIF associated with cauda equina have been reported but are exceedingly rare [43].

On examination, point tenderness over the distal aspect of the lumbar spine and sacrum may be present, though it is not frequently encountered [44]. Stability of the pelvic ring must be assessed given the frequent association between SIF and additional pelvic fractures. Provocative testing of the sacrum and sacroiliac joints including flexion-abduction-external rotation (FABER) and simultaneous maximal hip flexion and contralateral hip extension while supine (Gaenslen' test) will often illicit significant pain but are poorly tolerated in the acute setting and have poor specificity for SIF. If the patient is able to ambulate, gait testing will be significant for a slowed, antalgic gait with poor overall mobility [13].

Imaging

Given the nonspecific presentation of SIF and its association with low back pain, initial imaging is frequently focused on the lumbar spine and/or pelvis. This may lead to delayed recognition and diagnosis [10, 45]. Imaging techniques useful in the diagnosis of SIF include radiographs, MRI, bone scintigraphy, and CT scans.

Plain Radiographs

The initial diagnostic workup includes plain film radiographs, which consists of anterior posterior (AP) views of the pelvis and possibly AP and lateral views of the lumbar spine depending on symptomology. Supplemental radiographs including pelvic inlet and outlet views may be ordered to better assess the pelvic ring. However, insufficiency fractures are difficult to detect on radiograph, and frequently plain X-rays are not sensitive and inadequate [11]. This is particularly true in the acute setting prior to calcification at the fracture site. Additionally, overlying bowel gas, calcified iliac arteries, demineralization of the surrounding bone, and SI joint arthritis can obscure visualization making diagnosis difficult

[46]. Less than 15–20% of injuries are detected on initial evaluation, and after retrospective review of patients with SIF confirmed on CT or bone scintigraphy, only 30–50% of injuries can be detected on plain radiographs [16, 47].

When present, SIF usually present as vertical lines of sclerosis lateral to the neural foramina (Fig. 19.3) [11] . This is best appreciated in subacute or chronic injuries after the initiation of fracture healing. Typically, there are no distinct fracture lines, but subtle anterior cortical disruptions can be detected (Fig. 19.4) [48]. A review of 20 patients with SIF found that that fracture lines were evident in 12.5% of cases, and sclerosis was only noted in 57% of cases [6]. The onset and resolution of sclerosis at the fracture site is variable and ranges from 1 to 13 months after initial presentation [49].

Computed Tomography (CT)

Following plain radiographs, CT is often the next step in the diagnostic workup for possible SIF and is a useful adjunct to advance imaging such as MRI or bone scintigraphy. Compared to X-rays, CT has a greater sensitivity with reported rates of 60–75% [50, 51]. Characteristic findings include cortical disruption over the anterior sacral cortex in Zone 1 of the sacrum consistent with vertical fractures (Figs. 19.5 and 19.6). Additionally, compression of the sacral ala medial to the SI joint may be appreciated. In these instances, CT relies on the presence of cortical irregularities for appropriate diagnosis, but in cases of occult fracture especially in an atraumatic setting, CT may be negative. Given these subtle findings, SIF are often overlooked or misinterpreted on the initial reading [47].

Magnetic Resonance Imaging (MRI)

Magnetic resonance imaging (MRI) is the most sensitive imaging technique for SIF with reported sensitivities of 98–100% [48]. Its application in

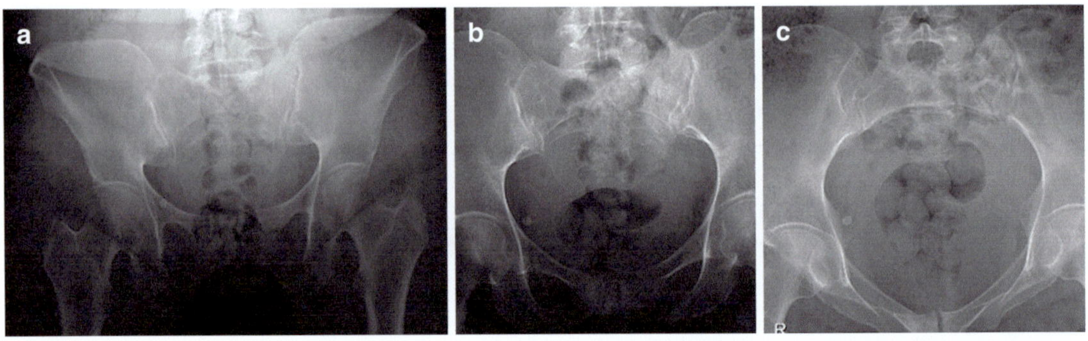

Fig. 19.3 Plain radiographs including (**a**) AP pelvis and (**b**, **c**) pelvic views demonstrating sclerosis in the left sacral ala suggestive of SIF

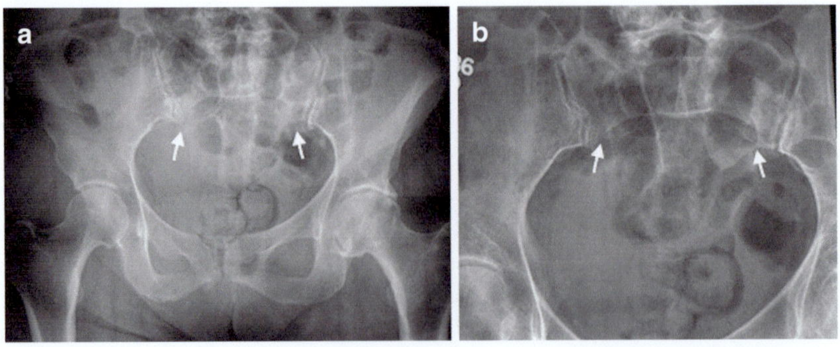

Fig. 19.4 Plain radiographs including (**a**) AP pelvis and (**b**) sacral view demonstrating bilateral anterior cortical disruption (arrows) indicative of bilateral vertical SIF

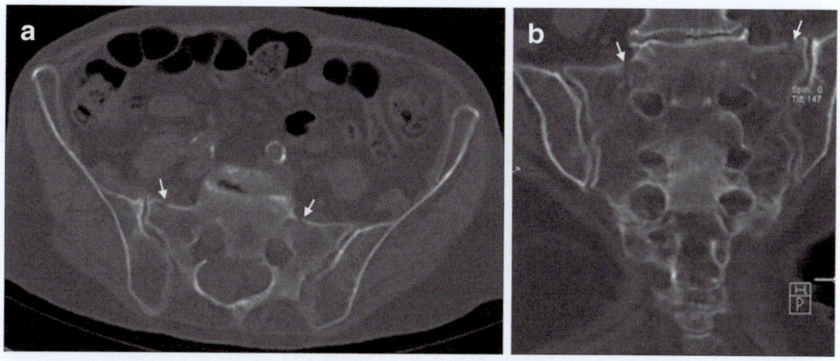

Fig. 19.5 Computed tomography (CT) including (**a**) axial and (**b**) coronal views demonstrating bilateral vertical SIF (arrows)

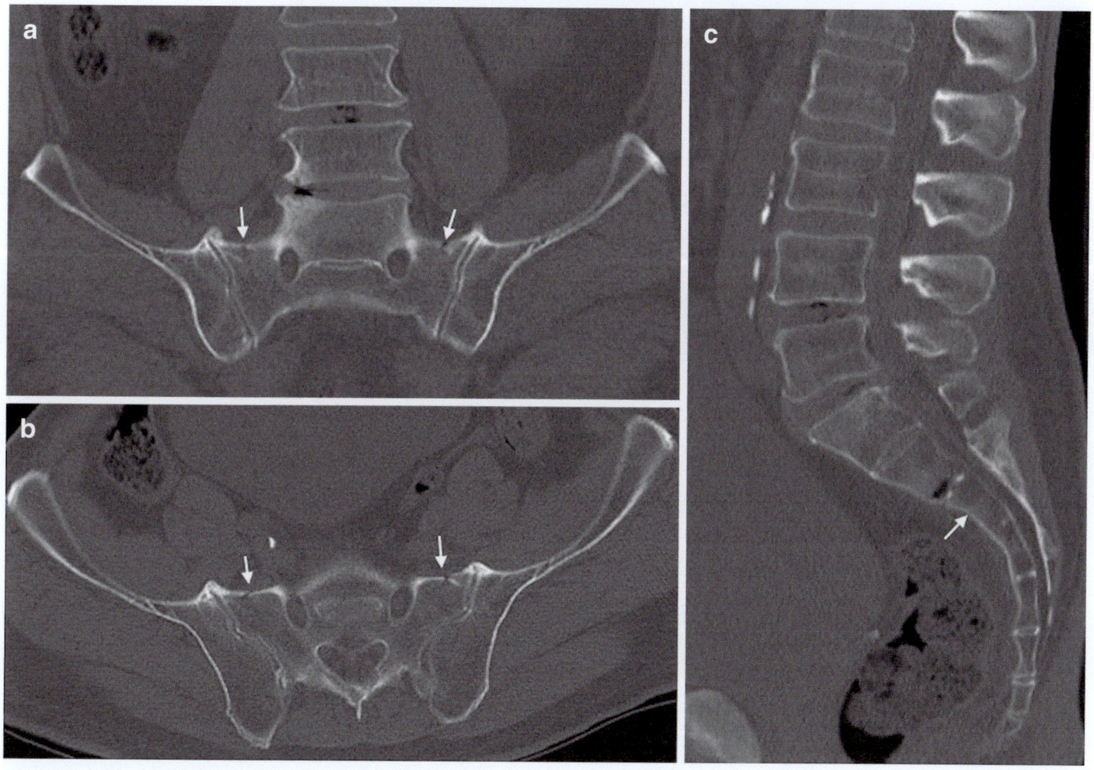

Fig. 19.6 CT including (**a**, **b**) coronal and (**c**) sagittal views demonstrating bilateral vertical SIF with horizontal component at S2 (arrows)

early injuries can detect marrow edema representative of post-traumatic bone hemorrhage related to SIF as early as 18 days after the initial symptoms. Case reports have described the presence of SIF on CT with negative MRI; however, this imaging was conducted in the acute setting possibly prior to the onset of early signal changes [52]. The marrow edema associated with SIF appears as low signal intensity on T1-weighted imaging and increased signal intensity on T2-weighted or short tau inversion recovery (STIR) series (Figs. 19.7 and 19.8) [51, 53]. Patterns of signal change will often mimic the fracture morphology as bands of abnormal signal paralleling the SI joint. These signal changes are also associated with other pathologic and non-pathologic processes including stress reactions, malignancy, nutrient vessels, and hyperplastic

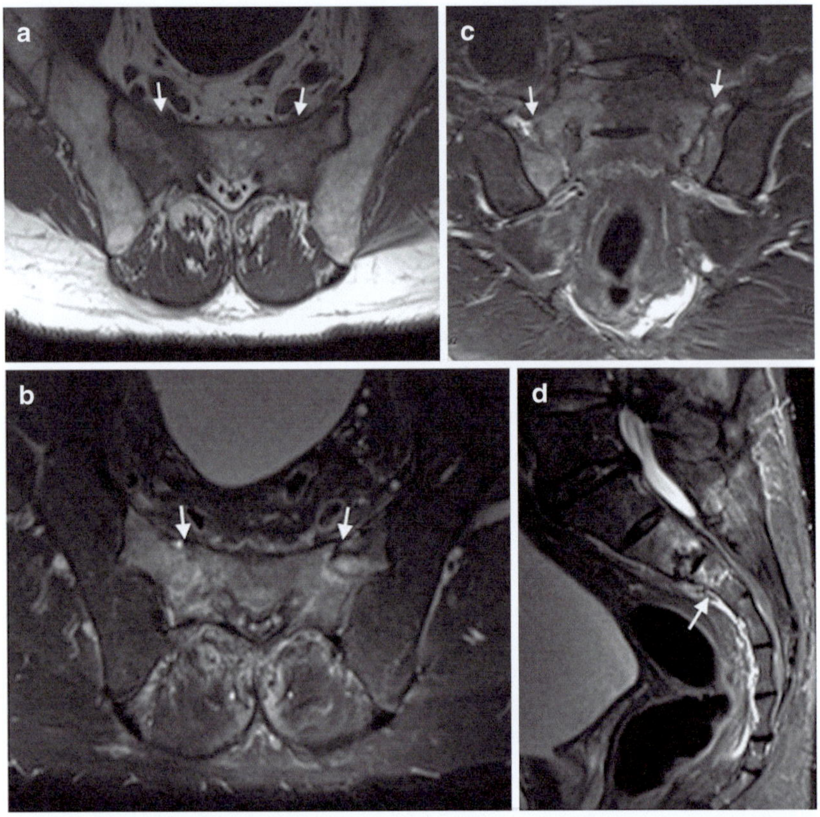

Fig. 19.7 MRI including (**a**) T1 axial, (**b**) T2 axial, (**c**) STIR axial, and (**d**) T2 sagittal series demonstrating bilateral SIF with horizontal component at S2 (arrows)

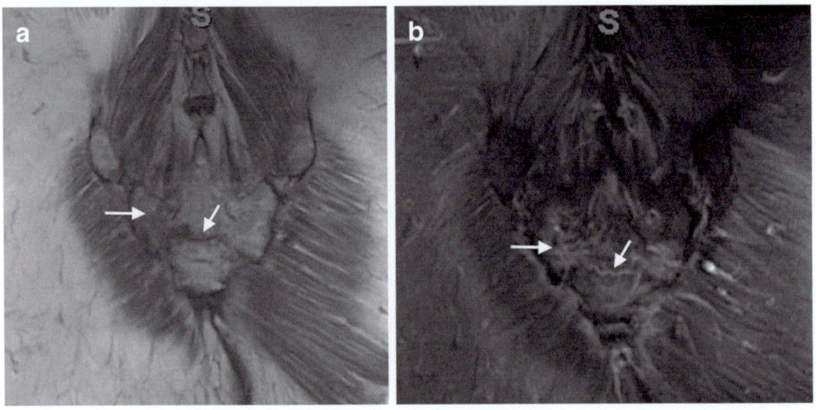

Fig. 19.8 MRI including sagittal (**a**) T1 and (**b**) T2 series demonstrating right vertical SIF with horizontal component

bone marrow [54]. This is of particular importance with SIF given their association with malignancy and pelvic irradiation, which can sometimes mislead the diagnosis.

In addition to signal changes within the sacral ala, a distinct fracture line may be present but is not required for diagnosis. Cabbarus et al. noted that in at least 7% of SIF, there was not a clearly discernable fracture. Adjacent soft tissue edema was present in approximately one-third of cases compared to 65% of pubic rami fractures [51]. When present, fracture lines can be seen as hypo-intense signal changes on T1-weighted imaging.

Bone Scintigraphy

Bone scintigraphy with technetium-99 m medronate methylene diphosphonate (MDP) is considered an important diagnostic tool for SIF given its high sensitivity; however, with increasing accessibility to MRI and inability to discern SIF from possible metastases, this imaging modality is now uncommonly used. For select patients, it has a sensitivity and positive predictive value of 96% and 92%, respectively [17]. The classical pattern of radiotracer uptake consists of the "H-type" pattern or a "Honda" sign (Fig. 19.9) [55]. When correlated to clinical symptoms consistent with SIF, this pattern is considered to be diagnostic. However, "H-type" fractures may not always be present and have been reported on bone scan in only 40–60% of cases [17, 22]. Radiotracer uptake may also be obscured by surrounding structures including the pubic bone, spine, and SI joints [17].

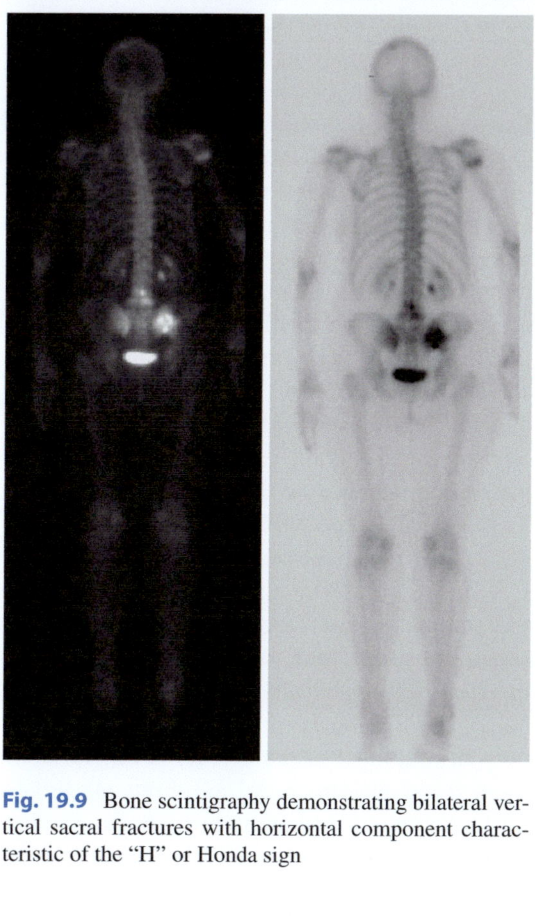

Fig. 19.9 Bone scintigraphy demonstrating bilateral vertical sacral fractures with horizontal component characteristic of the "H" or Honda sign

Treatment Options

Conservative Management

Initial management for the vast majority of SIF consists of conservative measures including limited rest, analgesia, and weight-bearing as pain allows using ambulation aides (cane, walker) with an emphasis on early mobilization as pain allows. Previously, some authors advocated for strict bed rest for pain control until symptom improvement. More recently, others have reported the importance of early mobilization and activity modification in a supervised environment to stimulate osteoblastic activity and prevent deconditioning [6, 9, 13, 56–58]. Assistive devices such as walkers, canes, or crutches can be used to offload weight-bearing on the affected sacrum allowing for early rehabilitation [13].

Symptom resolution with conservative therapy can take up to 1 year, though reported rates of recovery have varied from 4 to 15 months [11]. During this period, immobilization can be morbid, especially in an elderly population with SIF who may have preexisting comorbidities limiting their functional reserve. One particular concern is thromboembolic disease, with reported rates of deep vein thrombosis ranging from 29% to 61% and pulmonary embolism from 2% to 12% in patients with pelvic insufficiency fractures [58]. Additional well-known consequences include deleterious effects on muscle conditioning, the cardiopulmonary system, decubitus ulcers, and pneumonia [11].

Functional outcomes following SIF treated with conservative therapy are variable. However, these fractures are often a significant source of morbidity. Compared to displaced fractures of the pelvis, insufficiency fractures in the elderly have similar short-term and 2-year outcomes [59]. One series reviewed 60 patients aged 65 years or older found to have pelvic insufficiency fractures including 16 SIF who were managed with conservative therapy. They noted an overall mortality rate of 14.3%, with 25% of patients being institutionalized following the injury and 50% never returning to their former level of self-sufficiency [60]. In another smaller series of 20 patients with SIF, 17 were noted to have complete symptom resolution within 9 months with no patients reporting decreased independence in their daily activities [6].

Medical Management

Medical therapy in patients with SIF focuses on the underlying primary or secondary osteoporosis that predisposes to insufficiency fractures. While oral calcium and vitamin D supplements remain a mainstay of osteoporosis prevention, there is limited data to support their use in preexisting SIF, and additional supplementation may have limited efficacy in the setting of advanced osteoporosis [16]. Similarly, bisphosphonates are a common treatment of osteoporosis that act by inhibiting bone resorption and have been found to increase bone mineral density of the spine and hip [61, 62]. However, longtime use may negatively affect bone metabolism by inhibiting normal bone turnover, thereby predisposing to insufficiency fractures [63]. Once an insufficiency fracture has been identified, continuation of bisphosphonates remains controversial [42].

Newer anabolic agents are also being used in the setting of osteoporotic fractures. Teriparatide or recombinant human PTH has been used for insufficiency fractures, atypical fractures, and nonunions with promising results [64–66]. Its effect may increase bone mineral density and trabecular and cortical thickness thereby aiding fracture healing and preventing subsequent pathology [42]. Yoo et al. compared 21 patients with SIF who received daily teriparatide injections to 20 patients with SIF who did not receive additional medical therapies. They found that those treated with teriparatide had earlier time to mobilization (1.2 weeks vs 2.0 weeks) and faster bony healing with all patients receiving teriparatide demonstrating healed fractures by 8 weeks [67]. This is consistent with smaller case series that have shown improved SIF healing following the administration of teriparatide [68]. Alternatively, the use of PTH has also shown to have benefits in the setting of SIF. In one series five patients with SIF were treated with PTH and compared to ten cases of SIF without the use PTH. The treatment group receiving PTH was found to have shorter duration until bony union and improved VAS scores [69].

Surgical Management

Given the potential morbidity associated with immobility from intractable pain, operative stabilization has gained increasing popularity in the treatment of SIF in patients with displaced fractures or who have failed conservative therapy. The mainstay of surgical intervention previously consisted of screw fixation either via a minimally invasive or percutaneous approach. However, in recent years minimally invasive augmentation with cement, or sacroplasty, has gained wider spread use. While vertebroplasty has been well described for osteoporotic fractures of the vertebral column, this analogous procedure involving injection of bone cement into the pathologic sacrum is now being used to treat patients with persistent symptoms and/or disability [70–72].

Screw Fixation

Operative fixation of sacral fractures has evolved significantly over time with a shift away from open exposures toward minimally invasive techniques. However, in significantly displaced fractures, open reduction may be required with the use of spinopelvic fixation. Various methods of fixation have been described including iliosacral screws, transsacral bars, and posterior tension banding [73–76]. Regardless, fracture morphology, displacement, and areas of instability dictate the appropriate method of fixation.

Iliosacral screw fixation has been well described in the treatment of posterior ring injuries and is a useful method of osteosynthesis in the setting of SIF. Done in either a prone or supine position, one or two screws can be inserted percutaneously into the S1 and/or S2 body [77, 78]. The use of two screws may help to prevent rotational instability; however, variability in sacral anatomy may limit screw placement [79]. Another consideration is bone quality, which is likely to be poor in elderly patients with insufficiency fractures. In order to optimize screw purchase, iliosacral screws can be advanced to the midline of the vertebral body where the density of cancellous bone is higher relative to the sacral ala [80]. Additional augmentation with washers or PMMA (polymethylmethacrylate) cement has also been described to improve fixation [81, 82].

Another percutaneous approach is transsacral-transiliac screw fixation. This technique is useful in the setting of bilateral posterior ring injuries with poor bone quality and may help to overcome weak screw purchase if used in the sacrum alone [83]. These constructs consist of a partially threaded 6.5 or 7.3 mm single or double transsacral-transiliac screw that traverses the sacrum through either the S1 or S2 body [84]. Screw size and location are dictated by the sacral anatomy and therefore require careful preoperative planning. When passing the screws, the goal is to insert them through safe anatomic pathways in the sacrum called transsacral corridors, which vary in size and location [79]. Sanders et al. recently reported on 11 patients who underwent transsacral-transiliac screw fixation for SIF following failed non-operative management. They found all patients went onto fracture healing with significant improvements in VAS and Oswestry Low Back Disability Index scores following surgery, with no surgical complications [84].

Sacroplasty

First described by Garant, sacroplasty has evolved from the principles of vertebroplasty used for insufficiency fractures in the thoracic and lumbar spine [85]. Early attempts at cement injection into the sacrum were used for painful metastases, and since then the technique has evolved for use with SIF. It has gained increased popularity, especially in cases of nondisplaced SIF refractory to non-operative management. This percutaneous procedure involves the forceful injection of PMMA cement into the fractures site, which is then distributed throughout the area of injury. Once hardened, the cement acts to stabilize the fracture allowing for pain relief and early mobilization. Various percutaneous methods have been described and will be detailed below, including the use of CT with or without fluoroscopic guidance.

The biomechanical principles of sacroplasty have not been well elucidated. Compared to vertebroplasty, where cement acts to resist compressive forces along the axis of the spine, sacroplasty must counteract shear forces along vertically oriented fracture lines in the sacrum [50]. The proposed advantage of this technique is that injecting cement stabilizes the fracture and prevents continued micromotion, thereby improving pain. This has been supported by finite element analysis (FEA) in cadaveric models that have demonstrated that PMMA injection with sacroplasty decreases fracture propagation by 93% and micromotion at the fracture site by 48% [86]. This stabilization may only occur locally at the fracture site, as additional FEA models have showed increases in overall sacral stiffness by only 1–4% vs 40–60% at the site of cement-bone interface [87]. However, cadaveric testing has failed to show restoration of strength or stiffness following cement injection, regardless of the volume injected or the approach used [88, 89].

Multiple basic approaches have been described for needle introduction into the fracture site and include a posterior or short-axis, long-axis, and midline approach. The two primary approaches consist of a posterior (short-axis) or long-axis approach, while a midline approach is typically used if additional injections are needed into a horizontal fracture component [11]. In the short-axis approach, the needle is placed in the posterior-to-anterior direction versus a long-axis approach where the needle is introduced in the caudal-cephalad direction [90]. The long-axis approach has the potential benefit of using a single cannula, injecting cement directly along a vertically oriented fracture line, and decreased risk of ventral perforation/extravasation [91]. In either case there is the potential risk of perforating the anterior or superior cortex and entering the sacral foramen [92].

Posterior (Short-Axis) Technique

The patient is positioned prone in a radiologic suite and a lateral scout CT, or fluoroscopic imaging is taken for localization. The choice of posterior puncture site is dependent on fracture

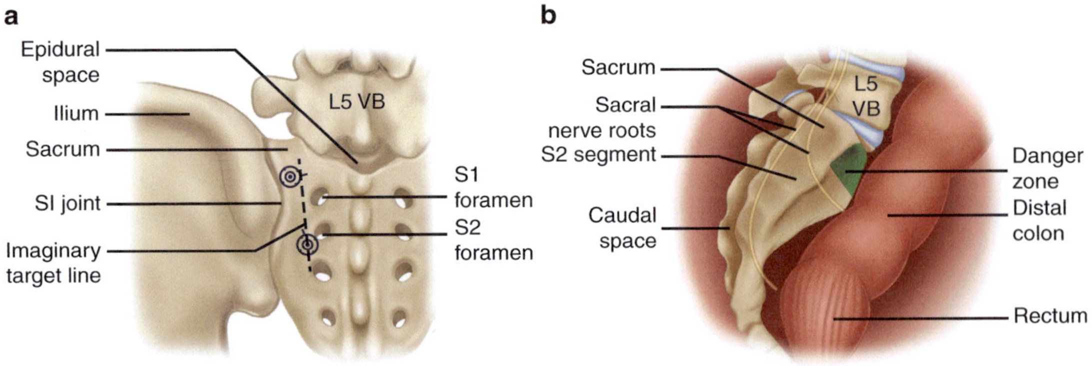

Fig. 19.10 Short-axis technique for percutaneous sacroplasty. (**a**) Appropriate start point in coronal plane lateral to sacral foramina at S1 and S2 and (**b**) needle position in the sagittal plane. Tip should not extend into anterior 1/3 of S1 body to prevent anterior perforation

location and morphology. Traditionally a posterolateral approach is used, which begins at a point centered on the S1 or S2 vertebral body, halfway between the dorsal aspect of the sacral foramina and SI joint (Fig. 19.10). Alternatively, an oblique central posterior approach can be used, which is centered over the sacral ala but angles medially between the spinal canal and sacral foramina. Once the appropriate approach has been determined, a small incision is made, and the needle is introduced into the posterior cortex of the sacrum and advanced 2–3 mm. Location is confirmed with CT or fluoroscopic imaging. After necessary adjustments are made, the needle is advance in small 5–10 mm intervals with manual pressure or with a mallet, checking position with localizing images. Final position of the needle should be within 10 mm to the anterior sacral cortex; however, care must be taken not to penetrate the anterior cortex. If using fluoroscopy, optimal needle position on lateral films will be within the anterior aspect of the middle third of the vertebral body. On AP imaging, confirmation of needle placement lateral to the sacral foramina must be achieved.

Once the needle is in appropriate position, the cement is prepared. When choosing cement, it should preferentially contain opacifiers to allow for visualization and have a long setting time. Cement is then injected in 0.5 mL aliquots, with repeat imaging after each injection. Between injections, the needle is removed along the fracture line in 1 cm intervals, but if cement extravasation is noted, injection through that needle should cease. The total volume of cement injected ranges from 3 to 8 mL per side and varies on fracture pattern, location, and morphology. Once the cement has hardened, the needles can be removed and surgical site is dressed. Postoperatively, patients are monitored for neurologic change. They are made weight-bearing as tolerated, given appropriate analgesia, and can be discharged on the same day.

Long-Axis Technique [90]

The patient is positioned prone on the radiologic procedure table, and the imaging beam is canted cephalad to align the image with the L5-S1 disk space and is oriented perpendicular to the long-axis of the sacrum. Localization is used to mark the starting point at the midpoint between the inferior aspect of the SI joint and lateral aspect of S3 foramen. A spinal needle is inserted, and positioning is checked on AP and lateral images. On lateral imaging, the needle is pointed toward the center of S1. Once the needle position is confirmed, the cannula is advanced into the posterior cortex approximately 1 cm. Position is confirmed on AP and lateral imaging. The cannula is advanced in 5–10 mm intervals, checking with localizing imaging at each interval. The final position should demonstrate the cannula tip 1 cm inferior to the geometric center of the S1 body. If the needle has advanced past this point, it should be withdrawn given the high risk of cephalad perforation.

After confirming the cannula position, cement is mixed and injected into the sacrum under fluoroscopic visualization. As the S1 body is filled, the cannula is withdrawn in 1 cm increments along the fracture line. Once the needle approaches the inferior aspect of the SI joint, cement injection is stopped. Approximately 3–8 mL of cement is injected. After the injection is completed, final imaging is done to confirm cement filling and evaluate for extravasation. The cannula sites are dressed and the patient is monitored for neurologic changes, made weight-bearing as tolerated with expected same-day discharge.

Long-term outcome data following sacroplasty is limited; early reports from multiple cases series have demonstrated favorable results with pain improvement. Dougherty et al. reported on 57 patients undergoing percutaneous sacroplasty and found that 76% of patients experienced at least 30% decrease in pain scores and 60% endorsed decrease opioid usage [93]. These improvements occur almost immediately following the procedure and persist at 1-year follow-up [94]. Another series by Gupta et al. consisting of 53 patients undergoing sacroplasty found significant improvements in VAS, Functional Mobility Scale, and Analgesic Scale scores with 93% reporting complete resolution or improvement in overall pain [95]. The largest series to date consists of 243 patients undergoing sacroplasty for SIF or sacral lesions. Preoperative VAS scores improved significantly from 9.2 ± 1.1 points to 1.9 ± 1.7 following CT-guided percutaneous sacroplasty [96]. By improving pain, the procedure may also allow for improved mobilization and decreased disability. Onen et al. found a decrease in ODI scores from 44 [38–46] preoperatively to 14 [11–22] postoperatively in patients undergoing sacroplasty [97]. Similarly, significant improvements in clinical mobility scale scores have been reported at 4, 24, and 48 weeks postoperatively [98].

While sacroplasty is considered a safe procedure, complications can result from extravasation of cement outside of the sacrum with neurologic compromise being the most concerning. Few reported cases of cement leakage into the sacral foramina have been reported with an overall frequency of PMMA extravasation of 7.4% [92, 94, 96, 98, 99]. The most commonly affected location is the S1 foramen resulting in S1 neuritis, which may improve with targeted epidural steroid injections [94]. However, in cases where the neuritis is refractory to conservative therapy, surgical decompression may be required to remove the cement and allow for nerve root decompression [99]. Additional potential complications include extravasation into the spinal canal, pulmonary emboli, and infection though no cases have been reported in the literature to date.

References

1. Lourie H. Spontaneous osteoporotic fracture of the sacrum. An unrecognized syndrome of the elderly. JAMA. 1982;248(6):715–7.
2. Pentecost RL, Murray RA, Brindley HH. Fatigue, insufficiency, and pathologic fractures. JAMA. 1964;187:1001–4.
3. Rommens PM, Hofmann A. Comprehensive classification of fragility fractures of the pelvic ring: Recommendations for surgical treatment. Injury. 2013;44(12):1733–44.
4. Mathis JM, Golovac S. Image-guided spine interventions. 2nd ed. New York: Springer; 2010. xii, 403 p. p.
5. Burge R, Dawson-Hughes B, Solomon DH, Wong JB, King A, Tosteson A. Incidence and economic burden of osteoporosis-related fractures in the United States, 2005–2025. J Bone Miner Res. 2007;22(3):465–75.
6. Gotis-Graham I, McGuigan L, Diamond T, Portek I, Quinn R, Sturgess A, et al. Sacral insufficiency fractures in the elderly. J Bone Joint Surg Br. 1994;76(6):882–6.
7. Hatzl-Griesenhofer M, Pichler R, Huber H, Maschek W. The insufficiency fracture of the sacrum. An often unrecognized cause of low back pain: results of bone scanning in a major hospital. Nuklearmedizin. 2001;40(6):221–7.
8. Wat SY, Seshadri N, Markose G, Balan K. Clinical and scintigraphic evaluation of insufficiency fractures in the elderly. Nucl Med Commun. 2007;28(3):179–85.
9. Weber M, Hasler P, Gerber H. Insufficiency fractures of the sacrum. Twenty cases and review of the literature. Spine (Phila Pa 1976). 1993;18(16):2507–12.

10. Tamaki Y, Nagamachi A, Inoue K, Takeuchi M, Sugiura K, Omichi Y, et al. Incidence and clinical features of sacral insufficiency fracture in the emergency department. Am J Emerg Med. 2017;35(9):1314.
11. Lyders EM, Whitlow CT, Baker MD, Morris PP. Imaging and treatment of sacral insufficiency fractures. AJNR Am J Neuroradiol. 2010;31(2):201–10.
12. Denis F, Davis S, Comfort T. Sacral fractures: an important problem. Retrospective analysis of 236 cases. Clin Orthop Relat Res. 1988;227:67–81.
13. Lin JT, Lane JM. Sacral stress fractures. J Womens Health (Larchmt). 2003;12(9):879–88.
14. Aresti N, Murugachandran G, Shetty R. Cauda equina syndrome following sacral fractures: a report of three cases. J Orthop Surg (Hong Kong). 2012;20(2):250–3.
15. Byrnes DP, Russo GL, Ducker TB, Cowley RA. Sacrum fractures and neurological damage. Report of two cases. J Neurosurg. 1977;47(3):459–62.
16. Schindler OS, Watura R, Cobby M. Sacral insufficiency fractures. J Orthop Surg (Hong Kong). 2007;15(3):339–46.
17. Fujii M, Abe K, Hayashi K, Kosuda S, Yano F, Watanabe S, et al. Honda sign and variants in patients suspected of having a sacral insufficiency fracture. Clin Nucl Med. 2005;30(3):165–9.
18. Linstrom NJ, Heiserman JE, Kortman KE, Crawford NR, Baek S, Anderson RL, et al. Anatomical and biomechanical analyses of the unique and consistent locations of sacral insufficiency fractures. Spine (Phila Pa 1976). 2009;34(4):309–15.
19. Cooper KL, Beabout JW, Swee RG. Insufficiency fractures of the sacrum. Radiology. 1985;156(1):15–20.
20. Wild A, Jaeger M, Haak H, Mehdian SH. Sacral insufficiency fracture, an unsuspected cause of low-back pain in elderly women. Arch Orthop Trauma Surg. 2002;122(1):58–60.
21. Yoder K, Bartsokas J, Averell K, McBride E, Long C, Cook C. Risk factors associated with sacral stress fractures: a systematic review. J Man Manip Ther. 2015;23(2):84–92.
22. Finiels H, Finiels PJ, Jacquot JM, Strubel D. Fractures of the sacrum caused by bone insufficiency. Meta-analysis of 508 cases. Presse Med. 1997;26(33):1568–73.
23. West SG, Troutner JL, Baker MR, Place HM. Sacral insufficiency fractures in rheumatoid arthritis. Spine (Phila Pa 1976). 1994;19(18):2117–21.
24. Hoshino Y, Doita M, Yoshikawa M, Hirayama K, Sha N, Kurosaka M. Unstable pelvic insufficiency fracture in a patient with rheumatoid arthritis. Rheumatol Int. 2004;24(1):46–9.
25. Fukunishi S, Fukui T, Nishio S, Imamura F, Yoshiya S. Multiple pelvic insufficiency fractures in rheumatoid patients with mutilating changes. Orthop Rev (Pavia). 2009;1(2):e23.
26. Peh WC, Gough AK, Sheeran T, Evans NS, Emery P. Pelvic insufficiency fractures in rheumatoid arthritis. Br J Rheumatol. 1993;32(4):319–24.
27. Negishi H, Kobayashi M, Nishida R, Yamada H, Ariga S, Sasaki F, et al. Primary hyperparathyroidism and simultaneous bilateral fracture of the femoral neck during pregnancy. J Trauma. 2002;52(2):367–9.
28. Henry AP, Lachmann E, Tunkel RS, Nagler W. Pelvic insufficiency fractures after irradiation: diagnosis, management, and rehabilitation. Arch Phys Med Rehabil. 1996;77(4):414–6.
29. Stabler A, Beck R, Bartl R, Schmidt D, Reiser M. Vacuum phenomena in insufficiency fractures of the sacrum. Skeletal Radiol. 1995;24(1):31–5.
30. Peris P, Navasa M, Guanabens N, Monegal A, Moya F, Brancos MA, et al. Sacral stress fracture after liver transplantation. Br J Rheumatol. 1993;32(8):702–4.
31. Schulman LL, Addesso V, Staron RB, McGregor CC, Shane E. Insufficiency fractures of the sacrum: a cause of low back pain after lung transplantation. J Heart Lung Transplant. 1997;16(10):1081–5.
32. Aretxabala I, Fraiz E, Perez-Ruiz F, Rios G, Calabozo M, Alonso-Ruiz A. Sacral insufficiency fractures. High association with pubic rami fractures. Clin Rheumatol. 2000;19(5):399–401.
33. Blomlie V, Rofstad EK, Talle K, Sundfor K, Winderen M, Lien HH. Incidence of radiation-induced insufficiency fractures of the female pelvis: evaluation with MR imaging. AJR Am J Roentgenol. 1996;167(5):1205–10.
34. Abe H, Nakamura M, Takahashi S, Maruoka S, Ogawa Y, Sakamoto K. Radiation-induced insufficiency fractures of the pelvis: evaluation with 99mTc-methylene diphosphonate scintigraphy. AJR Am J Roentgenol. 1992;158(3):599–602.
35. Igdem S, Alco G, Ercan T, Barlan M, Ganiyusufoglu K, Unalan B, et al. Insufficiency fractures after pelvic radiotherapy in patients with prostate cancer. Int J Radiat Oncol Biol Phys. 2010;77(3):818–23.
36. Ikushima H, Osaki K, Furutani S, Yamashita K, Kishida Y, Kudoh T, et al. Pelvic bone complications following radiation therapy of gynecologic malignancies: clinical evaluation of radiation-induced pelvic insufficiency fractures. Gynecol Oncol. 2006;103(3):1100–4.
37. Vavken P, Krepler P. Sacral fractures after multi-segmental lumbosacral fusion: a series of four cases and systematic review of literature. Eur Spine J. 2008;17(Suppl 2):S285–90.
38. Khan MH, Smith PN, Kang JD. Sacral insufficiency fractures following multilevel instrumented spinal fusion: case report. Spine (Phila Pa 1976). 2005;30(16):E484–8.
39. Klineberg E, McHenry T, Bellabarba C, Wagner T, Chapman J. Sacral insufficiency fractures caudal to instrumented posterior lumbosacral arthrodesis. Spine (Phila Pa 1976). 2008;33(16):1806–11.
40. Meredith DS, Taher F, Cammisa FP Jr, Girardi FP. Incidence, diagnosis, and management of sacral fractures following multilevel spinal arthrodesis. Spine J. 2013;13(11):1464–9.
41. Waites MD, Mears SC, Mathis JM, Belkoff SM. The strength of the osteoporotic sacrum. Spine (Phila Pa 1976). 2007;32(23):E652–5.

42. Tsiridis E, Upadhyay N, Giannoudis PV. Sacral insufficiency fractures: current concepts of management. Osteoporos Int. 2006;17(12):1716–25.
43. Muthukumar T, Butt SH, Cassar-Pullicino VN, McCall IW. Cauda equina syndrome presentation of sacral insufficiency fractures. Skeletal Radiol. 2007;36(4):309–13.
44. Rawlings CE 3rd, Wilkins RH, Martinez S, Wilkinson RH Jr. Osteoporotic sacral fractures: a clinical study. Neurosurgery. 1988;22(1 Pt 1):72–6.
45. Grangier C, Garcia J, Howarth NR, May M, Rossier P. Role of MRI in the diagnosis of insufficiency fractures of the sacrum and acetabular roof. Skeletal Radiol. 1997;26(9):517–24.
46. White JH, Hague C, Nicolaou S, Gee R, Marchinkow LO, Munk PL. Imaging of sacral fractures. Clin Radiol. 2003;58(12):914–21.
47. Schneider R, Yacovone J, Ghelman B. Unsuspected sacral fractures: detection by radionuclide bone scanning. AJR Am J Roentgenol. 1985;144(2):337–41.
48. Blake SP, Connors AM. Sacral insufficiency fracture. Br J Radiol. 2004;77(922):891–6.
49. De Smet AA, Neff JR. Pubic and sacral insufficiency fractures: clinical course and radiologic findings. AJR Am J Roentgenol. 1985;145(3):601–6.
50. Wagner D, Ossendorf C, Gruszka D, Hofmann A, Rommens PM. Fragility fractures of the sacrum: how to identify and when to treat surgically? Eur J Trauma Emerg Surg. 2015;41(4):349–62.
51. Cabarrus MC, Ambekar A, Lu Y, Link TM. MRI and CT of insufficiency fractures of the pelvis and the proximal femur. AJR Am J Roentgenol. 2008;191(4):995–1001.
52. Fredericson M, Moore W, Biswal S. Sacral stress fractures: magnetic resonance imaging not always definitive for early stage injuries: a report of 2 cases. Am J Sports Med. 2007;35(5):835–9.
53. Brahme SK, Cervilla V, Vint V, Cooper K, Kortman K, Resnick D. Magnetic resonance appearance of sacral insufficiency fractures. Skeletal Radiol. 1990;19(7):489–93.
54. Spitz DJ, Newberg AH. Imaging of stress fractures in the athlete. Radiol Clin North Am. 2002;40(2):313–31.
55. Ries T. Detection of osteoporotic sacral fractures with radionuclides. Radiology. 1983;146(3):783–5.
56. Peh WC, Khong PL, Ho WY, Yeung HW, Luk KD. Sacral insufficiency fractures. Spectrum of radiological features. Clin Imaging. 1995;19(2):92–101.
57. Newhouse KE, el-Khoury GY, Buckwalter JA. Occult sacral fractures in osteopenic patients. J Bone Joint Surg Am. 1992;74(10):1472–7.
58. Babayev M, Lachmann E, Nagler W. The controversy surrounding sacral insufficiency fractures: to ambulate or not to ambulate? Am J Phys Med Rehabil. 2000;79(4):404–9.
59. Mears SC, Berry DJ. Outcomes of displaced and nondisplaced pelvic and sacral fractures in elderly adults. J Am Geriatr Soc. 2011;59(7):1309–12.
60. Taillandier J, Langue F, Alemanni M, Taillandier-Heriche E. Mortality and functional outcomes of pelvic insufficiency fractures in older patients. Joint Bone Spine. 2003;70(4):287–9.
61. Black DM, Cummings SR, Karpf DB, Cauley JA, Thompson DE, Nevitt MC, et al. Randomised trial of effect of alendronate on risk of fracture in women with existing vertebral fractures. Fracture Intervention Trial Research Group. Lancet. 1996;348(9041):1535–41.
62. McClung MR, Geusens P, Miller PD, Zippel H, Bensen WG, Roux C, et al. Effect of risedronate on the risk of hip fracture in elderly women. Hip Intervention Program Study Group. N Engl J Med. 2001;344(5):333–40.
63. Odvina CV, Zerwekh JE, Rao DS, Maalouf N, Gottschalk FA, Pak CY. Severely suppressed bone turnover: a potential complication of alendronate therapy. J Clin Endocrinol Metab. 2005;90(3):1294–301.
64. Im GI, Lee SH. Effect of teriparatide on healing of atypical femoral fractures: a systemic review. J Bone Metab. 2015;22(4):183–9.
65. Miyakoshi N, Aizawa T, Sasaki S, Ando S, Maekawa S, Aonuma H, et al. Healing of bisphosphonate-associated atypical femoral fractures in patients with osteoporosis: a comparison between treatment with and without teriparatide. J Bone Miner Metab. 2015;33(5):553–9.
66. Peichl P, Holzer LA, Maier R, Holzer G. Parathyroid hormone 1–84 accelerates fracture-healing in pubic bones of elderly osteoporotic women. J Bone Joint Surg Am. 2011;93(17):1583–7.
67. Yoo JI, Ha YC, Ryu HJ, Chang GW, Lee YK, Yoo MJ, et al. Teriparatide treatment in elderly patients with sacral insufficiency fracture. J Clin Endocrinol Metab. 2017;102(2):560–5.
68. Wu CC, Wei JC, Hsieh CP, Yu CT. Enhanced healing of sacral and pubic insufficiency fractures by teriparatide. J Rheumatol. 2012;39(6):1306–7.
69. Na WC, Lee SH, Jung S, Jang HW, Jo S. Pelvic insufficiency fracture in severe osteoporosis patient. Hip Pelvis. 2017;29(2):120–6.
70. Jensen ME, Evans AJ, Mathis JM, Kallmes DF, Cloft HJ, Dion JE. Percutaneous polymethylmethacrylate vertebroplasty in the treatment of osteoporotic vertebral body compression fractures: technical aspects. AJNR Am J Neuroradiol. 1997;18(10):1897–904.
71. Evans AJ, Jensen ME, Kip KE, DeNardo AJ, Lawler GJ, Negin GA, et al. Vertebral compression fractures: pain reduction and improvement in functional mobility after percutaneous polymethylmethacrylate vertebroplasty retrospective report of 245 cases. Radiology. 2003;226(2):366–72.
72. Barr JD, Barr MS, Lemley TJ, McCann RM. Percutaneous vertebroplasty for pain relief and spinal stabilization. Spine (Phila Pa 1976). 2000;25(8):923–8.
73. Comstock CP, van der Meulen MC, Goodman SB. Biomechanical comparison of posterior internal fixation techniques for unstable pelvic fractures. J Orthop Trauma. 1996;10(8):517–22.
74. Albert MJ, Miller ME, MacNaughton M, Hutton WC. Posterior pelvic fixation using a transiliac 4.5-

mm reconstruction plate: a clinical and biomechanical study. J Orthop Trauma. 1993;7(3):226–32.
75. Schildhauer TA, Josten C, Muhr G. Triangular osteosynthesis of vertically unstable sacrum fractures: a new concept allowing early weight-bearing. J Orthop Trauma. 1998;12(5):307–14.
76. Rommens PM, Wagner D, Hofmann A. Surgical management of osteoporotic pelvic fractures: a new challenge. Eur J Trauma Emerg Surg. 2012;38(5):499–509.
77. Routt ML Jr, Kregor PJ, Simonian PT, Mayo KA. Early results of percutaneous iliosacral screws placed with the patient in the supine position. J Orthop Trauma. 1995;9(3):207–14.
78. Tsiridis E, Upadhyay N, Gamie Z, Giannoudis PV. Percutaneous screw fixation for sacral insufficiency fractures: a review of three cases. J Bone Joint Surg Br. 2007;89(12):1650–3.
79. Wagner D, Kamer L, Rommens PM, Sawaguchi T, Richards RG, Noser H. 3D statistical modeling techniques to investigate the anatomy of the sacrum, its bone mass distribution, and the trans-sacral corridors. J Orthop Res. 2014;32(11):1543–8.
80. Kraemer W, Hearn T, Tile M, Powell J. The effect of thread length and location on extraction strengths of iliosacral lag screws. Injury. 1994;25(1):5–9.
81. Tjardes T, Paffrath T, Baethis H, Shafizadeh S, Steinhausen E, Steinbuechel T, et al. Computer assisted percutaneous placement of augmented iliosacral screws: a reasonable alternative to sacroplasty. Spine (Phila Pa 1976). 2008;33(13):1497–500.
82. Folsch C, Goost H, Figiel J, Paletta JR, Schultz W, Lakemeier S. Correlation of pull-out strength of cement-augmented pedicle screws with CT-volumetric measurement of cement. Biomed Tech (Berl). 2012;57(6):473–80.
83. Moed BR, Whiting DR. Locked transsacral screw fixation of bilateral injuries of the posterior pelvic ring: initial clinical series. J Orthop Trauma. 2010;24(10):616–21.
84. Sanders D, Fox J, Starr A, Sathy A, Chao J. Transsacral-transiliac screw stabilization: effective for recalcitrant pain due to sacral insufficiency fracture. J Orthop Trauma. 2016;30(9):469–73.
85. Garant M. Sacroplasty: a new treatment for sacral insufficiency fracture. J Vasc Interv Radiol. 2002;13(12):1265–7.
86. Whitlow CT, Yazdani SK, Reedy ML, Kaminsky SE, Berry JL, Morris PP. Investigating sacroplasty: technical considerations and finite element analysis of polymethylmethacrylate infusion into cadaveric sacrum. AJNR Am J Neuroradiol. 2007;28(6):1036–41.
87. Anderson DE, Cotton JR. Mechanical analysis of percutaneous sacroplasty using CT image based finite element models. Med Eng Phys. 2007;29(3):316–25.
88. Richards AM, Mears SC, Knight TA, Dinah AF, Belkoff SM. Biomechanical analysis of sacroplasty: does volume or location of cement matter? AJNR Am J Neuroradiol. 2009;30(2):315–7.
89. Waites MD, Mears SC, Richards AM, Mathis JM, Belkoff SM. A biomechanical comparison of lateral and posterior approaches to sacroplasty. Spine (Phila Pa 1976). 2008;33(20):E735–8.
90. Smith DK, Dix JE. Percutaneous sacroplasty: long-axis injection technique. AJR Am J Roentgenol. 2006;186(5):1252–5.
91. Binaghi S, Guntern D, Schnyder P, Theumann N. A new, easy, fast, and safe method for CT-guided sacroplasty. Eur Radiol. 2006;16(12):2875–8.
92. Bayley E, Srinivas S, Boszczyk BM. Clinical outcomes of sacroplasty in sacral insufficiency fractures: a review of the literature. Eur Spine J. 2009;18(9):1266–71.
93. Dougherty RW, McDonald JS, Cho YW, Wald JT, Thielen KR, Kallmes DF. Percutaneous sacroplasty using CT guidance for pain palliation in sacral insufficiency fractures. J Neurointerv Surg. 2014;6(1):57–60.
94. Frey ME, DePalma MJ, Cifu DX, Bhagia SM, Daitch JS. Efficacy and safety of percutaneous sacroplasty for painful osteoporotic sacral insufficiency fractures: a prospective, multicenter trial. Spine (Phila Pa 1976). 2007;32(15):1635–40.
95. Gupta AC, Chandra RV, Yoo AJ, Leslie-Mazwi TM, Bell DL, Mehta BP, et al. Safety and effectiveness of sacroplasty: a large single-center experience. AJNR Am J Neuroradiol. 2014;35(11):2202–6.
96. Kortman K, Ortiz O, Miller T, Brook A, Tutton S, Mathis J, et al. Multicenter study to assess the efficacy and safety of sacroplasty in patients with osteoporotic sacral insufficiency fractures or pathologic sacral lesions. J Neurointerv Surg. 2013;5(5):461–6.
97. Onen MR, Yuvruk E, Naderi S. Reliability and effectiveness of percutaneous sacroplasty in sacral insufficiency fractures. J Clin Neurosci. 2015;22(10):1601–8.
98. Talmadge J, Smith K, Dykes T, Mittleider D. Clinical impact of sacroplasty on patient mobility. J Vasc Interv Radiol. 2014;25(6):911–5.
99. Barber SM, Livingston AD, Cech DA. Sacral radiculopathy due to cement leakage from percutaneous sacroplasty, successfully treated with surgical decompression. J Neurosurg Spine. 2013;18(5):524–8.

20 Future Treatment Strategies

Hai Le, Umesh Metkar, Afshin E. Razi, and Stuart H. Hershman

Introduction

Osteoporotic vertebral compression fractures (VCFs) present tremendous challenges to treating providers and place substantial economic burden on our healthcare system [1]. In the United States, 700,000 osteoporotic VCFs are estimated to occur annually [2], while in Europe, an estimated 1.4 million osteoporotic VCFs occur annually [3]. This number is expected to rise dramatically over the next decade as the population ages [4]. As emphasized throughout this textbook, osteoporotic VCFs can cause significant pain, disability, and deformity, ultimately impairing patients' quality of life and ability to carry out their activities of daily living [5, 6]. The effective prevention and treatment of osteoporotic VCFs can greatly impact the life and health of patients [7]. Managing these fractures requires a comprehensive multidisciplinary approach utilizing different treatment modalities [8]. This chapter summarizes current screening, prevention, and treatment options while focusing on recent advances and future directions for the management of osteoporotic VCFs.

H. Le
Department of Orthopaedic Surgery, University of California – Davis, Davis, CA, USA
e-mail: haile@ucdavis.edu

U. Metkar
Department of Orthopaedic Surgery, Beth Israel Deaconess Medical Center, Harvard Medical School, Boston, MA, USA
e-mail: umetkar@bidmc.harvard.edu

A. E. Razi
Department of Orthopaedic Surgery, Maimonides Medical Center, Brooklyn, NY, USA

S. H. Hershman (✉)
Department of Orthopaedic Surgery, Massachusetts General Hospital, Harvard Medical School, Boston, MA, USA
e-mail: shhershman@mgh.harvard.edu

Screening Patients at Risk of Osteoporosis

Osteoporotic VCF is a fragility fracture and is, therefore, preventable. Successful prevention of osteoporotic VCFs relies strongly on identifying patients who are at risk of developing osteoporosis. Early diagnosis allows timely implementation of preventive and therapeutic measures.

Clinically, the diagnosis of osteoporosis is based on the criteria established by the World Health Organization (WHO). Osteoporosis is defined by any of the following:

1. A history of fracture of the hip or spine
2. A bone mineral density (BMD) in the osteoporosis range (T-score of ≤ -2.5)
3. A major osteoporotic fracture 10-year probability of $\geq$20% *or* a hip fracture 10-year probability $\geq$3%, calculated using the Fracture Risk Assessment Tool (FRAX®)

Screening recommendations vary to some extent between agencies. The US Preventive

A. E. Razi, S. H. Hershman (eds.), *Vertebral Compression Fractures in Osteoporotic and Pathologic Bone*, https://doi.org/10.1007/978-3-030-33861-9_20

Services Task Force (USPSTF) recommends screening in women ≥65 years and in postmenopausal women <65 years who are at increased risk for osteoporosis. The National Osteoporosis Foundation (NOF) also recommends screening in women ≥65 years [9]. According to the USPSTF, current evidence is insufficient to recommend screening for osteoporosis in men. However, osteoporosis is a concern in this group as well [10], with a reported incidence of osteoporotic VCFs as high as 5.7 per 1000 men per year [11]. For this reason, one of the main focuses moving forward is to design new screening tools that can better detect osteoporosis in both women and men.

Current and Future Screening Tests

The gold standard for osteoporosis screening is bone mineral density (BMD) assessment using dual-energy x-ray absorptiometry (DEXA), also known as bone densitometry. In simple terms, DEXA works by sending x-ray beams through the bones and detecting how much radiation energy is absorbed and how much passes through. Bones with greater BMD absorb more radiation, and therefore less energy is detected by the machine on the opposite side; the converse is true for bones with lower density. Other screening tests that similarly measure BMD include quantitative ultrasonography (QUS), quantitative computed tomography (QCT), and high-resolution peripheral quantitative computed tomography (HR-pQCT). Although CT-based measurement of Hounsfield units (HUs) can reliably determine regional BMD of the vertebral bodies [12], this method has been shown to be inaccurate in patients with adult spinal deformity [13].

The aforementioned studies all have specific advantages and disadvantages [14]. Most notably, these screening tests measure the quantity of bone (i.e., mineral composition) but provide little if any information on the actual quality. Bone strength, however, is a product of bone density and quality [15]. This explains why patients with normal BMD can still sustain fragility fractures and why not all patients with osteoporosis by WHO criteria go on to develop osteoporosis-related fractures. Additionally, there are many artefactual causes that can artificially increase BMD measurement; therefore a normal or high BMD may not necessarily indicate "normal" or "healthy" bone [16]. The presence of degenerative changes or spinal deformity, for example, may cause false elevation of BMD [13, 17]. Another drawback of BMD tests is that measurements are made under unloaded or static conditions. Bone, however, is a dynamic structure with anisotropic and viscoelastic properties. Bone fracture depends on the strength of the bone and the forces to which it is subjected (i.e., applied load) [18]. Thus, although BMD is a good predictor of fragility fractures, it is far from perfect. The best screening tests to detect osteoporosis and predict age-related fractures should measure both the quantity and quality of bone under in vivo loading.

Currently there are several techniques that are better able to determine bone strength but have limited use in the clinical setting [19]. One such innovation is bone microindentation testing (BMT), which measures the mechanical properties of bone (called bone material strength, or BMS) in vivo. BMT involves pressing a handheld probe against the cortical surface of the tibia, applying a test load, and then measuring how much this load indents the bone surface [20, 21]. Malgo et al. (2015) showed that BMS was decreased in patients with fragility fractures compared to those without fractures, even when BMD was similar between the two groups [22]. This suggests that BMS via microindentation may be a better predictor of fragility fractures than BMD. Other studies have focused on measuring dynamic bone quality using tools that subject bone to real-time in vivo loading [23, 24]. Bhattacharya et al. (2010) used accelerometers attached to the patient's specific bony prominences to measure bone shock absorption (BSA) during heel strike. BSA provides information on the bone's structural integrity. The authors showed that BSA was significantly lower in osteoporotic patients with VCFs compared to osteoporotic patients without VCFs [23]. Like BMS, BSA may better predict osteoporotic-related fractures than BMD. As previously stated, these new technologies have not yet been widely or routinely used for clinical diagnosis.

As we better understand bone biology and the pathogenesis of osteoporosis, there has been a growing interest in utilizing biochemical markers to diagnose osteoporosis and monitor response to therapy [25]. These biomarkers are measured in the serum or urine and include markers of bone formation (e.g., bone-specific alkaline phosphatase, osteocalcin, procollagen type I N-propeptide and C-propeptide) and markers of bone resorption (e.g., type I collagen N-telopeptide and C-telopeptide, deoxypyridinoline) [25–27]. These biomarkers have been primarily used for research purposes, and further research is needed to determine the clinical application of these tests in the management of osteoporosis [28].

Finally, genome-wide association studies (GWASs) have identified specific single nucleotide polymorphisms (SNPs) that are associated with osteoporosis [29]. The gene encoding the low-density lipoprotein receptor-related protein 5 (LRP5) is one of the most well-studied genes. LRP5 polymorphisms have been shown to be closely linked to osteoporosis [30, 31] and predict BMD [32, 33] and osteoporosis-related fractures [34, 35]. As research intensifies and technology becomes more sophisticated, efforts should concentrate on identifying different genetic determinants of osteoporosis and developing validated genetic screening tests for this condition.

Preventing Osteoporotic Vertebral Compression Fractures

Early diagnosis and treatment of osteoporosis is the foundation for various treatment strategies for osteoporotic VCFs. Osteoporosis prevention includes eating a balanced diet with adequate calcium and vitamin D intake. Bone health can be maintained by making healthy lifestyle modifications such as exercise and smoking cessation. Additionally, patients should avoid taking medications that can have adverse effects on bone metabolism including glucocorticoids, antiepileptics, antidepressants, and antiretrovirals [36].

Current and Future Medical Therapies

Patients with osteoporosis should be cared for and followed closely by their primary care physician, rheumatologist, or endocrinologist. Pharmacologic therapy should be initiated in patients with osteoporosis and in those who are at high risk of developing osteoporosis. Current FDA-approved pharmacologic agents either slow down bone turnover (antiresorptive) or promote bone formation (anabolic). Antiresorptive agents include bisphosphonates (e.g., alendronate, risedronate, ibandronate, zoledronate), selective estrogen receptor modulators (SERMs) such as raloxifene, estrogen or estrogen-progestin hormone therapy, receptor activator of nuclear factor kappa-B ligand (RANKL) inhibitor (i.e., denosumab), and calcitonin [9]. Teriparatide (parathyroid hormone 1-34) and abaloparatide (parathyroid hormone-related protein (PTHrP) analogue) are the only FDA-approved anabolic agents [37].

As we better understand the molecular mechanisms of bone formation and breakdown, new therapies are emerging that specifically target these pathways to prevent and/or treat osteoporosis. One major pathway is the Wnt/β-catenin signaling pathway, which is essential for the regulation of bone metabolism and remodeling. Briefly, Wnt is a glycoprotein ligand that binds to frizzled, a transmembrane receptor. Coreceptors LRP5/6 then bind to the Wnt-frizzled complex. This ultimately leads to translocation of β-catenin into the nucleus to upregulate gene transcription important in osteogenesis [38]. Sclerostin is a molecule that binds to LRP5/6 and inhibits Wnt/β-catenin signaling [39]. Loss-of-function mutations of the SOST gene encoding sclerostin leads to a sclerosing bone dysplasia genetic disorder called sclerosteosis. Researchers have taken advantage of this knowledge to develop romosozumab, a monoclonal antibody that inhibits sclerostin. Studies have shown its effectiveness in promoting bone formation and preventing bone resorption [40]. McClung et al. (2014) showed that romosozumab increases BMD in postmenopausal women [41]. This pharmacologic agent is not yet FDA-approved, however [37].

Another group of agents currently being investigated are the cathepsin K inhibitors. Cathepsin K is a collagenase enzyme involved in osteoclast-mediated bone resorption; therefore, inhibitors of cathepsin K such as odanacatib can slow this process [42, 43]. There is currently no FDA-approved cathepsin K inhibitor for the treatment of osteoporosis. Future research efforts should focus on elucidating the cell signaling pathways responsible for bone metabolism to identify new molecular targets for osteoporosis therapy.

Treating Osteoporotic Vertebral Compression Fractures

For patients with osteoporotic VCFs, management includes both non-operative and operative options. Non-operative modalities have been discussed in great detail in this textbook and generally consist of activity modification, physical therapy, bracing, and pharmacotherapy for pain control and osteoporosis [44]. This section focuses primarily on the surgical management of osteoporotic VCFs.

Current and Future Surgical Options

While the pharmacotherapy of osteoporosis is continually evolving, the surgical management of osteoporotic VCFs has remained relatively unchanged over the past three decades. Current surgical options concentrate on addressing the fractured vertebra through cement augmentation techniques. The goals of these vertebral augmentation procedures are to decrease pain and prevent progressive kyphosis. Vertebroplasty was initially introduced by Galibert et al. in 1984 and described in the literature in 1987 [45]. The technique consists of injection of structural cement such as polymethyl methacrylate (PMMA) into the collapsed vertebral body to restore height, improve fatigue resistance, and maintain spinal stability. In addition to unreliable vertebral body height restoration, the principal drawbacks of vertebroplasty are cement embolization and extravasation of cement outside the confines of the vertebral body during injection [46, 47]. Kyphoplasty was subsequently developed to address the collapsed vertebra. The technique focuses on insertion and subsequent inflation of a balloon to create a void prior to cement injection. This allows the cement to be injected at a lower pressure and therefore decreases the likelihood of extravasation. Many systematic reviews have shown a significant decrease in cement extravasation with kyphoplasty compared to vertebroplasty [48, 49].

The effectiveness of vertebroplasty has recently been challenged. Buchbinder et al. (2009) and Kallmes et al. (2009) independently published the results of their randomized controlled trials (RCTs) in the New England Journal of Medicine (NEJM) and concluded that vertebroplasty did not do any better than a simulated procedure [50, 51]. In a 2010 guideline and evidence report published by the American Academy of Orthopaedic Surgeons (AAOS) titled "The Treatment of Symptomatic Osteoporotic Spinal Compression Fractures," the AAOS counseled:

- *We recommend against vertebroplasty for patients who present with an osteoporotic spinal compression fracture on imaging with correlating clinical signs and symptoms and who are neurologically intact.*
- *Kyphoplasty is an option for patients who present with an osteoporotic spinal compression fracture on imaging with correlating clinical signs and symptoms and who are neurologically intact.*

In contrast, the North American Spine Society (NASS) maintained their strong support for these vertebral augmentation procedures [52], which should be done in selected cases. The authors of this chapter uphold this position, as there have been dozens, if not hundreds of subsequent studies supporting the procedures' benefit in patients with osteoporotic VCFs who have failed medical management [53–56]. This discussion exposes the controversies that exist in the medical community regarding the use of vertebral augmentation to treat osteoporotic VCFs. Vertebroplasty and kyphoplasty have specific complications, and therefore future treatment strategies should focus on making them safer for patients.

One unsettled issue in vertebroplasty and kyphoplasty is determining which is the optimal filling cement or cement substitute for augmentation. Although PMMA is the most commonly used filling cement, other biodegradable bone cement substitutes have been evaluated including calcium phosphate cement (CPC) [57] and calcium sulfate cement (CSC) [58]. Certain bone putties such as MONTAGE® may be suitable filling agents for vertebral augmentation because they interdigitate into surrounding trabeculae, quickly harden after application, and fully resorb with fracture remodeling. Currently there are no level I randomized controlled trials comparing these different filling options. There are many vertebral augmentation systems available today such as Kyphon (Medtronic Inc.), Spasy (Joimax Inc.), AVAmax (Carefusion Inc.), and Ky/Spine (Ackermann Inc.) and Stabilit (Dfine Inc.) [59]. These systems were developed with the same principal goal: to safely deliver cement percutaneously into the vertebral body while minimizing extravasation.

A new system, the Kiva® VCF Treatment System by Benvenue Medical, Inc., was recently FDA-approved for VCFs. Unlike previous systems in which only cement is injected, the Kiva® system is implant-based. That is, a flexible cylindrical polyetheretherketone (PEEK) implant is first inserted percutaneously into the vertebral body to provide structural support. Cement is subsequently injected for additional vertebral augmentation and is contained within the implant. According to the KAST (Kiva Safety and Effectiveness Trial) randomized control study, patients with painful osteoporotic VCFs who received treatment using this implant-based system had improved pain (visual analogue scale score, or VAS) and function (Oswestry Disability Index, or ODI). The authors reported no device-related serious adverse events in 153 cases and concluded that the Kiva system was as effective and safe as traditional balloon kyphoplasty [60].

Recently, several studies evaluated the efficacy of a novel craniocaudal expandable titanium implant (SpineJack® by Vexim, France) used in the treatment of painful osteoporotic VCFs [61–63]. A prospective, multicentered European study examined the outcome of 108 fractures in 103 consecutive patients treated with the SpineJack® device. These patients were then followed for a period of 1 year. Approximately three quarters of the treated fractures were traumatic in nature, and one quarter of the fractures were secondary to osteoporosis. At a time point of 48 hours after the procedure, there was a mean reduction in the VAS score by 5.5 points, which was statistically significant ($p < 0.001$). At the 3-month and 12-month post-surgery time points, the reduction in VAS scores was maintained. Similar statistically significant improvements in pain and quality of life were seen in the Oswestry Disability Index (ODI) and EuroQol-VAS scores. In addition, there was a significant decrease in the number of patients requiring narcotics 48 hours after the procedure. No implant-related adverse events were noted during the study, and no device required removal. The authors concluded that the SpineJack® device was a safe and effective treatment for use in osteoporotic VCFs [62]. At this time, the SpineJack® device is currently approved for use in Europe; however, it is not yet available in the United States.

In summary, future technological innovations in the surgical management of osteoporotic VCFs are on the horizon. Current strategies seem to be focused on three main objectives: (1) developing new filling agents which are better able to interdigitate into the surrounding trabeculae, (2) introducing new ways to safely deliver augmentation agents while minimizing or preventing extravasation, and (3) designing new implant-based vertebral augmentation systems. While these avenues are exciting and show early promise, long-term data is lacking; multicentered, placebo-controlled trials should investigate these new techniques and innovations further.

References

1. Orsini LS, Rousculp MD, Long SR, et al. Health care utilization and expenditures in the United States: a study of osteoporosis-related fractures. Osteoporos Int. 2005;16:359–71.
2. Ensrud KE, Schousboe JT. Clinical practice. Vertebral fractures. N Engl J Med. 2011;364:1634–42.
3. Johnell O, Kanis JA. An estimate of the worldwide prevalence and disability associated with osteoporotic fractures. Osteoporos Int. 2006;17:1726–33.
4. Burge R, Dawson-Hughes B, Solomon DH, et al. Incidence and economic burden of osteoporosis-related fractures in the United States, 2005–2025. J Bone Miner Res. 2007;22:465–75.
5. Edidin AA, Ong KL, Lau E, et al. Life expectancy following diagnosis of a vertebral compression fracture. Osteoporosis Int. 2013;24:451–8.
6. Riggs BL, Melton LJ. The worldwide problem of osteoporosis: insights afforded by epidemiology. Bone. 1995;17:S505–11.
7. Jung HJ, Park YS, Seo HY, et al. Quality of life in patients with osteoporotic vertebral compression fractures. J Bone Metab. 2017;24:187–96.
8. Prather H, Watson JO, Gilula LA. Nonoperative management of osteoporotic vertebral compression fractures. Injury. 2007;38:S40–8.
9. Cosman F, de Beur SJ, LeBoff MS, et al. Clinician's guide to prevention and treatment of osteoporosis. Osteoporos Int. 2014;25:2359–81.
10. Kenny A, Taxel P. Osteoporosis in older men. Clin Cornerstone. 2000;2:45–51.
11. European Prospective Osteoporosis Study (EPOS) Group, Felsenberg D, Silman AJ, et al. Incidence of vertebral fracture in Europe: results from the European Prospective Osteoporosis Study (EPOS). J Bone Miner Res. 2002;17:716–24.
12. Schreiber JJ, Anderson PA, Rosas HG, et al. Hounsfield units for assessing bone mineral density and strength: a tool for osteoporosis management. J Bone Joint Surg Am. 2011;93:1057–63.
13. Kohan EM, Nemani VM, Hershman S, et al. Lumbar computed tomography scans are not appropriate surrogates for bone mineral density scans in primary adult spinal deformity. Neurosurg Focus. 2017;43:E4.
14. Sisodia GB. Methods of predicting vertebral body fractures of the lumbar spine. World J Orthop. 2013;4:241–7.
15. Licata A. Bone density vs bone quality: what's a clinician to do? Cleve Clin J Med. 2009;76:331–6.
16. Gregson CL, Hardcastle SA, Cooper C, et al. Friend or foe: high bone mineral density on routine bone density scanning, a review of causes and management. Rheumatology (Oxford). 2013;52:968–85.
17. Tenne M, McGuigan F, Besjakov J, et al. Degenerative changes at the lumbar spine--implications for bone mineral density measurement in elderly women. Osteoporos Int. 2013;24:1419–28.
18. Bouxsein ML. Biomechanics of osteoporotic fractures. Clin Rev Bone Miner Metabol. 2006;4:143–53.
19. Torres-del-Pliego E, Vilaplana L, Güerri-Fernández R, et al. Measuring bone quality. Curr Rheumatol Rep. 2013;15:373.
20. Arnold M, Zhao S, Ma S, et al. Microindentation: a tool for measuring cortical bone stiffness? A systematic review. Bone Joint Res. 2017;6:542–9.
21. Bridges D, Randall C, Hansma PK. A new device for performing reference point indentation without a reference probe. Rev Sci Instrum. 2012;83:044301.
22. Malgo F, Hamdy NA, Papapoulos SE, et al. Bone material strength as measured by microindentation in vivo is decreased in patients with fragility fractures independently of bone mineral density. J Clin Endocrinol Metab. 2015;100:2039–45.
23. Bhattacharya A, Watts NB, Davis K, et al. Dynamic bone quality: a noninvasive measure of bone's biomechanical property in osteoporosis. J Clin Densitom. 2010;13:228–36.
24. Bhattacharya A, Watts NB, Dwivedi A, et al. Combined measures of dynamic bone quality and postural balance: a fracture risk assessment approach in osteoporosis. J Clin Densitom. 2016;19:154–64.
25. Garnero P. Biomarkers for osteoporosis management: utility in diagnosis, fracture risk prediction and therapy monitoring. Mol Diagn Ther. 2008;12:157–70.
26. Garnero P. Markers of bone turnover for the prediction of fracture risk. Osteoporos Int. 2000;11:S55–65.
27. Szulc P, Delmas PD. Biochemical markers of bone turnover: potential use in the investigation and management of postmenopausal osteoporosis. Osteoporos Int. 2008. 2008;19:1683–704.
28. Cabral HW, Andolphi BF, Ferreira BV, et al. The use of biomarkers in clinical osteoporosis. Rev Assoc Med Bras (1992). 2016;62:368–76.
29. Duncan EL, Brown MA. Genetic studies in osteoporosis: the end of the beginning. Arthritis Res Ther. 2008;10:214.
30. Richards JB, Rivadeneira F, Inouye M, et al. Bone mineral density, osteoporosis, and osteoporotic fractures: a genome-wide association study. Lancet. 2008;371:1505–12.
31. van Meurs JB, Trikalinos TA, Ralston SH, et al. Large-scale analysis of association between LRP5 and LRP6 variants and osteoporosis. JAMA. 2008;299:1277–90.
32. Koay MA, Tobias JH, Leary SH, et al. The effect of LRP5 polymorphisms on bone mineral density is apparent in childhood. Calcif Tissue Int. 2007;81:1–9.
33. Mizuguchi T, Furuta I, Watanabe Y, et al. LRP5, low density lipoprotein receptor related protein 5, is a determinant for bone mineral density. J Hum Genet. 2004;49:80–6.
34. Bollerslev J, Wilson SG, Dick IM, et al. LRP5 gene polymorphisms predict bone mass and incident fractures in elderly Australian women. Bone. 2005;36:599–606.
35. van Meurs JB, Rivadeneira F, Jhamai M, et al. Common genetic variation of the low-density lipoprotein receptor-related protein 5 and 6 genes determines

fracture risk in elderly white men. J Bone Miner Res. 2006;21:141–50.
36. Watts NB. Adverse bone effects of medications used to treat non-skeletal disorders. Osteoporos Int. 2017;28:2741–6.
37. Canalis E. Management of endocrine disease: novel anabolic treatments for osteoporosis. Eur J Endocrinol. 2018;178(2):R33. [Epub ahead of print]
38. Krishnan V, Bryant HU, Macdougald OA. Regulation of bone mass by Wnt signaling. J Clin Invest. 2006;116:1202–9.
39. Li X, Zhang Y, Kang H, et al. Sclerostin binds to LRP5/6 and antagonizes canonical Wnt signaling. J Biol Chem. 2005;280:19883–7.
40. Li X, Ominsky MS, Warmington KS, et al. Sclerostin antibody treatment increases bone formation, bone mass, and bone strength in a rat model of postmenopausal osteoporosis. J Bone Miner Res. 2009;24:578–88.
41. McClung MR, Grauer A, Boonen S, et al. Romosozumab in postmenopausal women with low bone mineral density. N Engl J Med. 2014;370:412–20.
42. Brömme D, Lecaille F. Cathepsin K inhibitors for osteoporosis and potential off-target effects. Expert Opin Investig Drugs. 2009;18:585–600.
43. Stoch SA, Wagner JA. Cathepsin K inhibitors: a novel target for osteoporosis therapy. Clin Pharmacol Ther. 2008;83:172–6.
44. Parreira PCS, Maher CG, Megale RZ, et al. An overview of clinical guidelines for the management of vertebral compression fracture: a systematic review. Spine J. 2017;17:1932. [Epub ahead of print].
45. Galibert P, Deramond H, Rosat P, et al. Preliminary note on the treatment of vertebral angioma by percutaneous acrylic vertebroplasty. Neurochirurgie. 1987;33:166–8.
46. McCall T, Cole C, Dailey A. Vertebroplasty and kyphoplasty: a comparative review of efficacy and adverse events. Curr Rev Musculoskelet Med. 2008;1:17–23.
47. Venmans A, Klazen CA, Lohle PN, et al. Percutaneous vertebroplasty and pulmonary cement embolism: results from VERTOS II. AJNR Am J Neuroradiol. 2010;31:1451–3.
48. Hulme PA, Krebs J, Ferguson SJ, et al. Vertebroplasty and kyphoplasty: a systematic review of 69 clinical studies. Spine. 2006;31:1983–2001.
49. Taylor RS, Taylor RJ, Fritzell P. Balloon kyphoplasty and vertebroplasty for vertebral compression fractures: a comparative systematic review of efficacy and safety. Spine. 2006;31:2747–55.
50. Buchbinder R, Osborne RH, Ebeling PR, et al. A randomized trial of vertebroplasty for painful osteoporotic vertebral fractures. N Engl J Med. 2009;362:557–68.
51. Kallmes DF, Comstock BA, Heagerty PJ, et al. A randomized trial of vertebroplasty for osteoporotic spinal fractures. N Engl J Med. 2009;361:569–79.
52. Bono CM, Heggeness M, Mick C, et al. North American Spine Society: newly released vertebroplasty randomized controlled trials: a tale of two trials. Spine J. 2010;10:238–40.
53. Alvarez L, Alcaraz M, Pérez-Higueras A, et al. Percutaneous vertebroplasty: functional improvement in patients with osteoporotic compression fractures. Spine (Phila Pa 1976). 2006;31:1113–8.
54. Grafe IA, Da Fonseca K, Hillmeier J, et al. Reduction of pain and fracture incidence after kyphoplasty: 1-year outcomes of a prospective controlled trial of patients with primary osteoporosis. Osteoporos Int. 2005;16:2005–12.
55. Kasperk C, Grafe IA, Schmitt S, et al. Three-year outcomes after kyphoplasty in patients with osteoporosis with painful vertebral fractures. J Vasc Interv Radiol. 2010;21:701–9.
56. Klazen CA, Lohle PN, de Vries J, et al. Vertebroplasty versus conservative treatment in acute osteoporotic vertebral compression fractures (Vertos II): an open-label randomised trial. Lancet. 2010;376:1085–92.
57. Nakano M, Hirano N, Zukawa M, et al. Vertebroplasty using calcium phosphate cement for osteoporotic vertebral fractures: study of outcomes at a minimum follow-up of two years. Asian Spine J. 2012;6:34–42.
58. Perry A, Mahar A, Massie J, et al. Biomechanical evaluation of kyphoplasty with calcium sulfate cement in a cadaveric osteoporotic vertebral compression fracture model. Spine J. 2005;5:489–93.
59. Papanastassiou ID, Filis A, Gerochristou MA, et al. Controversial issues in kyphoplasty and vertebroplasty in osteoporotic vertebral fractures. Biomed Res Int. 2014;2014:934206.
60. Tutton SM, Pflugmacher R, Davidian M, et al. KAST study: the Kiva system as a vertebral augmentation treatment – a safety and effectiveness trial: a randomized, noninferiority trial comparing the Kiva system with balloon kyphoplasty in treatment of osteoporotic vertebral compression fractures. Spine (Phila Pa 1976). 2015;40:865–75.
61. Noriega DC, Ramajo RH, Lite IS, et al. Safety and clinical performance of kyphoplasty and SpineJack(®) procedures in the treatment of osteoporotic vertebral compression fractures: a pilot, monocentric, investigator-initiated study. Osteoporos Int. 2016;27:2047–55.
62. Noriega D, Maestretti G, Renaud C, et al. Clinical performance and safety of 108 SpineJack implantations: 1-year results of a prospective multicentre single-arm registry study. Biomed Res Int. 2015;2015:173872.
63. Renaud C. Treatment of vertebral compression fractures with the cranio-caudal expandable implant SpineJack®: technical note and outcomes in 77 consecutive patients. Orthop Traumatol Surg Res. 2015;101:857–9.

Index

A
Adult spinal deformity (ASD), 191
Alcohol consumption, 60
American Academy of Orthopaedic Surgeons (AAOS) guidelines, 111, 224
  multi-centered study, 111
  placebo-controlled study, 111
  post guidelines, 111, 112
  pre-AAOS guideline evidence, 110, 111
Anterior wedge fractures, 50, 51

B
Balloon-assisted vertebroplasty, 120
Biconcave fracture patterns, 51, 52
Bone physiology
  age related changes, 6, 7
  categories, 1
  cortical osteons, 1
  growth and remodeling, 2–4
  Haversian systems, 1
  inorganic bone matrix, 4, 5
  lamellae, 1
  leptin, 5
  neurohormonal regulation, 5
  neuropeptide Y (NPY), 5
  organic bone matrix, 4
  osteoblasts, 2
  osteoclast function, 5
  osteoclasts, 1, 2
  osteocytes, 1, 2
  preosteoclasts, 5
  regulators of G-protein (RGS), 5
  removal and replacement, 1

C
Calcitonin, 109
Camptocormia, 145
Centers for Medicaid and Medicare Services (CMS), 26
Cruciform Anterior Spinal Hyperextension (CASH) Brace, 104
Crush type fracture patterns, 52

D
Denosumab, 41, 148
Dual energy x-ray absorptiometry (DEXA), 34, 147

E
European Vertebral Osteoporosis Study (EVOS), 32
EuroQol-VAS scores, 225

F
Fibril-associated collagen with interrupted triple helices (FACIT), 4
Five-time sit-to-stand (FTSTS) test, 146
Fosamax® therapy, 43
Fracture Intervention Trial (FIT), 43
Fracture Intervention Trial Long-term Extension (FLEX), 43
Fracture Risk Assessment Tool (FRAX®), 35, 36
FRActure study in postmenopausal woMen with ostEoporosis (FRAME) trial, 42
Fragility fracture, 31

H
Haversian systems, 1
HORIZON-Pivotal Fracture Trial (PFT), 43

I
International Society for Clinical Densitometry (ISCD), 34
International Spine Research Consortium, 155

A. E. Razi, S. H. Hershman (eds.), *Vertebral Compression Fractures in Osteoporotic and Pathologic Bone*, https://doi.org/10.1007/978-3-030-33861-9

J
Jewett Brace, 104

K
Kiva Safety and Effectiveness Trial (KAST), 225
Kiva® VCF Treatment System, 225
Kümmel disease, 145
Kyphoplasty, 26, 53
Kyphoplasty cement augmentation technique
  anesthesia, 138
  balloon catheter insertion, 140
  bone cement, 140
  bone scan, 137
  cement delivery systems, 140, 141
  cement injection, 141, 142
  complications, 142, 143
  contraindications, 137
  disadvantage, 141
  indications, 137
  learning curve, 142
  MRI, 137
  multilevel compression fractures, 142
  office based procedure, 138
  patient positioning, 138
  radiation exposure, 142
  radiographic imaging, 137
  STIR imaging, 137
  toradol injection, 138
  trocar positioning, 139, 140
  unilateral pedicle approach, 138

L
Low bone mass, 59
Lumbar degenerative disc disease, 59
Lumbar spinal stenosis, 59

M
Male hypogonadism, 14
Metastatic disease, 63, 64
Microphthalmia-associated transcription factor (MITF), 2
MONTAGE®, 225

N
National Osteoporosis Foundation (NOF), 21, 36, 73
Neuropeptide Y (NPY), 5
New England Journal of Medicine (NEJM), 111, 224
North American Spine Society (NASS), 224
Nuclear factor of activated T-cells cytoplasmic-1 (NFAT-1), 2

O
One-size-fits-all approach, 36
Osteoporosis
  adult spinal deformity (ASD), 191
  biomechanics, 11
  bisphospohantes *vs.* teriparatide, 193, 194
  bone mineral density (BMD), 21, 191, 198
  bone quality, 199
  bone structure, 10
  calcium levels, 13
  cellular signaling, 12
  cement augmentation, 196–198
  chronic inflammatory diseases, 15
  cortical bone trajectory (CBT) technique, 195, 196
  CSF-1 receptor (c-Fms), 12
  definition, 9, 10
  DEXA (T-score) *vs.* spinal computed tomography, 191–193
  diabetes mellitus, 15, 16
  Dickkopf-related protein 1 (DKK-1), 12
  direct costs and indirect cost, 22–25
  epidemiology, 14
  estrogen deficiency, 13, 14
  female hypogonadism, 15
  glucocorticoid excess, 16
  hematologic diseases, 15
  human immunodeficiency virus, 16
  incidence and prevalence, 22
  instrumentation systems, 198, 199
  in-vitro biomechanical study, 198
  kyphoplasty-type technique/transpedicular prefilling augmentation technique, 197
  lifestyle factors, 17
  long screws fixation, 195, 196
  macrophage- colony stimulating factor (M-CSF), 12
  male hypogonadism, 14
  medical management, 194
  medications
    acid suppressive medications, 16
    anti-epileptic drugs, 17
    aromatase inhibitors, 16
    exogenous steroids, 16
    selective serotonin uptake inhibitors (SSRIs), 17
  osteoporotic pedicles, 197
  pathophysiology, 9
  pedicle screw augmentation, 197
  pedicle screws fixation, 195
  physiological changes, 21
  pre-operative radiological imaging, 191
  prevalence, 21, 26, 27, 191
  proximal junction kyphosis (PJK), 199–201
  pullout analysis, 197
  receptor activator of nuclear factor kappa-B ligand (RANKL), 11, 12
  sclerostin, 12
  screening, 17, 18
  supplemental fixation, 22
  surgical management, 201, 202
  thyrotoxicosis, 15
  treatment, 25–27
  trocar and prefilling augmentation technique, 197
  tumor necrosis factor (TNF) receptor, 11
  vertebral compression fracture (VCF), 22
  vitamin D3, 13
  weaker vertebral endplates, 22
  Wnt signal pathway, 12

World Health Organization (WHO), 21
Osteoporotic vertebral compression fractures (OVCFs)
adjacent segment disease, 188
advantages and disadvantages, 59
anti-osteoporotic drugs, 60
body mass index (BMI), 59
bracing, 104, 105
chronic oral glucocorticoid therapy, 58
complications, 187
cost, 57
DEXA scores, 58
epidural steroid injections, 58
frailty, 58
FRAX, 60
incidence and prevalence, 57
initial management, 101
injections, 103
lumbar decompression surgery, 59
medical managament, 184–186
medication, 58
minimally invasive techniques, 187
multidisciplinary care, 57
neurological manifestations, 59
pharmacologic treatment, 101, 102, 187
physical activity, 60
pre-operative and post-operative interventions, 187
prevention and treatment, 221, 223, 224, 225
prophylactic vertebral cement augmentation, 188
proximal junctional fracture, 183
biomechancial, 183, 184
cellular level, 184
psychological treatment, 101, 105
radiographic studies, 58
risk factor, 58–60, 184
sagittal spinal alignment, 183
screening, 58, 221–223
surgical managament, 186, 187
symptoms, 58
systemic corticosteroids, 58
T-score, 58, 60
type I, 57
type II, 57
type III, 57
United States Preventative Services Task Force (USPSTF), 58
vertebroplasty, 59
vitamin D deficiency, 60
Z-score, 58
Osteoprotegrin (OPG) functions, 2
Oswestry Disability Index (ODI), 26, 200, 225
Oswestry Low Back Disability Index scores, 215

P

Pathologic vertebral compression fracture (pVCF)
diagnosis, 63
etiologies, 63
history, 64
imaging, 65, 66
management, 63, 66, 67
physical examination, 64, 65

R

Raloxifene (Evista®), 42
Roland-Morris Disability Questionnaire, 26

S

Sacral insufficiency fractures (SIF)
anatomy and biomechanics, 206–208
bone scintigraphy, 213
clinical presentation and evaluation, 209
conservative management, 213, 214
CT, 210, 211
fatigue fractures, 205
incidence, 205, 206
insufficiency fracture, 205
medical management, 214
MRI, 210, 212
plain radiographs, 209, 210
risk factors, 205, 208, 209
surgical management
long-axis technique (90), 216, 217
minimally invasive augmentation, 214
morbidity, 214
posterior (short-axis) technique, 215, 216
sacroplasty, 215
screw fixation, 214, 215
vertebroplasty, 214
Secreted protein acid which is rich in cysteine (SPARC), 4
Sphingosine-1 phosphate (S1P), 5
Spinal column tumors
after SRS, 154–158
cement augmentation, 154
cervicothoracic junction (CTJ), 160
clinical characteristics, 158
clinical significance, 154
cranio-vertebral junction (CVJ), 158, 159
imaging studies, 154
incidence, 153, 154
management, 154
NOMS algorithm, 158
pathological fractures, 153
radiographic diagnosis, 160–162
spinal instability neoplastic score (SINS), 162, 163
subaxial cervical spine, 160
surgical management
cervical spine and cervico-thoracic junction, 164, 165
chemotherapy and radiation, 164
fenestrated pedicle screws (FPS), 171, 172
indications and contraindications, 164
less invasive approaches, 164
minimally invasive surgery (MIS), 172, 175
personalized treatment, 164
pre-operative evaluation, 164
surgical CVJ stabilization, 165–169
thoracic and lumbar spine metastases, 168, 170–174
vertebroplasty and kyphoplasty, 165
surgical optimization, 158
symptoms, 158, 159
thoracic and lumbar spine, 160

Spinal deformity management
evaluation, 145, 146
medical management, 147, 148
postoperative care, 151, 152
radiographic examination, 146–148
surgical management
anterior and posterior thoracolumbar approaches, 149
anterior column reconstruction, 149
bicortical placement, 149
bone mineral density, 149
cement augmentation, 151
complications, 149
dorsal and posterolateral fusion, 150
goals, 149
hemilaminectomy, 149
iliac instrumentation, 150
lower instrumented vertebra (LIV), 151
patient factors, 148, 149
short segment fixation, 150
spinal stenosis, 149
three-column osteotomies, 149
vacuum phenomenon, 150
Spinal Instability in Neoplasm Score (SINS), 66
Spinal Proprioception Extension Exercise Dynamic (SPEED) program, 186
SpineJack® device, 225
Spine Oncology Study Group (SOSG), 162
Stereotactic spine radiosurgery (SRS), 154–158

T
Teriparatide, 147
Thoracolumbarsacaral orthosis (TLSO), 104

U
United States Preventative Services Task Force (USPSTF), 58
U.S. healthcare, 21

V
Vertebral compression fractures (VCF)
acute radiculopathy, 71
anabolic agents, 42, 43
anterior wedge fractures, 50, 51
benign and pathologic VCFs, 80, 81
biconcave fracture patterns, 51, 52
biochemical bone turnover markers (BTMs), 73
BMD testing, 34
bone biopsy, 73
calcium, 37
chemical shift imaging, 88
chronicity, 77–80
classification system, 51
clinical consequences, 95
clinical presentation, 95
conventional radiography and scintigraphy, 80
cortex, 82
creep deformity and fatigue failure, 50
crush type fracture patterns, 52
DEXA scan, 69
diagnosis, 34–36
diagnostic evaluation, 70
diet, 37
differential diagnosis, 69, 72
diffusion weighted imaging, 86–88
discogenic/spondylotic pain, 70
dynamic contrast enhanced MRI, 88, 89
18F FDG PET/CT, 89–91
epidemiology, 31, 32
estrogen agonist/antagonist, 42
etiology, 70
excessive kyphosis, 71
extravertebral features
distant osseous findings, 86
paraspinal soft tissue, 84, 86
FRAX® tool, 35
initial radiologic evaluation, 76
intervertebral disc, 50
laboratory evaluation, 72, 73
malignant features, 86
marrow signal intensity
contrast enhancement, 84
marrow edema and inflammation, 83–85
morphologic features, 86
mechanism of pain, 52, 53
medical management, 38, 39
medication, 73
microstructure, 49, 50
morphologic features, 86
morphologic imaging, 89
morphology, 80
MRI, 77, 80
multidetector computed tomography (MDCT), 77
muscular/spondylotic pain, 70
NOF guidelines, 73
oral bisphosphonates, 40, 41
pain, 96
patient history, 70, 71
pharmacologic management, 39, 40
physical consequences, 97, 98
physical examination, 71, 72
positron emission tomography (PET)/CT, 80
qualitative evaluation, 86
qualitative/semi-quantitative imaging assessment, 77
rank ligand inhibition, 41, 42
red flag symptoms, 70
risk factors, 32, 33, 36, 37, 69, 70, 98
societal impact, 33, 34
symptoms, 71
Technetium 99m hydroxymethylene diphosphonate (Tc-99m HMDP), 89
trabecula, 82
treatment, 69
vacuum cleft/fluid sign, 83
Vertebral Fracture Assessment (VFA) software, 35
vertebral imaging, 35
VERT trial, 98

vertebral body contour, 81
vitamin D, 37, 38
Vertebral Efficacy with Risedronate Therapy (VERT) trial, 98
Vertebroplasty, 53
Vertebroplasty cement augmentation technique
advantages, 120
analgesics, 116
aseptic technique, 121
bone cements, 126, 127
bone demineralization, 116
bone density test, 117
bone needles, 124
cement augmentation, 120, 121
cement injection, 127–129
clinical feature, 117
complications, 129–133
CT, 118, 119
description, 121
early intervention, 117
fluoroscopy, 119, 120
goal, 120
heating pads, 116
image-guided percutaneous vertebroplasty, 117
image-guided vertebroplasty procedures, 115
imaging, 117
indications and contraindications, 117, 120
informed consent, 121
intravenous antibiotics, 121
invasive treatment strategies, 117
kyphotic deformity, 116
laboratory parameters, 121
medical management, 116
Medicare database, 115
MRI, 118
multilevel vertebroplasty, 128
needle placement, 122, 124–126
non-invasive treatments, 116
osteoporosis therapy, 129
pain relief and mobility improvement, 128
patient co-morbidities, 121
patient outcomes, 122
patient positioning, 122
patient selection, 117, 121
patient's pain diagram, 117
physical examination, 117
physical therapy, 116
radiographic evaluation, 118
for rotatory scoliosis, 129
spine brace, 129
temporary balloon tamp inflation, 120
treatment decision, 129
for vertebra plana deformity, 129
Vitamin D deficiency, 12, 13
Vitamin D receptor (VDR), 13

Z

Zoledronic acid (Reclast®), 41

MIX
Papier aus verantwortungsvollen Quellen
Paper from responsible sources
FSC® C105338

If you have any concerns about our products,
you can contact us on
ProductSafety@springernature.com

In case Publisher is established outside the EU,
the EU authorized representative is:
Springer Nature Customer Service Center GmbH
Europaplatz 3, 69115 Heidelberg, Germany

Printed by Libri Plureos GmbH
in Hamburg, Germany